Clinical Research Advances in Congenital Heart Disease

Editors

Raffaele Giordano
Massimiliano Cantinotti

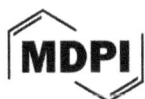

Basel • Beijing • Wuhan • Barcelona • Belgrade • Novi Sad • Cluj • Manchester

Editors
Raffaele Giordano
University of Naples Federico II
Naples, Italy

Massimiliano Cantinotti
Fondazione Toscana Gabriele
Monasterio
Pisa, Italy

Editorial Office
MDPI
St. Alban-Anlage 66
4052 Basel, Switzerland

This is a reprint of articles from the Special Issue published online in the open access journal *Journal of Clinical Medicine* (ISSN 2077-0383) (available at: https://www.mdpi.com/journal/jcm/special_issues/congenital_heart).

For citation purposes, cite each article independently as indicated on the article page online and as indicated below:

Lastname, A.A.; Lastname, B.B. Article Title. *Journal Name* **Year**, *Volume Number*, Page Range.

ISBN 978-3-0365-9432-3 (Hbk)
ISBN 978-3-0365-9433-0 (PDF)
doi.org/10.3390/books978-3-0365-9433-0

© 2023 by the authors. Articles in this book are Open Access and distributed under the Creative Commons Attribution (CC BY) license. The book as a whole is distributed by MDPI under the terms and conditions of the Creative Commons Attribution-NonCommercial-NoDerivs (CC BY-NC-ND) license.

Contents

About the Editors vii

Abdelhak El Bouziani, Lars S. Witte, Berto J. Bouma, Monique R. M. Jongbloed, Daniëlle Robbers-Visser, Bart Straver, et al.
Catheter-Based Techniques for Addressing Atrioventricular Valve Regurgitation in Adult Congenital Heart Disease Patients: A Descriptive Cohort
Reprinted from: *J. Clin. Med.* **2023**, *12*, 4798, doi:10.3390/jcm12144798 1

Massimiliano Cantinotti, Colin Joseph McMahon, Pietro Marchese, Martin Köstenberger, Marco Scalese, Eliana Franchi, et al.
Echocardiographic Parameters for Risk Prediction in Borderline Right Ventricle: Review with Special Emphasis on Pulmonary Atresia with Intact Ventricular Septum and Critical Pulmonary Stenosis
Reprinted from: *J. Clin. Med.* **2023**, *12*, 4599, doi:10.3390/jcm12144599 15

Katharina Meinel, Felicitas Korak, Martin Dusleag, Tanja Strini, Daniela Baumgartner, Ante Burmas, et al.
Mild Acquired von Willebrand Syndrome and Cholestasis in Pediatric and Adult Patients with Fontan Circulation
Reprinted from: *J. Clin. Med.* **2023**, *12*, 1240, doi:10.3390/jcm12031240 27

Agnieszka Bartczak-Rutkowska, Lidia Tomkiewicz-Pająk, Katarzyna Kawka-Paciorkowska, Natalia Bajorek, Aleksandra Ciepłucha, Mariola Ropacka-Lesiak and Olga Trojnarska
Pregnancy Outcomes in Women after the Fontan Procedure
Reprinted from: *J. Clin. Med.* **2023**, *12*, 783, doi:10.3390/jcm12030783 39

Zeming Zhou, Yuanrui Gu, Hong Zheng, Chaowu Yan, Qiong Liu, Shiguo Li, et al.
Interventional Occlusion of Large Patent Ductus Arteriosus in Adults with Severe Pulmonary Hypertension
Reprinted from: *J. Clin. Med.* **2023**, *12*, 354, doi:10.3390/jcm12010354 49

Marian Pop, Zsófia Kakucs and Simona Coman
CT Detection of an Anomalous Left Circumflex Coronary Artery from Pulmonary Artery (ALXCAPA) in 81-Year-Old Female Patient
Reprinted from: *J. Clin. Med.* **2023**, *12*, 226, doi:10.3390/jcm12010226 61

Laura Lang, Jennifer Gerlach, Anne-Christine Plank, Ariawan Purbojo, Robert A. Cesnjevar, Oliver Kratz, et al.
Becoming a Teenager after Early Surgical Ventricular Septal Defect (VSD) Repair: Longitudinal Biopsychological Data on Mental Health and Maternal Involvement
Reprinted from: *J. Clin. Med.* **2022**, *12*, 7242, doi:10.3390/jcm11237242 67

Yashendra Sethi, Neil Patel, Nirja Kaka, Ami Desai, Oroshay Kaiwan, Mili Sheth, et al.
Artificial Intelligence in Pediatric Cardiology: A Scoping Review
Reprinted from: *J. Clin. Med.* **2022**, *11*, 7072, doi:10.3390/jcm11237072 91

Flaminia Vena, Lucia Manganaro, Valentina D'Ambrosio, Luisa Masciullo, Flavia Ventriglia, Giada Ercolani, et al.
Neuroimaging and Cerebrovascular Changes in Fetuses with Complex Congenital Heart Disease
Reprinted from: *J. Clin. Med.* **2022**, *11*, 6740, doi:10.3390/jcm11226740 125

Zsófia Kakucs, Erhard Heidenhoffer and Marian Pop
Detection of Coronary Artery and Aortic Arch Anomalies in Patients with Tetralogy of Fallot Using CT Angiography
Reprinted from: *J. Clin. Med.* **2022**, *11*, 5500, doi:10.3390/jcm11195500 . . . . **135**

Massimiliano Cantinotti, Pietro Marchese, Marco Scalese, Eliana Franchi, Nadia Assanta, Martin Koestenberger, et al.
Atrial Function Impairments after Pediatric Cardiac Surgery Evaluated by STE Analysis
Reprinted from: *J. Clin. Med.* **2022**, *11*, 2497, doi:10.3390/jcm11092497 . . . . **147**

About the Editors

Raffaele Giordano

Raffaele Giordano was born in Salerno (Italy) in 1981. He received his Medicine Degree at the Second University of Naples (cum laude) in 2007 and Cardiac Surgery Specialist Degree at University of Naples "Federico II" (cum laude) in 2013. He was a Pediatric Cardiac Surgeon at the Heart Center of Massa, Tuscany Foundation "G. Monasterio", National Center of Research (CNR), from June 2013 to June 2016, consultant in Cardiac Surgery at University of Naples Federico II from July 2016 to November 2019, adjunct Professor of Cardiac Surgery at University of Naples Federico II from November 2019 and Associate Professor from November 2022 to date. He received his Ph.D in Biomorphological and Surgical Sciences at the University of Naples "Federico II". Prof. Giordano was an elected member of the National Council of the Italian Society of Cardiac Surgery, section of pediatric cardiac surgery and congenital heart disease, from November 2012 to 2014. To date, he is a member of Italian Pediatric Cardiology and Cardiac Surgery, organizer and member of the scientific secretariat of several conferences and training courses, and speaker at numerous conferences, seminars and refresher courses. He also cooperates with prestigious international Universities (John Hopkins, London, Cambridge, Gratz, etc.).

Massimiliano Cantinotti

Massimiliano Cantinotti has been a Consultant since 2008 in the Pediatric and Adult Congenital Heart Disease Department of "Fondazione CNR-Regione Toscana G. Monasterio (Massa and Pisa, Italy)", a prestigious tertiary Italian Research Institute for the care of heart problems of all the ages. From 2017, he has ran the echocardiography lab. His main fields of interest are cardiac imaging and research. He is the author of more than 150 indexed articles, mainly as the first author. His main fields of research are normal echocardiographic values, new imaging techniques (strain imaging, vortex imaging, 3D), sport cardiology, lung ultrasound, and cardiac biomarkers. He has won more than EUR 1 million in prizes for research projects. He also cooperates with prestigious international Universities (John Hopkins, London, Cambridge, Gratz, etc.). He is an active member of AEPC (European Association of Pediatric Cardiology).

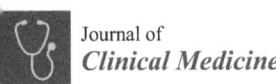

Article

Catheter-Based Techniques for Addressing Atrioventricular Valve Regurgitation in Adult Congenital Heart Disease Patients: A Descriptive Cohort

Abdelhak El Bouziani [1,†], Lars S. Witte [1,†], Berto J. Bouma [1], Monique R. M. Jongbloed [2,3], Daniëlle Robbers-Visser [1], Bart Straver [1], Marcel A. M. Beijk [1], Philippine Kiès [2], David R. Koolbergen [4], Frank van der Kley [2], Martin J. Schalij [2], Robbert J. de Winter [1] and Anastasia D. Egorova [2,*]

1. Department of Cardiology, CAHAL, Centre for Congenital Heart Disease Amsterdam-Leiden, Amsterdam University Medical Centres, AMC, Meibergdreef 9, 1105 AZ Amsterdam, The Netherlands
2. Department of Cardiology, CAHAL, Centre for Congenital Heart Disease Amsterdam-Leiden, Leiden University Medical Centre, 2300 RC Leiden, The Netherlands
3. Department of Anatomy and Embryology, Leiden University Medical Center, 2300 RC Leiden, The Netherlands
4. Department of Congenital Cardiothoracic Surgery, CAHAL, Centre for Congenital Heart Disease Amsterdam-Leiden, Leiden University Medical Centre, 2300 RC Leiden, The Netherlands
* Correspondence: a.egorova@lumc.nl; Tel.: +31-71-529-9098
† These authors contributed equally to this work.

Abstract: Introduction: Increasing survival of adult congenital heart disease (ACHD) patients comes at the price of a range of late complications—arrhythmias, heart failure, and valvular dysfunction. Transcatheter valve interventions have become a legitimate alternative to conventional surgical treatment in selected acquired heart disease patients. However, literature on technical aspects, hemodynamic effects, and clinical outcomes of percutaneous atrioventricular (AV) valve interventions in ACHD patients is scarce. Method: This is a descriptive cohort from CAHAL (Center of Congenital Heart Disease Amsterdam-Leiden). ACHD patients with severe AV valve regurgitation who underwent a transcatheter intervention in the period 2020–2022 were included. Demographic, clinical, procedural, and follow-up data were collected from patient records. Results: Five ACHD patients with severe or torrential AV valve regurgitation are described. Two patients underwent a transcatheter edge-to-edge repair (TEER), one patient underwent a valve-in-valve procedure, one patient received a Cardioband system, and one patient received both a Cardioband system and TEER. No periprocedural complications occurred. Post-procedural AV valve regurgitation as well as NYHA functional class improved in all patients. The median post-procedural NYHA functional class improved from 3.0 (IQR [2.5–4.0]) to 2.0 (IQR [1.5–2.5]). One patient died 9 months after the procedure due to advanced heart failure with multiorgan dysfunction. Conclusion: Transcatheter valve repair is feasible and safe in selected complex ACHD patients. A dedicated heart team is essential for determining an individualized treatment strategy as well as pre- and periprocedural imaging to address the underlying mechanism(s) of AV regurgitation and guide the transcatheter intervention. Long-term follow-up is essential to evaluate the clinical outcomes of transcatheter AV valve repair in ACHD patients.

Keywords: adult congenital heart disease (ACHD); transcatheter valve repair; atrioventricular (AV) regurgitation; hybrid; transcatheter edge-to-edge repair (TEER); Cardioband; valve-in-valve (ViV)

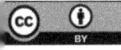

1. Introduction

Congenital heart disease (CHD) has an estimated prevalence of about 1% in the general population [1]. CHD patients have demonstrated an increasing survival over the past decades due to improved diagnostic imaging modalities as well as advances in surgical, pharmacological, and transcatheter management strategies. This aging group of CHD patients is, however, frequently confronted with a range of late complications such as arrhythmias, heart failure, and valvular dysfunction [2,3]. Transcatheter valve interventions have developed rapidly during the past decade and have become a legitimate alternative to conventional surgical treatment in selected patients [4]. In contrast to non-CHD adults suffering from functional atrioventricular (AV) valve regurgitation, adults with congenital heart disease (ACHD) are typically younger and often have several mechanisms contributing to AV valve dysfunction. Furthermore, the surgical risk in ACHD patients is increased due to complex anatomy, myocardial fibrosis due to the underlying condition, previous surgical interventions and cannulations, and intrathoracic and pericardial adhesions and collateral vessels. Literature on technical aspects, hemodynamic effects, and clinical outcomes of percutaneous AV valve interventions in CHD patients is scarce and these aspects have only been described in several case reports or series [5–7]. This descriptive cohort reports the recent experience of transcatheter valve therapies in complex ACHD patients in a large tertiary referral center.

2. Methods

This two-center observational, retrospective cohort study was performed at the departments of Cardiology of the Amsterdam University Medical Center and Leiden University Medical Center, united in the center of Congenital Heart Disease Amsterdam-Leiden (CAHAL). Consecutive ACHD patients with hemodynamically severe AV valve lesions (accessed in accordance with the 2021 ESC/EACTS Guidelines for the management of valvular heart disease) who underwent a catheter-based intervention to address the AV valve dysfunction between 2020 and 2022 were included in this cohort [8]. All patients were discussed by the multidisciplinary heart team which included an ACHD specialist, an interventional and an imaging cardiologist, a congenital cardiothoracic surgeon, a pediatric cardiologist, and a specialized nurse. Demographic, clinical, procedural, and follow-up data were collected from patient medical records.

Statistical Analysis

Descriptive statistics were utilized to summarize data. Normally distributed continuous data are displayed as mean ± standard deviation (SD) and non-normally distributed continuous data are displayed as median and 95% and the first and third interquartiles [IQ1–IQ3]. Categorical data are presented as numbers. Statistical analyses were performed with IBM SPSS Statistics for Windows, version 28 (IBM Corp., Armonk, NY, USA).

3. Results

Five complex ACHD patients (two women), median age 52 years (44–74), with severe or torrential symptomatic AV regurgitation were included in this descriptive cohort; Table 1. Three patients had a morphologically systemic left ventricle and two patients had a systemic right ventricle supporting the systemic circulation. Furthermore, in three out of five patients, the AV valve regurgitation was of the subpulmonary ventricle. All patients had a history of previous cardiac operations with a median of two [1.5–2] operations. At baseline two patients were in NYHA functional class IV, two patients were in NYHA functional class III, and one patient was in NYHA functional class II [2.5–4.0]. Four patients underwent a percutaneous intervention and one patient had a hybrid procedure. Two patients received a transcatheter edge-to-edge repair (TEER), one patient underwent a transcatheter valve-in-valve procedure, one patient received a Cardioband system, and one patient received a Cardioband system as well as a TEER.

Table 1. Demographic and clinical patient characteristics at baseline and latest follow-up.

	Patient A	Patient B	Patient C	Patient D	Patient E
Age (years)	75	40	48	52	72
Sex	male	female	male	male	female
CHD diagnosis and surgical history	BAV with severe aortic regurgitation, Ross at the age of 25 and ascending aorta replacement and AVR bioprosthesis due to autograft failure at the age of 65	M. Ebstein with severe tricuspid regurgitation right-left shunt over an open PFO, TV annuloplasty followed by replacement with a bioprosthesis at the age of 31	Left isomerism, DORV-Fallot type, hypoplastic left ventricle, mitral valve atresia, right modified Blalock–Taussig shunt at the age of 1, left modified Blalock–Taussig shunt at the age of 13, aorto-pulmonary shunt to the right pulmonary artery at the age of 20 because of occlusion of the left Blalock–Taussig shunt	Left isomerism, DORV-TGA, large ASD, PS, right-sided aortic arch, persistent left SVC, bilateral bi-directional Glenn anastomosis at the age of 31	Tetralogy of Fallot, Blalock shunt at the age of 4 and surgical correction at the age of 22, pulmonary homograft implantation at the age of 58, numerous ablation procedures for atrial fibrillation and flutters, chronic RV pacing due to a high degree AV-block
Concomitant cardiac lesions and diagnoses	Paroxysmal atrial fibrillation	None	Multiple systemic to pulmonary artery shunts, abnormal venous return with hemiazygos continuation of the IVC and a persistent left SVC, paroxysmal atrial fibrillation	Persistence of left SVC, abnormal venous return with azygos continuation of the IVC, permanent accepted atrial fibrillation, endocarditis	Permanent accepted atrial fibrillation
Number of previous cardiac surgeries	2	2	3	1	3
Non-cardiac comorbidities	Bilateral pulmonary embolism, hypertenstion	-	-	Epilepsy	Epilepsy
Morphology of the systemic ventricle	left	left	right	right	left
Pre-procedural NYHA class	III	II	IV	III	IV
Morphology of the regurgitant AV valve	TV (subpulmonary)	TV (subpulmonary)	TV (systemic)	common AV-valve (systemic)	TV (subpulmonary)
Severity of AV valve regurgitation	IV+/torrential	IV/severe	IV+/torrential	IV/severe	IV/severe
(Dominant) mechanism of AV valve regurgitation	Annulus dilatation	Bioprosthesis degeneration	Annulus dilatation	Annulus dilatation	Annulus dilatation, impingement by device lead
Main imaging findings	Moderately reduced left and right ventricular function, dilated RV, severe/torrential TR and right atrial dilatation, estimated filling pressures 20 mmHg	Moderately reduced right ventricular function	Dilated ventricle with impaired systolic function, severely dilated functional mono-atrium	Severely dilated functional mono-atrium, extensive network of coronary fistulae, Moderalety reduced systolic and diastolic systemic ventricular function	Preserved right ventricular function
Renal function (eGFR)	63 mL/min/1.73 m^2	85 mL/min/1.73 m^2	38 mL/min/1.73 m^2	>90 mL/min/1.73 m^2	89 mL/min/1.73 m^2
Cardiac pharmacotherapy	Vitamin K antagonist, sotalol, ACE-inhibitor, aldosterone receptor antagonist, loop diuretic, calcium antagonist, statin	None	Amiodarone, DOAC, aldosterone receptor antagonist, loop diuretic	Aldosterone receptor antagonist, DOAC, loop diuretic	Vitamin K antagonist, sotalol, aldosterone receptor antagonist, loop diuretic
Vascular access	Right femoral venous access	Right femoral venous access	Right transjugular venous access	Right lateral thoracotomy through the 5th intercostal space	Right femoral venous access

Table 1. Cont.

	Patient A	Patient B	Patient C	Patient D	Patient E
Intervention	Annuloplasty (Cardioband)	Valve-in-valve implantation (Sapien 3)	TEER (Triclip), two XTW clips between A-S leaflets	Hybrid TEER (MitraClip), two XTW clips between A-P leaflets	Annuloplasty (Cardioband) TEER (Triclip), two XTW clips
Procedural complications	None	None	None	None	None
Post-procedural AVVR grade	II	<I	II	II	I-II
Post-procedural NYHA class	I-II	I	III	II	II
NYHA class at latest follow-up	I-II	I	III	IV	II

ACE = angiotensin-converting enzyme; ASD = atrial septal defect; AVR = aortic valve replacement; AV = atrioventricular; AVVR = atrioventricular valve regurgitation; BAV = bicuspid aortic valve; CHD = congenital heart disease; DOAC = direct oral anticoagulants; DORV = double outlet right ventricle; eGFR = estimated glomerular filtration rate; IVC = inferior caval vein; NYHA = New York Heart Association; PFO = patent foramen ovale; PS = pulmonary stenosis; RV = SVC = superior caval vein; TEER = transcatheter edge-to-edge repair; TGA = transposition of the great arteries; TV = tricuspid valve.

All procedures were performed under general anesthesia with transesophageal (TEE) and/or fluoroscopic guidance, except for one case, which was performed under local anesthesia. No periprocedural complications were reported. Post-procedural AV valve regurgitation improved significantly in all patients (Figure 1). The median follow-up period was 17 months [12.5–23.0]. The median of the post-procedural NYHA functional class was II [1.5–2.5]. At latest follow-up, one patient was in NYHA functional class I, two patients were in NYHA functional class II, and one patient was in NYHA functional class III. One patient (patient D) was in NYHA functional class IV at latest follow-up and died 9 months after the procedure (Figure 2).

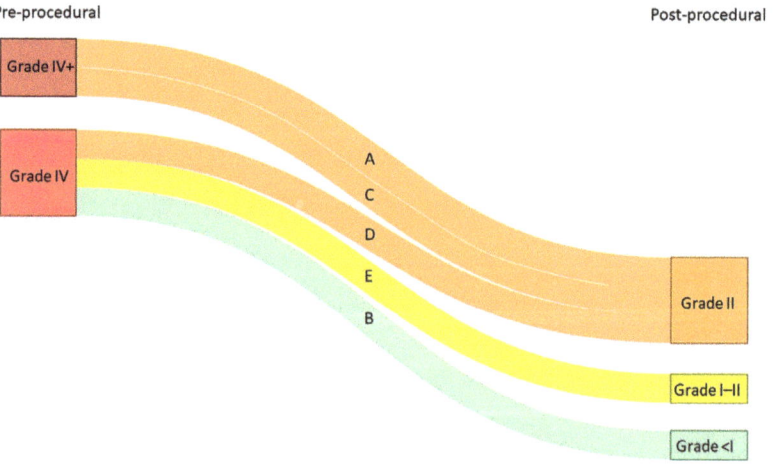

Figure 1. Atrioventricular (AV) valve regurgitation before and after transcatheter valve intervention Each line represents a single patient (A–E corresponding to patient A–E, respectively).

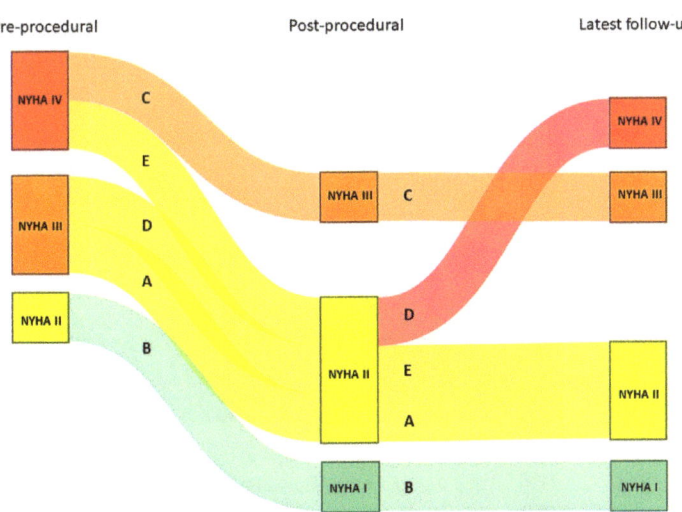

Figure 2. NYHA functional class before and after the transcatheter valve intervention, as well as at latest available follow-up. Each line represents a single patient (A–E corresponding to patient A–E, respectively).

3.1. Patient A

A 76-year-old male with a history of a Ross procedure due to severe regurgitation of a bicuspid aortic valve at the age of 25 years, ascending aorta replacement and aortic bioprosthesis implantation at the age of 65 and atrial fibrillation (AF), presented to the emergency department with complaints of dyspnea and progressive weight gain. He was documented to have persistent AF with inadequate rate-control and signs of moderate left- and right-sided decompensation. He was treated with loop diuretics and underwent successful cardioversion to sinus rhythm after recompensation. Transthoracic echocardiography (TTE) revealed moderately reduced left and right ventricular function, normal function of the aortic bioprosthesis (peak gradient < 30 mmHg, mean gradient < 20 mmHg, no regurgitation and pulmonary homograft (peak gradient 25 mmHg, mean gradient 14 mmHg, trivial regurgitation), trivial mitral regurgitation, and torrential tricuspid regurgitation (TR) with elevated filling pressures (peak TR gradient 50 mmHg, estimated right atrial pressures 10–15 mmHg) (Figure 3A–D). Laboratory analysis showed preserved renal function (eGFR 63 mL/min/1.73 m^2) and elevated levels of NT-proBNP (9652 ng/L, upper reference limit 520 ng/L). Despite pharmacological escalation, the patient remained in NYHA functional class III and experienced frequent recurrences of symptomatic AF. The severe functional TR due to annulus dilatation and progressive decline in systolic function of the overloaded right ventricle was deemed to be the cause. The perioperative risk of surgery involving a third thoracotomy in a septuagenarian was high, and therefore percutaneous options were evaluated. Given the malcoaptation and the dilated tricuspid valve (TV) annulus of 62 × 54 mm (Figure 3C), the heart team deemed transcatheter annular reduction with the Cardioband system (Edwards Lifesciences, Santa Ana, CA, USA) to be the best approach.

The patient underwent a successful Cardioband annular reduction using right venous femoral access under general anesthesia with fluoroscopic (selective cannulation of the right coronary artery) and TEE guidance (Figure 3E–H). A total of 18 anchors were placed between the anteroseptal and posteroseptal commissure reducing the annulus dimensions to 45 × 36 mm. The torrential TR (two jets) was reduced to moderate TR (Figure 3E,H). At two years follow-up, the patient was in NYHA functional class I-II and no heart-failure-related admissions occurred. His NT-proBNP serum levels decreased to 2762 ng/L and at echocardiography he had a stable moderately reduced RV function and moderate TR.

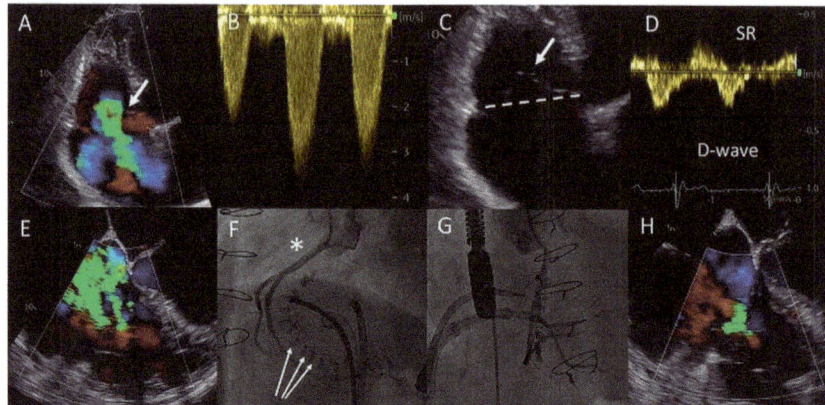

Figure 3. (**A**) Color Doppler apical four-chamber view shows torrential tricuspid regurgitation (TR) with a wide vena contracta (arrow) and flow disturbance filling the enlarged right atrium. (**B**) Continuous wave doppler showing a dense TR signal with elevated right ventricular pressures. (**C**) Noncoaptation of the tricuspid valve (TV) leaflets (arrow) and annulus dilatation (dash line, 53 mm) is seen. (**D**) The hepatic vein Doppler demonstrates a pattern in atrial fibrillation with a prominent and late peaking systolic reversal (SR) wave. The only forward flow is evident in diastole (D-wave). (**E**) Two TR jets (a vena contracta of 4 and 7 mm, respectively, ERO of 90 mm^2, regurgitant volume of 98 mL) are evident during transesophageal imaging. (**F**) Left anterior oblique and (**G**) right superior oblique fluoroscopic views showing patent right coronary artery (asterisk) and 18 anchors (arrows) between the two TV commissures allowing the Cardioband to significantly reduce the annulus dimensions. (**H**) Transesophageal echocardiography showing significant reduction in TR after the Cardioband annulus reduction procedure (appreciate the difference with panel (**E**), vena contracta of 3 and 5 mm, respectively, ERO 35 mm^2, regurgitant volume of 41 mL).

3.2. Patient B

A 40-year-old female born with Ebstein's anomaly of the TV who had previously undergone a surgical annuloplasty and a TV replacement with a bioprosthesis (TVR, 33 mm Sorin-Pericarbon MoreTM, Sorin Biomedica, Italy) and had two uncomplicated pregnancies afterwards was seen at the outpatient clinic with progressive complaints of reduced exercise tolerance, currently in NYHA functional class II. TTE revealed severe regurgitation and significant stenosis of the TVR bioprosthesis with progressively worsening right ventricular (RV) function and a giant right atrium (RA) partially compressing the left atrial compartment (Figure 4A–E). She was not using any pharmacotherapy, and had preserved renal function and elevated levels of NT-proBNP (670 ng/L, upper reference limit 247 ng/L). Magnetic resonance imaging confirmed preserved left ventricular function (EF 52%) and at least a moderately reduced RV function (EF 40%), likely overestimated in the setting of severe TR (44% regurgitant fraction). Given the significantly reduced RV function and the risks of a third thoracotomy, the heart team deemed a valve-in-valve transcatheter TV implantation to be feasible and lower risk (short-term), allowing the RV function to recover whilst the patient would still be eligible for a surgical re-TVR after the failure of this valve-in-valve prosthesis in the future. As a mother of two young children, the patient opted to defer surgery and pursue a transcatheter valve procedure.

This was successfully performed under local anesthesia, by means of right femoral access and fluoroscopy and TTE guidance. A temporary pacemaker wire was placed in the left ventricle and the AgilisTM steerable introducer (Abbott, IL, USA) was used to safely access the RA, given the relatively sharp angle between the vena cava-RA and the RA-RV axis (Figure 4F). The Edwards eSheath TM (Edwards Lifesciences, USA) was then used to implant a 29 mm Edwards SAPIEN 3 valve (Edwards Lifesciences) in the TVR bioprosthesis under rapid pacing (Figure 4G,H). Normal function of the new valve-in-valve bioprosthesis was confirmed by transthoracic echocardiography (Figure 4I–L). The periprocedural course was uneventful. At 22 months follow-up, the patient is in NYHA functional class I with moderately reduced (yet significantly improved) RV function and normal function of the bioprosthesis.

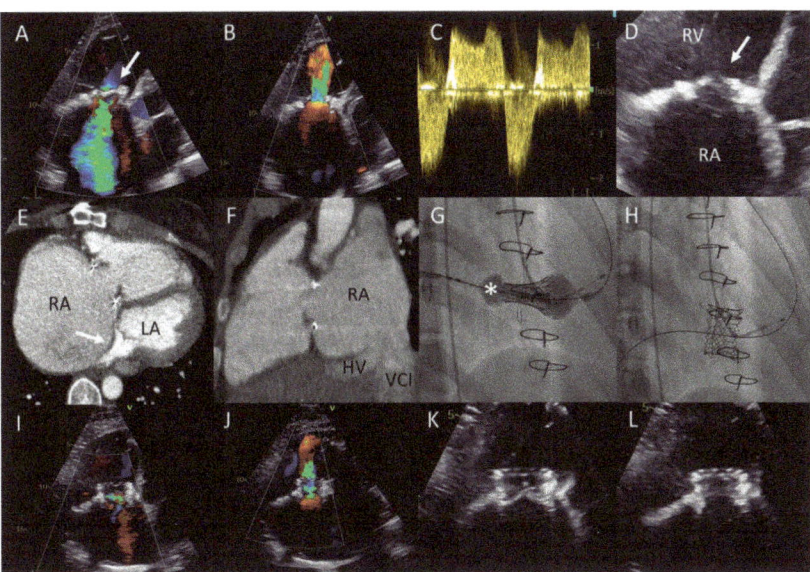

Figure 4. (**A**) Color Doppler apical four-chamber view shows severe tricuspid regurgitation (TR) with a wide vena contracta (arrow) and a systolic jet reaching the roof of the enlarged right atrium (RA). (**B**) Color Doppler showing turbulent inflow through the tricuspid valve (TV) bioprosthesis and aliasing, mean gradient was elevated at 4–5 mmHg. (**C**) Continuous wave Doppler showing a dense TR signal with low velocity. (**D**) Calcified and degenerated tricuspid bioprosthesis (arrow). (**E**) Axial slice through a computed tomography (CT) scan at the level of the right ventricle shows a giant RA and an intra-atrial septum deviation towards the left atrium (arrow), partially suppressing it. (**F**) Sagittal CT slice shows the inflow angle of the inferior vena cava-right RA and the RA-TV. Note the distended hepatic vein (HV). (**G,H**) Right anterior oblique fluoroscopy projections show the expansion of the Sapien 3 valve (asterisk) using the ring of the degenerated bioprosthesis as the reference and the final result, respectively. (**I,J**) Apical four-chamber color Doppler views showing normal function of the valve-in-valve bioprosthesis (appreciate the difference with (**A,B**), respectively). (**K,L**) View of the valve-in-valve bioprosthesis in systole (closed) and diastole (open), respectively.

3.3. Patient C

A 48-year-old male born with complex cyanotic congenital heart disease (left isomerism, Fallot type double outlet right ventricle (DORV), mitral valve atresia, large ventricular septal defect (VSD), functionally univentricular heart with a hypoplastic left ventricle) was palliated using multiple Blalock–Taussig (BT) shunts. He had an abnormal systemic venous return with a hemiazygos continuation of the inferior caval vein (IVC) and a persistent left superior caval vein (SVC) (Figure 5A). The patient had multiple hospitalizations for heart failure with functional TR due to severely dilated functional mono-atrium and annulus (Figure 5B) and systemic right ventricular dilation with (moderately) impaired systolic function and a restrictive filling pattern. Laboratory analysis showed preserved renal function (eGFR 71 mL/min/1.73 m^2) and elevated levels of NT-proBNP (5592 ng/L, upper reference limit 121 ng/L). TTE and TEE (Figure 5D) showed a severely dilated functional mono-atrium and RV with torrential TR. Computed tomography (CT) was performed for pre-procedural assessment of the approach (i.e., the trajectory and the distance from the right internal jugular vein to the TV was accessed as a potential venous access route given the anatomy). Furthermore, the CT showed a dilated ventricle of 12 × 11cm in the axial view and multiple large venous collaterals. Surgery was deemed high risk due to three previous thoracotomies, pronounced collaterals, and the severely dilated ventricle with reduced systolic function. Because of the hemiazygos continuation of the IVC, transcatheter access via the femoral vein was not feasible. Therefore, a transjugular TriClip (Abbott, IL, USA) transcatheter valve repair of the TV was performed under TEE guidance. Two XTW clips were implanted capturing the anterior and septal leaflets.

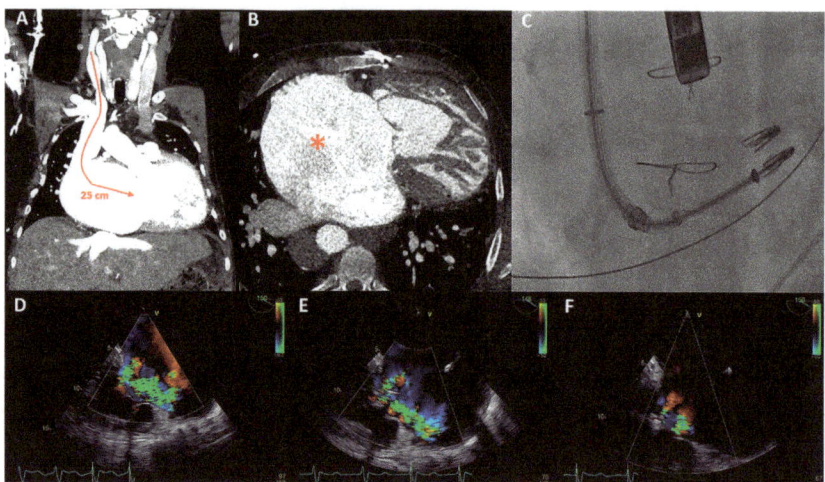

Figure 5. (**A**) Distance between the right internal jugular vein and tricuspid valve (TV) measured on a computed tomography (CT) scan in a coronal plane (arrow). (**B**) Severely dilated mono-atrium (asterisk) on CT scan in a sagittal plane. (**C**) Implantation of the second XTW clip (note the first XTW clip already released) under transesophageal echocardiography (TEE) guidance. (**D**) Preprocedural TEE imaging of the torrential (IV+) TR. (**E**) Periprocedural TEE showing TR after placing the first XTW clip. (**F**) TEE showing the significant reduction in TR after placing the second XTW clip to grade I–II.

As a result of the severely dilated annulus and tethering, the coaptation gap was large and simultaneous grasping of both leaflets was challenging. The TriClip system has the advanced option of independent leaflet grasping. First, the anterior leaflet (technically more challenging) was grasped and, subsequently, after minor device repositioning under TEE guidance, the septal leaflet was captured and the clip was released. The first clip was implanted near the commissure to narrow the coaptation gap so that the second clip could be implanted to treat the regurgitation (Figure 5C), which decreased to moderate (Figure 5E,F). Three weeks after the percutaneous procedure, at the outpatient clinic, the patient reported a decrease in orthopnea and exercise-induced dyspnea as the NYHA functional class was reduced from IV to III. At 17 months follow-up, the patient remained in NYHA functional class III. However, multiple heart-failure-related admissions occurred during follow-up (latest level of NT-proBNP was 8092 ng/L) and the patient developed atrial fibrillation (AF) which was treated with amiodarone.

3.4. Patient D

A 52-year-old man was born with left isomerism and a functionally univentricular heart. There was a large ASD, common AV valve, DORV with transposition position of the great arteries (TGAs), pulmonary stenosis, hypoplastic left ventricle, a right-sided aortic arch, a persistent left SVC, and an interrupted IVC (azygos continuation). At the age of 30, he received a bilateral bidirectional Glenn shunt. The patient was now admitted with peripheral edema and permanent AF with adequate rate control and had preserved renal function (eGFR 83 mL/min/1.73 m^2). Moderately reduced systolic and diastolic systemic ventricular function, severe atrial dilatation, and AV valve regurgitation were documented on TTE and TEE. Additional CT imaging showed a severely dilated functional mono-atrium in close proximity to the thoracic wall (Figure 6A), a patent bilateral SVC to pulmonary (Glenn) connection (Figure 6B), and an extensive network of coronary fistulae was noted. Subsequent catheterization confirmed connection of the azygos continuation of the IVC with the functional mono-atrium without a gradient, low pressures in the Glenn conduits, and moderate pulmonary stenosis. Cardiac decompensation with elevated levels of NT-proBNP (1314 ng/L, upper reference limit 121 ng/L) was adjudicated to the severe AV valve regurgitation and reduced systolic ventricular function (Figure 6C), and, despite escalating in diuretic treatment, the patient remained symptomatic (NYHA functional class III).

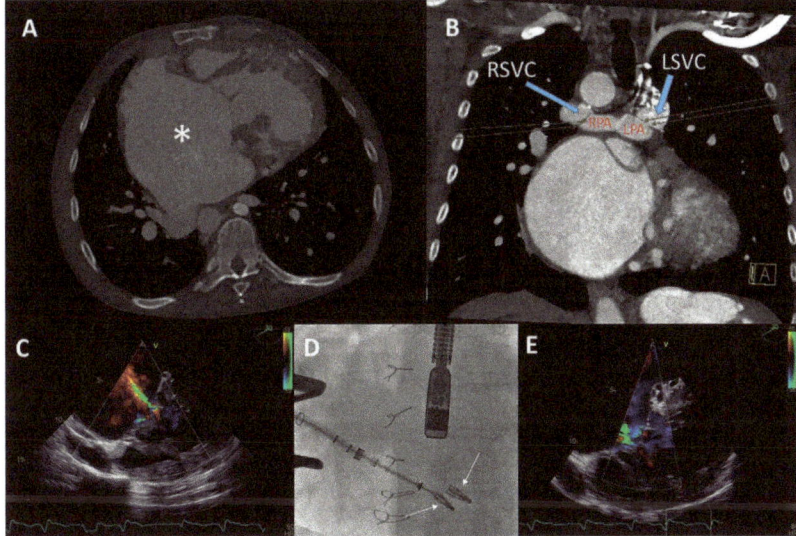

Figure 6. (**A**,**B**) Computed tomography (CT) scan of the thoracic cavity with the anatomical position of the dilated functional mono-atrium (asterisk) against the right thoracic wall (panel **A**) and bidirectional bilateral Glenn shunt (panel **B**) (LPA = left pulmonary artery, RPA = right pulmonary artery, LSVC = left superior vena cava, RSVC = right superior vena cava). (**C**) Pre-procedural transesophageal echocardiography (TEE) which visualized severe common atrioventricular (AV) valve regurgitation. (**D**) Anteroposterior fluoroscopic view of the two XTW MitraClips positioned in the AV valve. At the same time, it is appreciated that the delivery system is positioned through the fifth intercostal space after a right mini-lateral thoracotomy. (**E**) Moderate AV regurgitation after the hybrid procedure visualized with TEE.

Conventional surgical AV valve replacement or repair was considered extremely high risk due to the anatomical relation between the atrium and the thoracic wall, the extensive coronary fistulae, and the reduced ventricular function. Percutaneous AV valve replacement or repair was deemed non-feasible by the transvenous route due to interruption of the IVC with azygos continuation and sharp angulation into the mono-atrium (for a transfemoral approach). Furthermore, a transjugular approach was not feasible because of the bilateral Glenn connection. Therefore, it was decided that a hybrid procedure under general anesthesia with direct atrial access using a MitraClip delivery system (Abbott, IL, USA) was the best strategy.

The congenital cardiothoracic surgeon performed a right (mini) lateral thoracotomy in the fifth intercostal space to expose the giant mono-atrium. A double-purse string suture was placed and an incision was made to create an opening using a Safari wire for guidance and stability. The interventional cardiologist then placed two XTW clips under TEE guidance (Figure 6D), resulting in reduction in AV valve regurgitation to grade II (Figure 6E). Post-procedural TEE showed grade II regurgitation with stable position of the clips. No peri-procedural complications occurred. The patient could be discharged with adequate heart failure medication with an improvement in NYHA functional class (II). Unfortunately, the patient died after 9 months due to progressive ventricular dysfunction, worsening of the AV valve regurgitation, and heart-failure-related multi-organ dysfunction (NYHA functional class IV at the latest admission).

3.5. Patient E

A 72-year-old female born with Tetralogy of Fallot (TOF) and having undergone three previous thoracotomies (Blalock–Thomas–Tausig shunt at the age of 4, correction of TOF at the age of 22, and a pulmonary homograft implantation at the age of 58 years), numerous ablation procedures for atrial arrhythmias after which permanent AF was accepted, and a pacemaker implantation due to a high-degree AV block was evaluated at the outpatient clinic due to progressive complaints of dyspnea on exertion and a recent admission with right-sided decompensation. She was in NYHA functional class IV despite escalation in diuretic treatment.

Echocardiography showed severe TR with a regurgitant jet directed towards the inflow of the inferior vena cava and a progressive dilation of the RV with preserved systolic function (Figure 7A,B). The pulmonary homograft function was preserved. The mechanism of TR was considered to be multifactorial i.a. annulus dilatation in combination with impingement by the previous implanted RV pacing lead, leading to malcoaptation. The heart team deferred from surgical intervention on the TV due to high estimated peri-procedural risk in a septuagenarian with three previous thoracotomies. A two-step catheter-based approach was pursued: (1) Cardioband annulus reduction and (2) TriClip implantation to treat any hemodynamically significant residual TR.

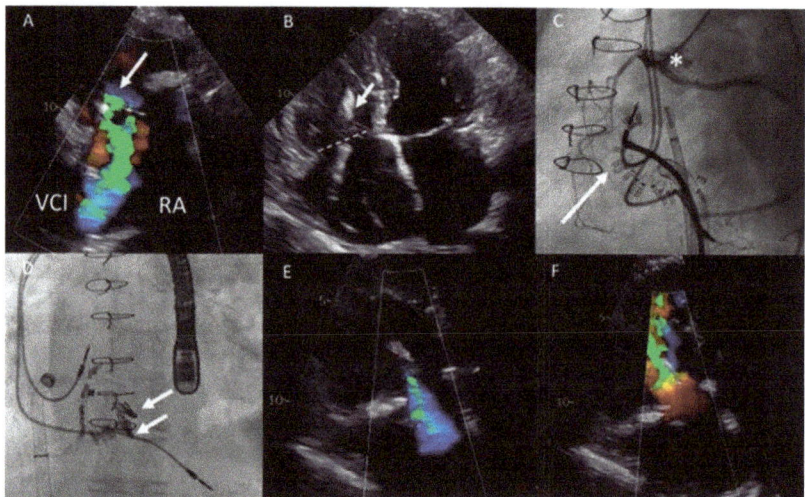

Figure 7. (**A**) Color Doppler modified parasternal right ventricular (RV) inflow view shows severe tricuspid regurgitation (TR) with a wide vena contracta (arrow) and leakage jet reaching the inferior vena cave (IVC). (**B**) Apical four-chamber view shows tricuspid valve (TV) annulus dilatation (dash line, 46 mm) and impingement by the RV pacemaker lead (arrow). (**C**) Left inferior oblique fluoroscopic view of the Cardioband (arrow) annulus reduction procedure (asterisk). (**D**) Anteroposterior fluoroscopic view shows the two XTW clips (arrows) implanted. (**E**,**F**) Modified apical four chamber color Doppler views showing mild (-moderate) residual TR and inflow through the TV (mean gradient of 3 mmHg).

Both procedures were performed in sequential order under general anesthesia, by means of right femoral access and fluoroscopy and transesophageal echocardiographic guidance (Figure 7C,D). A total of 15 anchors were used for the Cardioband annular reduction (Edwards Lifesciences, USA) reducing the annulus dimensions to 28 × 27 mm. Yet, moderate-severe TR persisted and the second procedure was planned for the patient. She underwent the placement of two TriClips (Abbott, IL, USA), resulting in reduction of TR to mild-moderate and a slightly elevated inflow gradient of 3 mmHg over de TV (Figure 7E,F). No periprocedural complications were documented. At 16 months follow-up, the patient remains in NYHA functional class II and is euvolemic. No heart-failure-related admissions occurred since the TV interventions.

4. Discussion

In this descriptive cohort, we report on the indication, methodology, and outcomes of transcatheter treatment of five consecutive ACHD patients with severe AV valve regurgitation in the setting of complex anatomical malformations: two patients underwent a TEER, one patient underwent a valve-in-valve procedure, one patient underwent a Cardioband system implantation, and one patient underwent a consecutive Cardioband implantation followed by TEER. In two out of five patients, the regurgitant AV valve was of the systemic ventricle (as opposed to three patients with AV valve regurgitation of the subpulmonary ventricle). Post-procedural AV valve regurgitation as well as NYHA functional class improved in all patients. This cohort is illustrative of the feasibility and the wide range of applications of transcatheter techniques in addressing AV valve lesions in ACHD patients and highlights the necessity of an individualized and anatomy-tailored approach.

4.1. Feasible and Patient Tailored Alternative to Surgery

All patients were discussed by a dedicated ACHD team and surgery was deemed to be too high risk for all patients reported. Lifetime rate of re-thoracotomies, extensive adhesions, unique anatomical challenges, hemorrhage prone collaterals, and multi-organ dysfunction are all recognized factors in this decision making favoring a transcatheter approach [9]. Many of these factors are not accurately accounted for by the EuroScore risk stratification and the validated ACHD specific cardiac surgery risk score is currently lacking. Shorter duration of hospitalization, avoidance of inflammatory response as a result of a cardiopulmonary bypass, and an overall shorter rehabilitation time are factors in favor of a transcatheter-based treatment.

However, despite the temptation of a less-invasive approach, it is important to recognize that data on procedural outcomes and long-term clinical results are scarce [5–7]. This calls for an international prospective registry addressing this gap in evidence in the heterogenous group of ACHD patients and a broad spectrum of valvular dysfunction. It is also important to be aware of the challenging vascular access sites and routes as well as specific intracardiac angulations (for which the standard delivery catheters are not optimized). The hemodynamic results of a (transcatheter) valve repair might not aways be as ideal as those of a replacement, and the tolerability and consequences of any residual lesions should always be considered in advance during heart team discussions. The increased risk of endocarditis after a majority of (right-sided) percutaneous interventions should also we weighed on a case-by-case basis.

The Cardioband system addresses the annular dilatation pathophysiology in a minimally invasive catheter delivered approach. Nickenig et al. conducted the TRI-REPAIR study in thirty patients with moderate or greater functional TR who received a Cardioband system. The implantation of a Cardioband resulted in sustained and significant TR reduction at two years follow-up with substantial improvement in NYHA functional class [10]. Gray et al. demonstrated similar results after one year follow-up [11]. To the best of our knowledge, the current manuscript describes for the first time the successful use of the Cardioband system to reduce TR in ACHD patients—one after numerous operations due to dysfunction of a bicuspid aortic valve and ascending aorta dilatation (patient A) and one late after TOF correction (patient E). The patients remain in NYHA functional class II 16 months and 2 years follow-up, respectively.

Valve-in-valve transcatheter TV replacement has previously been reported to be a good alternative to surgery in patients with severe TV regurgitation and high operative risk [12,13]. In line with this, we report a case of successful Edwards SAPIEN 3 valve implantation into a degenerated Sorin-Pericarbon MoreTM bioprosthesis in a patient with M. Ebstein, resulting in reduction of grade IV TR to trivial regurgitation and associated improvement in the NYHA class and RV function.

Furthermore, three patients underwent a successful TEER, where one patient had a systemic left ventricle whilst the two other patients had a systemic right ventricle. In particular, one of those patients had a functional mono-ventricle with reduced systolic function in the setting of a very complex anatomy, in which the implantation of the clips was feasible and safe (patient D). Despite best efforts, the patient died 9 months after the procedure due to progressive heart failure and concomitant multi-organ dysfunction. Ott et al. previously reported that TEER in congenitally corrected TGA was feasible and safe [14] and Schamroth Pravda et al. demonstrated successful TEER in ACHD patients with a range of primary defects [6].

Of particular interest for further studies remain the patients with a failing systemic right ventricle and TR (such as those late after Mustard/Senning repair or patients with congenitally corrected transposition of the great arteries), as well as the growing group of Fontan circulation patients with functional AV-valve regurgitation (REF + REF). These groups are at specifically high surgical risk and the potential of percutaneous AV valve therapies would be a welcome development to mitigate the risk of re-operations [15,16].

4.2. Dedicated ACHD Heart Team

The current series of patients illustrates the importance of a dedicated and experienced ACHD heart team in addressing AV valve dysfunction in this heterogenous patient group. Only after a thorough understanding of the mechanisms contributing to the valvular dysfunction, and careful consideration of the individual perioperative risks and the capability of a transcatheter technique in adequately addressing these mechanisms, can an individualized and weighted decision be made. Multidisciplinary expertise is essential and we advocate for all ACHD patients undergoing transcatheter AV valve repair or replacement to be discussed and treated in specialized centers by dedicated teams. As the vast majority of ACHD patients require a lifelong follow-up, the heart team can also be used as a forum to discuss treatment and follow-up strategies to ensure timely intervention (early enough to prevent irreversible remodeling and hemodynamic deterioration, yet late enough for the benefits of intervention to outweigh the lifetime risks of endocarditis and inevitable re-interventions).

4.3. Peri-Procedural Imaging and Potential for Virtual Reality

A comprehensive, multi-parametric, and multimodality approach is necessary to understand the underlying mechanism of AV valve regurgitation. This is essential to determine the optimal management strategy and timing of intervention. Given the current lack of robust data defining the optimal timing window for intervention for the vast majority of ACHD valvular lesions, and the often misleading seemingly "asymptomatic" status of the patients during long-term follow-up, serial imaging plays an essential role in timely detection of hemodynamic deterioration. Thorough review of patient records and focused imaging of the venous and arterial access and intracardiac connections is important, as many ACHD patients have concomitant vascular anatomy variants and venous return abnormalities and have undergone numerous vascular interventions, potentially compromising conventional vascular access routes. Patient C is illustrative of a transjugular venous access utilization and patient D required a hybrid procedure with surgical exposure of the functional mono-atrium and the common AV valve. Of note, several studies showed that pre-procedural planning using 3D modeling/virtual reality (VR) in pediatric cardiothoracic patients is feasible as there are some reports of the experience in ACHD patients [17–19]. VR utilization is increasing, with VR becoming more robust and accessible for daily practice [20]. VR is expected to play an important role in preprocedural planning and intraprocedural guidance, specifically for the ACHD cases with complex anatomy and challenging vascular access.

4.4. Study Limitations

This descriptive cohort is inherently limited by the small numbers of a heterogenous population and should therefore be interpreted in this context. It describes a two-center experience of an experienced ACHD interventional team and the techniques utilized might not be widely implemented in various settings. The follow-up period is limited and no data are available regarding the long-term (clinical) outcomes.

5. Conclusions and Clinical Implication

In conclusion, novel (hybrid) transcatheter valve therapies, including transcatheter edge-to-edge repair using a TriClip or MitraClip, transcatheter annulus reduction using a Cardioband, and valve-in-valve replacement techniques are feasible and can address AV valve regurgitation in highly selected complex ACHD patients. Comprehensive multimodality imaging and a dedicated ACHD heart team are essential in successfully implementing patient-tailored transcatheter techniques and deferring high risk surgery in selected patients. Long term data on hemodynamic and clinical outcomes are essential in evaluating the efficacy and durability of transcatheter AV valve interventions in ACHD.

Author Contributions: Conceptualization, A.E.B., L.S.W. and A.D.E.; methodology, A.E.B., L.S.W., R.J.d.W. and A.D.E.; software, A.E.B., L.S.W. and A.D.E.; validation. A.E.B., L.S.W., B.J.B., M.R.M.J., D.R.-V., B.S., M.A.M.B., P.K., D.R.K., F.v.d.K., M.J.S., R.J.d.W. and A.D.E.; formal analysis, not applicable; investigation, B.J.B., M.R.M.J., D.R.-V., B.S., M.A.M.B., P.K., D.R.K., F.v.d.K., M.J.S., R.J.d.W. and A.D.E.; resources, A.E.B., L.S.W. and A.D.E.; data curation, A.E.B., L.S.W. and A.D.E.; writing—original draft preparation, A.E.B., L.S.W. and A.D.E.; writing—review and editing, A.E.B., L.S.W., B.J.B., M.R.M.J., D.R.-V., B.S., M.A.M.B., P.K., D.R.K., F.v.d.K., M.J.S., R.J.d.W. and A.D.E.; visualization, A.E.B., L.S.W. and A.D.E.; supervision, R.J.d.W. and A.D.E.; project administration, A.E.B., L.S.W. and A.D.E.; funding acquisition, not applicable. All authors have read and agreed to the published version of the manuscript.

Funding: This research received no external funding.

Institutional Review Board Statement: All tests and procedures performed involving the human participants were in accordance with the ethical standards of the institutional and/or national research committees and with the 2013 Helsinki declaration or comparable ethical standards. The institutional medical ethics approval has been waived by the scientific board of the department of Cardiology, LUMC, in accordance with the local regulations, due to the retrospective nature of the study reporting results obtained by regular medical care and the small number of patients involved.

Informed Consent Statement: All the patients provided consent for publication of this descriptive cohort.

Data Availability Statement: All data relevant to the study are included in the article. Additional data are available on reasonable request.

Conflicts of Interest: The authors declare no conflict of interests.

Disclosures: The Department of Cardiology of the Leiden University Medical Center received unrestricted research grants from Abbott Vascular, Bayer, Bioventrix, Biotronik, Boston Scientific, Edwards Lifesciences, GE Healthcare and Medtronic. The Department of Cardiology of the Amsterdam University Medical Center received unrestricted research grant from Abbott Vascular.

References

1. Bouma, B.J.; Mulder, B.J. Changing Landscape of Congenital Heart Disease. *Circ. Res.* **2017**, *120*, 908–922. [CrossRef] [PubMed]
2. Erikssen, G.; Liestøl, K.; Seem, E.; Birkeland, S.; Saatvedt, K.J.; Hoel, T.N.; Døhlen, G.; Skulstad, H.; Svennevig, J.L.; Thaulow, E.; et al. Achievements in congenital heart defect surgery: A prospective, 40-year study of 7038 patients. *Circulation* **2015**, *131*, 337–346. [CrossRef] [PubMed]
3. Mutluer, F.O.; Çeliker, A. General Concepts in Adult Congenital Heart Disease. *Balk. Med. J.* **2018**, *35*, 18–29. [CrossRef] [PubMed]
4. Tan, W.; Stefanescu Schmidt, A.C.; Horlick, E.; Aboulhosn, J. Transcatheter Interventions in Patients with Adult Congenital Heart Disease. *J. Soc. Cardiovasc. Angiogr. Interv.* **2022**, *1*, 100438. [CrossRef]
5. Barry, O.M.; Bouhout, I.; Kodali, S.K.; George, I.; Rosenbaum, M.S.; Petit, C.J.; Kalfa, D. Interventions for Congenital Atrioventricular Valve Dysfunction: JACC Focus Seminar. *J. Am. Coll. Cardiol.* **2022**, *79*, 2259–2269. [CrossRef] [PubMed]
6. Schamroth Pravda, N.; Vaknin Assa, H.; Sondergaard, L.; Bajoras, V.; Sievert, H.; Piayda, K.; Levi, A.; Witberg, G.; Shapira, Y.; Hamdan, A.; et al. Transcatheter Interventions for Atrioventricular Dysfunction in Patients with Adult Congenital Heart Disease: An International Case Series. *J. Clin. Med.* **2023**, *12*, 521. [CrossRef] [PubMed]
7. Silini, A.; Iriart, X. Percutaneous edge-to-edge repair in congenital heart disease: Preliminary results of a promising new technique. *Int. J. Cardiol. Congenit. Heart Dis.* **2022**, *8*, 100370. [CrossRef]
8. Vahanian, A.; Beyersdorf, F.; Praz, F.; Milojevic, M.; Baldus, S.; Bauersachs, J.; Capodanno, D.; Conradi, L.; De Bonis, M.; De Paulis, R.; et al. 2021 ESC/EACTS Guidelines for the management of valvular heart disease: Developed by the Task Force for the management of valvular heart disease of the European Society of Cardiology (ESC) and the European Association for Cardio-Thoracic Surgery (EACTS). *Eur. Heart J.* **2021**, *43*, 561–632. [CrossRef] [PubMed]
9. Alqahtani, F.; Berzingi, C.O.; Aljohani, S.; Hijazi, M.; Al-Hallak, A.; Alkhouli, M. Contemporary Trends in the Use and Outcomes of Surgical Treatment of Tricuspid Regurgitation. *J. Am. Heart Assoc.* **2017**, *6*, e007597. [CrossRef] [PubMed]
10. Nickenig, G.; Weber, M.; Schüler, R.; Hausleiter, J.; Nabauer, M.; von Bardeleben, R.S.; Sotiriou, E.; Schäfer, U.; Deuschl, F.; Alessandrini, H.; et al. Tricuspid valve repair with the Cardioband system: Two-year outcomes of the multicentre, prospective TRI-REPAIR study. *EuroIntervention* **2021**, *16*, e1264–e1271. [CrossRef] [PubMed]
11. Gray, W.A.; Abramson, S.V.; Lim, S.; Fowler, D.; Smith, R.L.; Grayburn, P.A.; Kodali, S.K.; Hahn, R.T.; Kipperman, R.M.; Koulogiannis, K.P.; et al. 1-Year Outcomes of Cardioband Tricuspid Valve Reconstruction System Early Feasibility Study. *JACC Cardiovasc. Interv.* **2022**, *15*, 1921–1932. [CrossRef] [PubMed]
12. Taggart, N.W.; Cabalka, A.K.; Eicken, A.; Aboulhosn, J.A.; Thomson, J.D.R.; Whisenant, B.; Bocks, M.L.; Schubert, S.; Jones, T.K.; Asnes, J.D.; et al. Outcomes of Transcatheter Tricuspid Valve-In-Valve Implantation in Patients with Ebstein Anomaly. *Am. J. Cardiol.* **2018**, *121*, 262–268. [CrossRef] [PubMed]
13. Hahn, R.T.; Kodali, S.; Fam, N.; Bapat, V.; Bartus, K.; Rodés-Cabau, J.; Dagenais, F.; Estevez-Loureiro, R.; Forteza, A.; Kapadia, S.; et al. Early Multinational Experience of Transcatheter Tricuspid Valve Replacement for Treating Severe Tricuspid Regurgitation. *JACC Cardiovasc. Interv.* **2020**, *13*, 2482–2493. [CrossRef] [PubMed]
14. Ott, I.; Rumpf, P.M.; Kasel, M.; Kastrati, A.; Kaemmerer, H.; Schunkert, H.; Ewert, P.; Tutarel, O. Transcatheter valve repair in congenitally corrected transposition of the great arteries. *EuroIntervention* **2021**, *17*, 744–746. [CrossRef] [PubMed]
15. Blusztein, D.; Moore, P.; Qasim, A.; Mantri, N.; Mahadevan, V.S. Transcatheter Edge-To-Edge Repair of Systemic Tricuspid Valve in Extracardiac Fontan Circulation. *J. Am. Coll. Cardiol. Case Rep.* **2022**, *4*, 221–225. [CrossRef] [PubMed]
16. Guerin, P.; Jalal, Z.; Le Ruz, R.; Cueff, C.; Hascoet, S.; Bouvaist, H.; Ladouceur, M.; Levy, F.; Hugues, N.; Malekzadeh-Milani, S.G.; et al. Percutaneous Edge-To-Edge Repair for Systemic Atrioventricular Valve Regurgitation in Patients with Congenital Heart Disease: The First Descriptive Cohort. *J. Am. Heart Assoc.* **2022**, *1*, e025628. [CrossRef] [PubMed]
17. Ghosh, R.M.; Jolley, M.A.; Mascio, C.E.; Chen, J.M.; Fuller, S.; Rome, J.J.; Silvestro, E.; Whitehead, K.K. Clinical 3D modeling to guide pediatric cardiothoracic surgery and intervention using 3D printed anatomic models, computer aided design and virtual reality. *3D Print. Med.* **2022**, *8*, 11. [CrossRef] [PubMed]
18. Ong, C.S.; Krishnan, A.; Huang, C.Y.; Spevak, P.; Vricella, L.; Hibino, N.; Garcia, J.R.; Gaur, L. Role of virtual reality in congenital heart disease. *Congenit. Heart Dis.* **2018**, *13*, 357–361. [CrossRef] [PubMed]
19. Rad, A.A.; Vardanyan, R.; Lopuszko, A.; Alt, C.; Stoffels, I.; Schmack, B.; Ruhparwar, A.; Zhigalov, K.; Zubarevich, A.; Weymann, A. Virtual and Augmented Reality in Cardiac Surgery. *Braz. J. Cardiovasc. Surg.* **2022**, *37*, 123–127. [CrossRef] [PubMed]
20. Mahtab, E.A.F.; Egorova, A.D. Current and future applications of virtual reality technology for cardiac interventions. *Nat. Rev. Cardiol.* **2022**, *19*, 779–780. [CrossRef] [PubMed]

Disclaimer/Publisher's Note: The statements, opinions and data contained in all publications are solely those of the individual author(s) and contributor(s) and not of MDPI and/or the editor(s). MDPI and/or the editor(s) disclaim responsibility for any injury to people or property resulting from any ideas, methods, instructions or products referred to in the content.

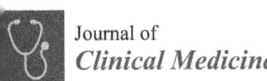

Review

Echocardiographic Parameters for Risk Prediction in Borderline Right Ventricle: Review with Special Emphasis on Pulmonary Atresia with Intact Ventricular Septum and Critical Pulmonary Stenosis

Massimiliano Cantinotti [1,2], Colin Joseph McMahon [3,4], Pietro Marchese [1,5], Martin Köstenberger [6], Marco Scalese [5], Eliana Franchi [1], Giuseppe Santoro [1], Nadia Assanta [1], Xander Jacquemyn [7], Shelby Kutty [7] and Raffaele Giordano [8,*]

1 Fondazione G. Monasterio CNR-Regione Toscana, 56124 Pisa, Italy; cantinotti@ftgm.it (M.C.); pmarchese@ftgm.it (P.M.); eliana.franchi@ftgm.it (E.F.); giuseppe.santoro@ftgm.it (G.S.); assanta@ftgm.it (N.A.)
2 Institute of Clinical Physiology, 56124 Pisa, Italy
3 Department of Pediatric Cardiology, Childrens Health Ireland, D12 N512 Dublin, Ireland; colin.mcmahon@olchc.ie
4 School of Medicine, University College Dublin, D04 V1W8 Dublin, Ireland
5 Istituto di Scienze Della Vita (ISV), Scuola Superiore Sant'Anna, 56127 Pisa, Italy; scalese@ifc.cnr.it
6 Department of Pediatrics, Division of Pediatric Cardiology, Medical University Graz, 8036 Graz, Austria; martin.koestenberger@medunigraz.at
7 Helen B. Taussig Heart Center, Department of Pediatrics, Johns Hopkins Hospital, Baltimore, MD 21205, USA; skutty1@jhmi.edu (X.J.); shelby.kutty@gmail.com (S.K.)
8 Adult and Pediatric Cardiac Surgery, Department Advanced Biomedical Sciences, University of Naples "Federico II", 80131 Naples, Italy
* Correspondence: r.giordano81@libero.it; Tel./Fax: +39-0817464702

Abstract: The aim of the present review is to highlight the strengths and limitations of echocardiographic parameters and scores employed to predict favorable outcome in complex congenital heart diseases (CHDs) with borderline right ventricle (RV), with a focus on pulmonary atresia with intact ventricular septum and critical pulmonary stenosis (PAIVS/CPS). A systematic search in the National Library of Medicine using Medical Subject Headings and free-text terms including echocardiography, CHD, and scores, was performed. The search was refined by adding keywords "PAIVS/CPS", Ebstein's anomaly, and unbalanced atrioventricular septal defect with left dominance. A total of 22 studies were selected for final analysis; 12 of them were focused on parameters to predict biventricular repair (BVR)/pulmonary blood flow augmentation in PAIVS/CPS. All of these studies presented numerical (the limited sample size) and methodological limitations (retrospective design, poor definition of inclusion/exclusion criteria, variability in the definition of outcomes, differences in adopted surgical and interventional strategies). There was heterogeneity in the echocardiographic parameters employed and cut-off values proposed, with difficultly in establishing which one should be recommended. Easy scores such as TV/MV (tricuspid/mitral valve) and RV/LV (right/left ventricle) ratios were proven to have a good prognostic accuracy; however, the data were very limited (only two studies with <40 subjects). In larger studies, RV end-diastolic area and a higher degree of tricuspid regurgitation were also proven as accurate predictors of successful BVR. These measures, however, may be either operator and/or load/pressure dependent. TV Z-scores have been proposed by several authors, but old and heterogenous nomograms sources have been employed, thus producing discordant results. In summary, we provide a review of the currently available echocardiographic parameters for risk prediction in CHDs with a diminutive RV that may serve as a guide for use in clinical practice.

Keywords: echocardiography; borderline right ventricles; scores; pediatrics

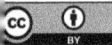

1. Background

Borderline right ventricle (RV) encompasses a wide spectrum of complex congenital heart diseases (CHDs) with neonatal presentation including pulmonary atresia with intact ventricular septum (IVS), critical pulmonary stenosis (CPS), [1–13] severe Ebstein's anomaly [14–22], and unbalanced atrioventricular septal defect (uAVSD) with left dominance [23–26]. Echocardiography is the foremost and often only imaging modality employed in the diagnosis and estimation of disease severity, which influences surgical/interventional planning in these complex defects. Despite this, echocardiographic parameters and scores for disease severity and risk prediction in complex CHDs with borderline RV are lacking and heterogeneous in nature. Several studies have tried to evaluate which echocardiographic measures were able to predict favorable outcomes including successful biventricular repair (BVR) and the need for pulmonary blood flow stabilization/re-intervention, in neonatal CHDs with borderline RV [1–26]. Most of the literature is focused on pulmonary atresia IVS and CPS [1–13], whereas very few studies are available for Ebstein's anomaly [18,21] and uAVSD with left dominance [25,26]. Consequently, our aim was to review echocardiographic parameters predictive of a favorable outcome in borderline RV, with special attention on those parameters most predictive for successful BVR. We also investigated which variables predicted the need for duct stenting/shunt palliation after percutaneous balloon pulmonary valvuloplasty in PAIVS and CPS.

2. Methods

In June 2022, we performed a systematic search in the National Library of Medicine for Medical Subject Headings and free-text terms including "echocardiography," "congenital heart disease", and "scores". The search was refined by adding keywords for "pulmonary atresia intact ventricular septum" and "critical pulmonary stenosis," "Ebstein's anomaly" and "uAVSD with left dominance". The titles and abstracts of articles identified were evaluated and excluded if: [1] the reports were written in languages other than English (1 study) and [2] studies did not report echocardiographic scores (25 studies).

3. Results

From 48 studies initially selected, 22 original studies [1–13,16–21,23,25,26] met the criteria established and were selected for analysis (Figure 1).

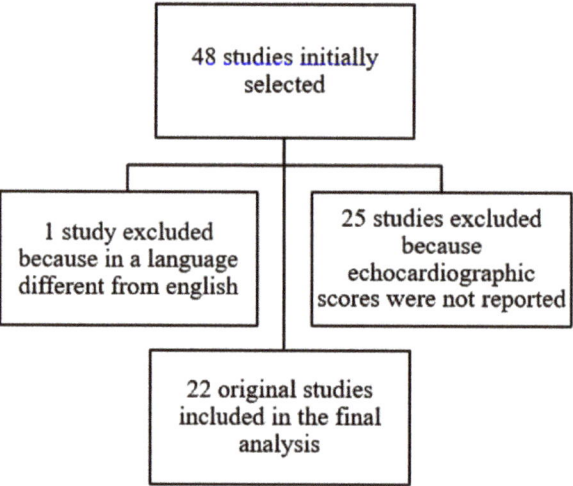

Figure 1. Study selection.

3.1. Pulmonary Atresia with Intact Ventricular Septum and Critical Pulmonary Stenosis

3.1.1. General Methodological Limitations

Echocardiographic parameters able to determine favorable immediate [2–4,6,10] and long-term outcome in neonates with PAIVS and CPS were analyzed [1,5,11]. All studies were retrospective in nature, and most comprised of single-center designs with limited exceptions [1,2,12]. Sample size was limited (varying from 22 to 36 subjects) [4,5,7,9,10] or relatively limited (varying from 53 to 99 subjects) [2,6,8,11].

Inclusion criteria were different in most studies, including only those children undergoing percutaneous balloon pulmonary valvuloplasty as an initial procedure [3–6,8–10]. Most of the studies were focused only on PA IVS undergoing percutaneous balloon pulmonary valvuloplasty (PBPV) [1,3,5,8,9,16], whereas some had more exhaustive inclusion criteria such as children treated with both PBPV and surgically with a Blalock–Thomas–Taussig shunt (BTT) [11] or those only [13] treated surgically, either with BTT or closed trans-ventricular valvulotomy [13]. Few studies also included CPS [3,4], whereas one was limited to children with CPS [6].

Endpoints were also different between studies, comprising of the need for PDA stenting or BTT [3,4,6,8] reintervention [2,6,10] and good biventricular outcome [1,5,11,13]. Whereas most of the authors evaluated only neonates [1,2,4,6,8–11], others additionally included older children [5,8,13] up to 8 years of age.

Exclusion criteria were often poorly defined, and when they were specified [2,8,11–14], they also varied between different authors. They consisted of decompression after the neonatal period [1,2], previous BTT [5], RV-dependent coronary circulation [3,5], unipartite RV [5] or diminutive RV [3,10], and muscular infundibular atresia [3,9]. Neonates with Ebstein's anomaly were excluded from four cohorts [1,2,5,10], whereas this was not specifically described in other studies [6,8,13]. The echocardiographic parameters evaluated also varied among different authors, as detailed in Table 1 and Supplementary Table S1.

Table 1. Major studies evaluating echocardiographic parameters for risk prediction in PA IVS/CPS.

	Population	End Point	Echo Predictors
Cho MJ 2013 South Corea [4]	9 PA IVS, 13 CPS Undergoing PBPV −10 need aPBF Age 4.89 ± 2.47 days Weight 2.98 ± 0.6 kg −10 do not need aPBF Age 10.10 ± 10.63 days Weight 3.3 ± 0.3 kg	Need of PDA stenting or shunt	TV z-score ≤ -0.74 (AUC 0.8; specificity 90%, sensitivity 77.8%, $p = 0.0189$) TV/MV ≤ 0.9, (AUC 0.939; specificity 90%, sensitivity 88.89%; $p < 0.0001$) z-score IVSD ≥ 2.37 (AUC 0.804; specificity 75%, sensitivity 85.71%; $p = 0.0222$)
Chen RHS 2018 Hong Kong [5]	36 PA IVS Undergoing PBPV −26 BVR Age 5 (1–83) days Weight 3.21 ± 0.55 kg −5 no BVR Age 4 (2–51) days Weight 2.8 ± 0.31	Good BVR outcome	TV/MV > 0.79 AUC 0.858 specificity 100%, sensitivity 70%, PPV 100%, NPV 50%)
Yucel IK, 2016 Turkey [6]	56 CPS Undergoing PBPV Age 7 (2–28) days. Weight 3.1 (1.6–4.5) kg NR 34 do not need aPBF Weight 3.07 ± 0.4 kg NR 21 need aPBF Weight 3.17 ± 0.4 kg	Need of PDA stenting or shunt Need of re-intervention	TV Z score < −1.93 (AUC = 0.696, specificity 84.4%, sensitivity 63.2%, $p = 0.022$) PV Z score < −1.69 (AUC = 0.72, specificity 64.7%, sensitivity 74%, $p = 0.008$) Bipartite RV (odds ratio 9.6).

Table 1. Cont.

	Population	End Point	Echo Predictors
Alwi M 2005 Malaysia [8]	53 PA IVS Undergoing PBPV −10 need aPBF Age 8 days (3 days–7 months) Weight 3.1 (2.4–6.8) kg −37 do not need aPBF Age 7 days (1 day–8 years) Weight 3.3 (2–18) kg	Need of PDA stenting or shunt	Lower TV z score TV Z-score −1.1 ± 1.47 Need of aPBF TV Z-score −0.58 ± 1.18 No need of aPBF
Drighil A, 2009, USA [9]	26 PA IVS Undergoing PBPV Age 6 (1–49) days −13 successful BVR Age 14.5 ± 9.0 days Weight 3.3 ± 0.6 kg −13 unsuccessful BVR Age 17.6 ± 15.3 days Weight 3.1 ± 0.6 kg	PBPV success	(1) RV/LV diameter > 0.76 predicts a 92.3% success rate. (2) RV/LV diameter ≤ 0.70 + RV/LV length ≤ 0.76 predicts 100% failure (3) RV/LV diameter ≤ 0.76 and RV/LV length > 0.70, 75% success rate
Schwartz MC, 2006, USA [10]	23 PA IVS undergoing RFV Age 2 (−16) days Weight 3.1 (2.1–4.1) kg	Need of re-intervention	Lower post-procedural PV PG ($p = 0.05$) TV z-score < −0.7 ($p = 0.08$)
Cleuziou J, 2010, Germany [11]	86 PA IVS 55 underwent PVVP (16 plus shunt) 26 underwent shunt. BVR in 56 Age 2.2 ± 4.8 years Shunt palliation in 13 UV in 17	Predictors of BVR Predictors of mortality	RV decompression ± shunt ($p < 0.001$), Tripartite RV ($p < 0.001$) No coronary fistulae ($p < 0.001$). At univariate analysis TV z score < 5, unipartite RV, coronary fistula, Ebstein's, RV dependent coronary circulation, connection of the fistula with LCA and RCA
Maskatia SA, 2018, USA [1]	81 PA IVS Undergoing PBPV Age 3 (2–4) days	BVR, RV growth	Baseline RV area ≥ 0.6 cm²/m² (Sensitivity 93%, specificity 80%, AUC 0.88, odds ratio 50.4) Follow-up RV area ≥ 0.8 cm²/m² sensitivity 100% specificity 100%, AUC 0.96, odds ratio 67) More than moderate TR
Minich LL, 2000, USA [13]	23 successful surgical BVR ° Age 11–20 days Weight 3.5 ± 0.6 kg 13 unsuccessful BVR Weight 2.9 ± 0.5 kg	BVR	Greater pre-op weight TV z score > −3, TV/MV > 0.5
Petit CJ, 2017, USA [2]	99 PA IVS undergoing PBPV Age 3 (2–5) days Weight 3.3 (2.7–3.7) kg	Primary: Reintervention post-RV decompression. Secondary: BVR	Virtual atresia (HR, 0.51; 95% CI, 0.28–091; $p = 0.027$), Smaller RV length (HR, 0.94; 95% CI, 0.89–0.99; $p = 0.027$), ≤Mild TR (HR, 3.58; 95% CI, 2.04–6.30; $p < 0.001$). ≤Mild TR (OR, 18.6; 95% CI, 5.3–5.2; $p < 0.001$) Lower RV area (OR, 0.81; 95% CI, 0.72–0.91; $p < 0.001$).
Giordano M, 2022, Italy [3]	55 PA IVS or CPS Age NR Weight 2.9 ± 5 kg 27 need aPBF Weight 3.0 ± 0.4 kg 28 do not need aPBF Weight 2.9 ± 0.6 KG	Need of PDA stenting or shunt	Composite score including TV < 8.8 mm, TV z-score ← 2.12, TV/MV <0.78, PV < 6.7 mm, PV z-score ←1.17, RVED area < 1.35 cm², RA area > 2.45 cm², % of PFO right-to-left shunt > 69.5%, moderate/severe TR, RV systolic pressure > 42.5 mmHg, tricuspid E/E' ratio > 6.6 A score ≥ 4 sensitivity 100% and specificity 86%

Legend to Table: aPBF = adjunctive pulmonary blood flow, AUC = area under the ROC curve, BVR = biventricular repair; CI = confidence interval, CPS = critical pulmonary stenosis, HR = hazard ratio, IVSD = end-diastolic interventricular septal thickness; LCA = left coronary artery; LV = left ventricle; MV = mitral valve; NR = number; OR = odds ratio; PDA = patent arterial duct, PFO = patent foramen ovale: PV = pulmonary valve, PG = pressure gradient, PBPV = percutaneous balloon pulmonary valvuloplasty, RCA = right coronary artery; RV = right ventricle; RVED = right ventricle end-diastolic; TR = tricuspid regurgitation; TV = tricuspid valve; ° closed trans-ventricular valvulotomy with and central shunt.

3.1.2. Echocardiographic Parameters Evaluated

The Tricuspid Valve

- Tricuspid valve Z-score

Many authors used TV Z-scores as an indicator for the need of PDA stenting or BTT [3,4,6], re-intervention [11], or BVR success [13]. The specific Z-scores employed, however, differed among various studies. Often the source of Z-score [27–32] was not provided [3,6,8,10], whereas a few authors used very old (e.g., Rowllat) [13,17] or old formulas (e.g., Daubeney) [4,5,28]. Only a few authors [1,2,4] used recently provided Z-scores (e.g., Pettersen) [31]. The use of different nomograms (especially older ones) may generate discordant ranges of normality, thus generating confusion in disease severity estimation. It is well known that nomograms employed for years have important limitations, providing a range of normality widely different from those obtained with the more recently proposed Z-scores [27,31,32]. To provide a practical example: in a baby of 3 kg and 50 cm with a given TV annulus of 10 mm, the Z-score varied from -3.8 using older Z-scores (Daubeney) [15], to -1.59 (Cantinotti) [27], to -1.24 (Pettersen) [31], and up to -0.55 (Lopez) [32] using more recent nomograms. Thus, it is not surprising that the range/cut-off values for the TV Z-score that indicated a higher risk for PA IVS/CPS varied greatly among different studies. For instance, in terms of the need for PDA stenting or surgical shunt, the critical TV Z-scores cut-off values varied from ≤ 0.7 to -2.12 [3–5,8,11] according to the different authors. Those authors who employed older Z-score sources [15] tended to overestimate the degree of hypoplasia [12], suggesting that even children with very low TV scores (up to -5) had the possibility for successful BVR. Authors who employed more recent nomograms (e.g., Pettersen) [31] demonstrated that even mild TV hypoplasia (a cut-off value TV Z-score ≤ 0.74 having a specificity of 90% and a sensitivity of 77.8%) [4] was predictive of the need for PDA stenting/shunt in 36 neonates and infants with PAIVS/CPS who underwent CPBP. Despite these findings, TV hypoplasia is considered a negative indicator [4,11]; Petit and colleagues [2] demonstrated that in 99 patients with PAIVS, a larger TV annulus was associated with a higher risk of reintervention for restenosis of the right ventricular outflow tract (RVOT) (hazard ratio, 1.20 per 1 mm increase; $p = 0.071$).

- TV/MV annular ratio

The use of the TV/MV annular ratio may overcome the issues related to the use of different Z-scores. The TV/MV annular ratio is an easy and very reproducible measurement, independent of external formulas, that has been employed by several authors [3–5,13] (Figure 2). Similar to TV Z-scores, the cut-offs indicated by different authors varied widely. A few studies demonstrated that children with mild [23] (e.g., TV/MV ratio > 0.79) or even moderate [13] TV hypoplasia (e.g., TV/MV ratio ≥ 0.5) could achieve a successful BVR. Paradoxically, other studies reported that even a very mild (e.g., TV/MV ratio ≤ 0.9) [4] or mild ratio (e.g., TV/MV ratio < 0.78) [3] was predictive of the need for PDA stenting or BT shunt to stabilize the pulmonary blood flow [3,4].

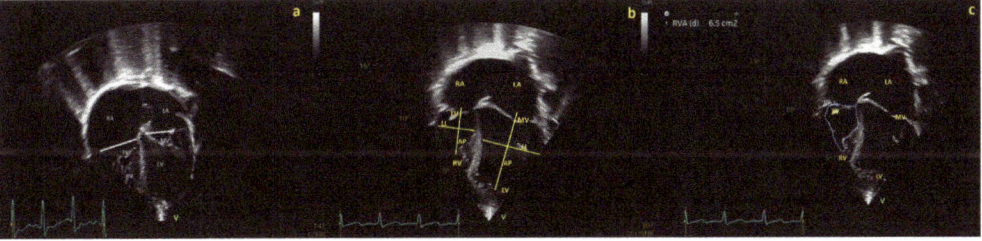

Figure 2. Four chamber view of a PAIVS with diminutive, hypertrophied RV. (**a**) Mitral valve (MV) and tricuspid valve (TV) diameters. (**b**) Base–apex and laterolateral diameters of the right (RV) and left ventricles (LV), (**c**) right ventricle end-diastolic (RVED) area.

- Tricuspid regurgitation

The degree of tricuspid regurgitation (TR) is an important indicator for successful BVR [1,2]. Maskatia et al. [1] found that in 81 neonates with PAIVS treated with PBPV, a greater than moderate TR was associated with RV growth. Similarly, mild or less than mild [2] TR was associated with the need for re-intervention and failing BVR in 99 neonates with PAIVS. Other authors [3] have indicated that the presence of moderate/severe TR was a risk factor for duct dependency of the pulmonary circulation. It is important to remember that the criteria for grading TR in the pediatric age by echocardiography, especially at younger neonatal ages, are not completely defined [33,34]. Consequently, different criteria to grade TR have been adopted by several authors. Maskatia et al. [1], graded the TR as none/mild or moderate/severe according to vena contracta, jet area, deceleration time, and flow reversal in pulmonary arteries; however, the cut-off values for inclusion in different categories are described to be not indicated [1]. Other studies [2,3] refer to respective guidelines, however, pediatric guidelines for the quantitative echocardiographic evaluation of TR are not currently available [33,34] and adult guidelines are often extrapolated to children without any validation [35].

Right Ventricle Size

Evaluation of RV size is difficult at echocardiography and may be even more difficult in hypoplastic, hypertrophied bipartite RV, such as those in neonates with PAIVS.

- RV diameters

An easy way to measure RV dimensions is to calculate the lateral diameter and base-apex length in the four-chamber view (Figure 2). The RV/LV lateral diameters ratio has been tested for prediction of BVR by Drighill and colleagues [10], who retrospectively evaluated 26 patients with PAIVS who underwent PBPV at a single institution (13 with successful BVR, 13 with unsuccessful BVR). The authors [10] demonstrated that an RV/LV diameter > 0.76 predicted a 92.3% success rate for BVR. When the RV/LV diameter was ≤ 0.76 and RV/LV length was >0.70, the success rate for BVR dropped to 75%. When both the RV/LV diameter was ≤ 0.70 and the RV/LV length was ≤ 0.76, there was a 100% probability of failure for BVR. Additionally, the RV length determined by the four-chamber view [2] was one of the major determinants for any re-intervention after decompression in 99 children with PAIVS undergoing PBPV (hazard ratio-HR-, 0.94; for 0.01 mm, 95% CI 0.89–0.99; $p = 0.027$) [2].

- Right ventricle end-diastolic (RVED) area

Another technique to measure RV size by echocardiography is to trace the end-diastolic area in the four-chamber view. However, the tracing of endocardial borders may be quite difficult in very hypertrophied, trabeculated RV such as those of neonates with PAIVS/CPS (Figure 2). RV areas and volumes in the neonatal age are greatly influenced by load and pressure conditions and may vary greatly from one moment to the other. Therefore, the cut-off for the RVED area proposed by different authors differed widely from 6 cm^2/m^2 for BVR [1] to 1.35 cm^2 for ductal dependency after PBPV [3]. Maskatia et al. [1] investigated 81 neonates who underwent PBPV for PAIVS and demonstrated that an RVED area at baseline ≥ 6 cm^2/m^2 had a sensitivity of 93% and a specificity of 80% in predicting BVR. Petit and colleagues [2] showed that the RVED area was lower in neonates with PAIVS who underwent univentricular palliation ($n = 17$) compared with those who underwent biventricular repair ($n = 82$) (mean 1.0 cm^2, range 0.9 to 1.2 cm^2 in UVP versus 2.1 cm^2, range 1.6 to 2.6 cm^2 in BVR, $p < 0.0001$). The RVED area had an odds ratio of 0.81 per 0.1 cm^2 increase (95% CI, 0.72–0.91; $p < 0.001$) for the prediction of BVR, however, cut-off values were not proposed (2). Lastly, Giordano et al. indicated a value for the RVED area of 1.35 cm^2 as a risk factor for duct-dependent pulmonary circulation after PBPV in PAIV [3].

- Composite scores and other indices

With the previously described limitations related to the use of Z-scores, both PV Z-scores [3,6] and interventricular septum diastolic thickness Z-scores [4] have been demonstrated to be other markers able to predict duct/shunt dependency of the pulmonary circulation in PA IVS/CPS. Giordano et al. [3] recently proposed a score using multiple echocardiographic measurements (e.g., TV < 8.8 mm, TV Z-score $\leq$ 2.12, TV/MV < 0.78, PV < 6.7 mm, PV Z-score $\leq$ 1.17, RVED area < 1.35 cm^2, right atrial (RA) area > 2.45 cm^2, % of PFO right-to-left shunt > 69.5%, moderate/severe TR, RV systolic pressure > 42.5 mmHg, tricuspid E/E' ratio > 6), each of them assigning one point if reaching the cut-off value. A score $\geq$ 4 had a 100% sensitivity and 86% specificity in predicting the need for PDA stenting/shunt in 55 neonates with PA-IVS/CPS (Table 1) [3].

4. Severe Ebstein's Anomaly

Despite the broad surgical literature on Ebstein's' anomaly [14–17], there are limited echocardiographic studies [18–21] aimed to evaluate the echocardiographic predictors for BVR in severe neonatal forms of Ebstein's anomaly.

Celermajer's index: In 1992 [18], Celermajer and colleagues published a famous score to grade Ebstein's disease severity based on simple echocardiographic data. The score is calculated as the ratio of RA + atrialized RV to the functional RV + left atrium (LA) + LV. The study included 50 neonates with Ebstein's anomaly evaluated in London from 1960 to 1990 [26]; however, only in 28 out of 50 cases were echocardiographic data available. Four neonates had a score of grade 1, who were all alive at a follow-up of 5 to 9 years; ten neonates had a score of grade 2, of which one died suddenly at 4 months; nine neonates had grade 3, of which five died (ranging from 4 months to 9 years of total life); and five neonates had grade 4, all of whom died within 18 months.

In 2013, Yu et al. [21] reviewed 59 cases of Ebstein's anomaly from South Korea, reporting a mortality rate of 23.7%; however, neither the Carpenter's classification (p = 0.175) nor the Celermajer's index (p = 0.958) was significantly related to death. Instead, univariate analysis revealed that fetal distress (p = 0.002), prematurity (p = 0.036), low birth weight (p = 0.003), diameter of the ASD (p = 0.002), and pulmonary stenosis/atresia (p = 0.001) were related to mortality. On multivariate analysis, however, only fetal distress (p = 0.004) and pulmonary atresia/stenosis (p < 0.001) remained significant determinants of outcome [21]. Both studies [18,21] suffered from methodological limitations including being single-center in origin, retrospective in design, and including all neonates diagnosed without clear inclusion and exclusion criteria (all neonates with Ebstein's anomaly regardless of the severity of the disease were included, including those with associated congenitally corrected transposition of the great arteries) [18,21]. Furthermore, surgical/interventional algorithms were not described but were certainly different from more recent ones. The study cohort in one paper [21] also had an uneven distribution of disease severity, with only eight (15.3%) and two neonates (3.8%) having grade II and grade IV of Celermajer's index and/or type C and D of Carpentier's classification, respectively [21].

In a retrospective surgical series from 2016 [17] on 12 neonates who were diagnosed with severe TR and pulmonary atresia related to Ebstein's anomaly (n = 9) or isolated TV dysplasia (n = 3), six underwent a BVR and three survived [17]. A TR flow velocity > 3.0 m/s was an indicator of successful BVR [17]. A study evaluating the characteristics of Ebstein's anomaly during fetal life revealed a series of independent predictors of mortality including gestational age < 32 weeks, TV Z-score, pulmonary regurgitation (all p < 0.001), and the presence of pericardial effusion (p = 0.04) [22].

5. Unbalanced AVSD

Unbalanced atrioventricular septal defect (UAVSD) with left dominance is usually defined when the atrioventricular valve index (AVVI) (left valve area/right valve area in subcostal view) is >0.6 [23–26]. Studies that assessed the ability of scores to predict successful BVR in UAVSD have excluded those with a left dominance [23], thus data for UAVSD with left dominance are extremely limited [25,26]. In 2015, Jegatheeswaran et al. [25] reviewed data from 58 patients with UAVSD (50 with right dominance and 8 with left dominance) treated at four different centers between 2000 and 2006. They observed that in patients with UAVSD with left dominance (e.g., AVVI of >0.6), surgical strategies varied and interim palliation (PA banding) and one-and-a-half ventricle repair strategies were preferred.

Later, Nathan et al. [26] reviewed 16 UAVSD cases (including 6 with left dominance) with prior single ventricle palliation who underwent conversion to BVR between 2003 and 2011 at the Children's Hospital, Boston. Primary BVR or initial pulmonary artery banding or shunting with subsequent conversion to BVR was recommended for those with a mild hypoplasia of the ventricle (LV or RV volumes > 30 mL/m^2) or AVVI (0.19 < AVVI < 0.39 or 0.61 < AVVI < 0.80. 60% to 80% overriding,) and apex-forming ventricles [26]. In contrast, in UAVSD patients with the same AVV characteristics but moderate ventricular hypoplasia (RV/LV 15 to 30 mL/m^2) and near apex-forming ventricles, single ventricle palliation and ventricular recruitment with subsequent staged biventricular conversion was advised, whereas univentricular palliation was advised only in UAVSD with severe ventricular hypoplasia (LV/RV < 15 mL/m^2, 0.19 < AVVI > 0.81, 80% overriding) [26].

6. Discussion

Although echocardiography is often the primary and sometimes only imaging modality for pre-surgical/interventional diagnosis in complex neonatal CHDs characterized by borderline RV, the echocardiographic indicators available for risk prediction in this cardiac lesion remain limited.

All the literature data reviewed herein showed significant methodological limitations, including a single-center design [3–13,18,21,25,26], retrospective design [3–11,13, 18,21,25,26], poor definition of inclusion/exclusion criteria [3–13,18,21,25,26], the lack of interventional algorithms, and a clearly limited [4,5,7,9,10] or relatively limited sample size [2,6,8,11]. Furthermore, studies [7,8,11–13,19] reviewing the surgeries/interventions of two or more decades ago may have little clinical relevance now.

A series of echocardiographic parameters have been proposed for BVR risk assessment in patients suffering from PAIVS/CPS [1–13]. However, it is difficult to establish which of the parameters proposed should be recommended for use in daily practice. TV/MV [4,5,13] and RV/LV [9] diameter ratio can be readily acquired and very reproducible indices that show a good accuracy for the prediction of successful BVR or the need for pulmonary blood flow augmentation after PBVP. However, data are very limited, with three studies enrolling less than 30 cases [3,5,9]. In larger studies [1–3] (up to 99 investigated cases), the RVED area has been demonstrated as an accurate predictor of BVR [1,2] or the need for pulmonary blood flow augmentation [3]. The RVED area, however, may be less reproducible and very dependent on load conditions, thus discordant cut-off values have been reported by different studies [1,3]. Similarly, it has been demonstrated that a higher degree of TR is favorable for BVR [1,2]. However, estimation of TR in the neonatal age is highly subjective and very dependent on load/pressure conditions, the pulmonary vascular bed, and ventilatory support. Data that focused on TV Z-scores [4,6,8,13] may have significant limitations, since the nomograms that were employed [28–31] are different from those currently employed [27,32]; thus, the cut-off values are poorly applicable in daily practice.

The use of composite scores with multiple markers, as recently proposed, seems to be a reasonable approach for future studies [3]. There is a need for large prospective studies with clear endpoints and clear inclusion/exclusion criteria. Furthermore, the timing of echocardiographic examination (before and/or after PBPV), measurement, and quantification techniques also needs to be standardized. Lastly, attention to confounders such as the strategies for pulmonary blood flow augmentation (BTM of duct stenting), criteria for re-intervention, and definition of a successful BVR need to be specified.

In summary, there is a shortage of echocardiographic studies clarifying prognostic indicators in other forms of borderline RV including Ebstein's anomaly (and other forms of tricuspid valve dysplasia) [18–21] and UAVSD [23–26]. Although widely used, the prognostic value of the Celermajer index [17] for BVR in severe neonatal Ebstein's anomaly has been poorly validated in clinical studies. The score may also present limitations due to the dependency on cardiac load and pressure [33,34] in chamber area. The level of agreement between the Celermajer score determined by echocardiography and that obtained through MRI is only moderate at best (kappa coefficient = 0.39, $p = 0.002$). Typically, echocardiography tends to overestimate the severity of Ebstein's anomaly, although underestimations can rarely occur [18].

The available literature describing UAVSD is extremely limited [25,26], since the studies aiming to investigate echocardiographic indicators for BVR in this specific population excluded or do not analyze UAVSD with left dominance. Additionally, data on rare defects, such as isolated RV hypoplasia [36], that may present with cyanosis in the neonatal age are also very limited [36].

7. Conclusions

Our review summarizes the strengths and limitations of the current echocardiographic indices to predict successful BVR and the need for reintervention/pulmonary blood flow stabilization in complex neonatal CHD with borderline RV, with a specific focus on PAIVS and CPS. Examining the echocardiographic evaluation of disease severity is crucial for complex CHD's encountered in daily practice and should serve as a guide for further research that would appear to be necessary based on the observations from this review.

Supplementary Materials: The following supporting information can be downloaded at: https://www.mdpi.com/article/10.3390/jcm12144599/s1. Table S1: Inclusion/exclusion criteria in major studies evaluating echocardiographic parameters for risk prediction in PA IVS/CPS. References [1–6,8–11,13] are cited in Supplementary Materials.

Author Contributions: All authors contributed to the study conception and design. Material preparation, data collection, and analysis were performed by R.G., P.M., E.F., M.S., G.S., M.K., C.J.M., X.J. and N.A. The first draft of the manuscript was written by M.C. and S.K. and all authors commented on previous versions of the manuscript. All authors have read and agreed to the published version of the manuscript.

Funding: This research received no external funding.

Institutional Review Board Statement: The study was conducted in accordance with the Declaration of Helsinki, and approved by the Institutional Review Board (Meyer CE 62/2016).

Informed Consent Statement: Not applicable.

Data Availability Statement: The data presented in this study are available on request from the corresponding author.

Conflicts of Interest: The authors declare no conflict of interest.

References

1. Maskatia, S.A.; Petit, C.J.; Travers, C.D.; Goldberg, D.J.; Rogers, L.S.; Glatz, A.C.; Qureshi, A.M.; Goldstein, B.H.; Ao, J.; Sachdeva, R. Echocardiographic parameters associated with biventricular circulation and right ventricular growth following right ventricular decompression in patients with pulmonary atresia and intact ventricular septum: Results from a multicenter study. *Congenit. Heart Dis.* **2018**, *13*, 892–902. [CrossRef] [PubMed]
2. Petit, C.J.; Glatz, A.C.; Qureshi, A.M.; Sachdeva, R.; Maskatia, S.A.; Justino, H.; Goldberg, D.J.; Mozumdar, N.; Whiteside, W.; Rogers, L.S.; et al. Outcomes After Decompression of the Right Ventricle in Infants with Pulmonary Atresia with Intact Ventricular Septum Are Associated with Degree of Tricuspid Regurgitation: Results from the Congenital Catheterization Research Collaborative. *Circ. Cardiovasc. Interv.* **2017**, *10*, e004428. [CrossRef] [PubMed]
3. Giordano, M.; Santoro, G.; Gaio, G.; Bigazzi, M.C.; Esposito, R.; Marzullo, R.; Di Masi, A.; Palladino, M.T.; Russo, M.G. Novel echocardiographic score to predict duct-dependency after percutaneous relief of critical pulmonary valve stenosis/atresia. *Echocardiography* **2022**, *39*, 724–731. [CrossRef] [PubMed]
4. Cho, M.-J.; Ban, K.-H.; Kim, M.-J.; Park, J.-A.; Lee, H.-D. Catheter-based Treatment in Patients with Critical Pulmonary Stenosis or Pulmonary Atresia with Intact Ventricular Septum: A Single Institute Experience with Comparison between Patients with and without Additional Procedure for Pulmonary Flow. *Congenit. Heart Dis.* **2013**, *8*, 440–449. [CrossRef]

5. Chen, R.H.S.; KT Chau, A.; Chow, P.C.; Yung, T.C.; Cheung, Y.F.; Lun, K.S. Achieving biventricular circulation in patients with moderate hypoplastic right ventricle in pulmonary atresia intact ventricular septum after transcatheter pulmonary valve perforation. *Congenit. Heart Dis.* **2018**, *13*, 884–891. [CrossRef]
6. Yucel, I.K.; Bulut, M.O.; Kucuk, M.; Balli, S.; Celebi, A. Intervention in Patients with Critical Pulmonary Stenosis in the Ducta Stenting Era. *Pediatr. Cardiol.* **2016**, *37*, 1037–1045. [CrossRef]
7. Kovalchin, J.P.; Forbes, T.J.; Nihill, M.R.; Geva, T. Echocardiographic Determinants of Clinical Course in Infants with Critical and Severe Pulmonary Valve Stenosis. *J. Am. Coll. Cardiol.* **1997**, *29*, 1095–1101. [CrossRef]
8. Alwi, M.; Kandavello, G.; Choo, K.-K.; Aziz, B.A.; Samion, H.; Latiff, H.A. Risk factors for augmentation of the flow of blood to the lungs in pulmonary atresia with intact ventricular septum after radiofrequency valvotomy. *Cardiol. Young* **2005**, *15*, 141–147 [CrossRef]
9. Drighil, A.; Aljufan, M.; Slimi, A.; Yamani, S.; Mathewson, J.; Alfadly, F. Echocardiographic determinants of successful balloor dilation in pulmonary atresia with intact ventricular septum. *Eur. Heart J. Cardiovasc. Imaging* **2009**, *11*, 172–175. [CrossRef]
10. Schwartz, M.C.; Glatz, A.C.; Dori, Y.; Rome, J.J.; Gillespie, M.J. Outcomes and Predictors of Reintervention in Patients with Pulmonary Atresia and Intact Ventricular Septum Treated with Radiofrequency Perforation and Balloon Pulmonary Valvuloplasty *Pediatr. Cardiol.* **2013**, *35*, 22–29. [CrossRef]
11. Cleuziou, J.; Schreiber, C.; Eicken, A.; Hörer, J.; Busch, R.; Holper, K.; Lange, R. Predictors for Biventricular Repair in Pulmonary Atresia with Intact Ventricular Septum. *Thorac. Cardiovasc. Surg.* **2010**, *58*, 339–344. [CrossRef]
12. Hanley, F.L.; Sade, R.M.; Blackstone, E.H.; Kirklin, J.W.; Freedom, R.M.; Nanda, N.C. Outcomes in neonatal pulmonary atresia with intact ventricular septum. A multiinstitutional study. *J. Thorac. Cardiovasc. Surg.* **1993**, *105*, 406–427. [CrossRef] [PubMed]
13. Minich, L.; Tani, L.Y.; Ritter, S.; Williams, R.V.; Shaddy, R.E.; Hawkins, J.A. Usefulness of the preoperative tricuspid/mitral valve ratio for predicting outcome in pulmonary atresia with intact ventricular septum. *Am. J. Cardiol.* **2000**, *85*, 1325–1328. [CrossRef] [PubMed]
14. Sainathan, S.; Silva, L.D.F.D.; da Silva, J.P. Ebstein's anomaly: Contemporary management strategies. *J. Thorac. Dis.* **2020**, *12* 1161–1173. [CrossRef] [PubMed]
15. Baek, J.S.; Yu, J.J.; Im, Y.M.; Yun, T.J. Outcomes of neonatal Ebstein's anomaly without right ventricular forward flow. *J. Thorac Cardiovasc. Surg.* **2016**, *152*, 516–521. [CrossRef]
16. Sano, S.; Fujii, Y.; Kasahara, S.; Kuroko, Y.; Tateishi, A.; Yoshizumi, K.; Arai, S. Repair of Ebstein's anomaly in neonates and small infants: Impact of right ventricular exclusion and its indications. *Eur. J. Cardiothorac. Surg.* **2014**, *45*, 549–555. [CrossRef]
17. Mizuno, M.; Hoashi, T.; Sakaguchi, H.; Kagisaki, K.; Kitano, M.; Kurosaki, K.; Yoshimatsu, J.; Shiraishi, I.; Ichikawa, H. Application of Cone Reconstruction for Neonatal Ebstein Anomaly or Tricuspid Valve Dysplasia. *Ann. Thorac. Surg.* **2016**, *101*, 1811–1817 [CrossRef]
18. Celermajer, D.S.; Cullen, S.; Sullivan, I.D.; Spiegelhalter, D.J.; Wyse, R.K.; Deanfield, J.E. Outcome in neonates with Ebstein's anomaly. *J. Am. Coll. Cardiol.* **1992**, *19*, 1041–1046. [CrossRef]
19. Cieplucha, A.; Trojnarska, O.; Bartczak-Rutkowska, A.; Kociemba, A.; Rajewska-Tabor, J.; Kramer, L.; Pyda, M. Severity Scores for Ebstein Anomaly: Credibility and Usefulness of Echocardiographic vs. Magnetic Resonance Assessments of the Celermajer Index *Can. J. Cardiol.* **2019**, *35*, 1834–1841. [CrossRef]
20. Prota, C.; Di Salvo, G.; Sabatino, J.; Josen, M.; Paredes, J.; Sirico, D.; Pernia, M.U.; Hoschtitzky, A.; Michielon, G.; Citro, R.; et al Prognostic value of echocardiographic parameters in pediatric patients with Ebstein's anomaly. *Int. J. Cardiol.* **2019**, *278*, 76–83 [CrossRef]
21. Yu, J.J.; Yun, T.-J.; Won, H.-S.; Im, Y.M.; Lee, B.S.; Kang, S.Y.; Ko, H.K.; Park, C.S.; Park, J.-J.; Gwak, M.; et al. Outcome of Neonates with Ebstein's Anomaly in the Current Era. *Pediatr. Cardiol.* **2013**, *34*, 1590–1596. [CrossRef] [PubMed]
22. Freud, L.R.; Escobar-Diaz, M.C.; Kalish, B.T.; Komarlu, R.; Puchalski, M.D.; Jaeggi, E.T.; Szwast, A.L.; Freire, G.; Levasseur, S.M. Kavanaugh-McHugh, A.; et al. Outcomes and Predictors of Perinatal Mortality in Fetuses with Ebstein Anomaly or Tricuspid Valve Dysplasia in the Current Era: A Multicenter Study. *Circulation* **2015**, *132*, 481–489. [CrossRef] [PubMed]
23. Cantinotti, M.; Marchese, P.; Giordano, R.; Franchi, E.; Assanta, N.; Koestenberger, M.; Jani, V.; Duignan, S.; Kutty, S.; McMahon C.J. Echocardiographic scores for biventricular repair risk prediction of congenital heart disease with borderline left ventricle: A review. *Heart Fail. Rev.* **2022**, *28*, 63–76. [CrossRef] [PubMed]
24. Cohen, M.S.; Jacobs, M.L.; Weinberg, P.M.; Rychik, J. Morphometric Analysis of Unbalanced Common Atrioventricular Canal Using Two-Dimensional Echocardiography. *J. Am. Coll. Cardiol.* **1996**, *28*, 1017–1023. [CrossRef]
25. Jegatheeswaran, A.; Pizarro, C.; Caldarone, C.A.; Cohen, M.S.; Baffa, J.M.; Gremmels, D.B.; Mertens, L.; Morell, V.O.; Williams, W.G.; Blackstone, E.H.; et al. Echocardiographic definition and surgical decision-making in unbalanced atrioventricular septal defect: A Congenital Heart Surgeons' Society multi-institutional study. *Circulation* **2010**, *122*, S209–S215. [CrossRef]
26. Nathan, M.; Liu, H.; Pigula, F.A.; Fynn-Thompson, F.; Emani, S.; Baird, C.A.; Marx, G.; Mayer, J.E.; del Nido, P.J. Biventricular Conversion after Single-Ventricle Palliation in Unbalanced Atrioventricular Canal Defects. *Ann. Thorac. Surg.* **2013**, *95*, 2086–2096 [CrossRef]
27. Cantinotti, M.; Scalese, M.; Giordano, R.; Assanta, N.; Marchese, P.; Franchi, E.; Viacava, C.; Koestenberger, M.; Jani, V.; Kutty, S. A statistical comparison of reproducibility in current pediatric two-dimensional echocardiographic nomograms. *Pediatr. Res.* **2020** *89*, 579–590. [CrossRef]

28. Daubeney, P.E.F.; Blackstone, E.H.; Weintraub, R.G.; Slavik, Z.; Scanlon, J.; Webber, S.A. Relationship of the dimension of cardiac structures to body size: An echocardiographic study in normal infants and children. *Cardiol. Young* **1999**, *9*, 402–410. [CrossRef]
29. Rowlatt, J.F.; Rimoldi, M.J.A.; Lev, M. The quantitative anatomy of the normal child's heart. *Pediatr. Clin. North Am.* **1963**, *10*, 499–588. [CrossRef]
30. Snider, A.R.; Serwer, G.A.; Ritter, S.B. *Echocardiography in Pediatric Heart Disease*; Mosby: St. Louis, MO, USA, 1997; pp. 137–142.
31. Pettersen, M.D.; Du, W.; Skeens, M.E.; Humes, R.A. Regression Equations for Calculation of Z Scores of Cardiac Structures in a Large Cohort of Healthy Infants, Children, and Adolescents: An Echocardiographic Study. *J. Am. Soc. Echocardiogr.* **2008**, *21*, 922–934. [CrossRef]
32. Lopez, L.; Frommelt, P.C.; Colan, S.D.; Trachtenberg, F.L.; Gongwer, R.; Stylianou, M.; Bhat, A.; Burns, K.M.; Cohen, M.S.; Dragulescu, A.; et al. Pediatric Heart Network Echocardiographic Z Scores: Comparison with Other Published Models. *J. Am. Soc. Echocardiogr.* **2020**, *34*, 185–192. [CrossRef] [PubMed]
33. Lopez, L.; Colan, S.D.; Frommelt, P.C.; Ensing, G.J.; Kendall, K.; Younoszai, A.K.; Lai, W.W.; Geva, T. Recommendations for Quantification Methods during the Performance of a Pediatric Echocardiogram: A Report from the Pediatric Measurements Writing Group of the American Society of Echocardiography Pediatric and Congenital Heart Disease Council. *J. Am. Soc. Echocardiogr.* **2010**, *23*, 465–495. [CrossRef] [PubMed]
34. Cantinotti, M.; Giordano, R.; Koestenberger, M.; Voges, I.; Santoro, G.; Franchi, E.; Assanta, N.; Valverde, I.; Simpson, J.; Kutty, S. Echocardiographic examination of mitral valve abnormalities in the paediatric population: Current practices. *Cardiol. Young* **2020**, *30*, 1–11. [CrossRef] [PubMed]
35. Zoghbi, W.A.; Adams, D.; Bonow, R.O.; Enriquez-Sarano, M.; Foster, E.; Grayburn, P.A.; Hahn, R.T.; Han, Y.; Hung, J.; Lang, R.M.; et al. Recommendations for noninvasive evaluation of native valvular regurgitation: A report from the american society of echocardiography developed in collaboration with the society for cardiovascular magnetic resonance. *J. Indian Acad. Echocardiogr. Cardiovasc. Imaging* **2020**, *4*, 58. [CrossRef]
36. Hirono, K.; Origasa, H.; Tsuboi, K.; Takarada, S.; Oguri, M.; Okabe, M.; Miyao, N.; Nakaoka, H.; Ibuki, K.; Ozawa, S.; et al. Clinical Status and Outcome of Isolated Right Ventricular Hypoplasia: A Systematic Review and Pooled Analysis of Case Reports. *Front. Pediatr.* **2022**, *10*, 794053. [CrossRef] [PubMed]

Disclaimer/Publisher's Note: The statements, opinions and data contained in all publications are solely those of the individual author(s) and contributor(s) and not of MDPI and/or the editor(s). MDPI and/or the editor(s) disclaim responsibility for any injury to people or property resulting from any ideas, methods, instructions or products referred to in the content.

Mild Acquired von Willebrand Syndrome and Cholestasis in Pediatric and Adult Patients with Fontan Circulation

Katharina Meinel [1], Felicitas Korak [2], Martin Dusleag [2], Tanja Strini [2], Daniela Baumgartner [1], Ante Burmas [1], Hannes Sallmon [3], Barbara Zieger [4], Axel Schlagenhauf [2,*] and Martin Koestenberger [1]

[1] Department of Pediatrics and Adolescent Medicine, Division of Pediatric Cardiology, Medical University of Graz, Auenbruggerplatz 34/2, 8036 Graz, Austria
[2] Department of Pediatrics and Adolescent Medicine, Division of General Pediatrics and Adolescent Medicine, Medical University of Graz, Auenbruggerplatz 34/2, 8036 Graz, Austria
[3] Department of Congenital Heart Disease/Pediatric Cardiology, Deutsches Herzzentrum der Charité (DHZC), Augustenburgerplatz 1, 13353 Berlin, Germany
[4] Department of Pediatrics and Adolescent Medicine, Division of Pediatric Hematology and Oncology, Faculty of Medicine, Medical Center—University of Freiburg, 79098 Freiburg, Germany
* Correspondence: axel.schlagenhauf@medunigraz.at; Tel.: +43-316-385-83336

Abstract: **Background:** Hemodynamic alterations in Fontan patients (FP) are associated with hemostatic dysbalance and Fontan-associated liver disease. Studies of other hepatopathologies indicate an interplay between cholestasis, tissue factor (TF), and von Willebrand factor (VWF). Hence, we hypothesized a relationship between the accumulation of bile acids (BA) and these hemostatic factors in FP. **Methods:** We included 34 FP (Phenprocoumon $n = 15$, acetylsalicylic acid (ASA) $n = 16$). BA were assessed by mass spectrometry. TF activity and VWF antigen (VWF:Ag) were determined by chromogenic assays. VWF collagen-binding activity (VWF:CB) was assessed via ELISA. **Results:** Cholestasis was observed in 6/34 FP (total BA ≥ 10 µM). BA levels and TF activity did not correlate ($p = 0.724$). Cholestatic FP had lower platelet counts ($p = 0.013$) from which 5/6 FP were not treated with ASA. VWF:Ag levels were increased in 9/34 FP and significantly lower in FP receiving ASA ($p = 0.044$). Acquired von Willebrand syndrome (AVWS) was observed in 10/34-FP, with a higher incidence in cholestatic FP (4/6) ($p = 0.048$). **Conclusions:** Cholestasis is unexpectedly infrequent in FP and seems to be less frequent under ASA therapy. Therefore, ASA may reduce the risk of advanced liver fibrosis. FP should be screened for AVWS to avoid bleeding events, especially in cholestatic states.

Keywords: Fontan circulation; Fontan-associated liver disease; cholestasis; bile acids; hemostasis; thromboprophylaxis; acquired von Willebrand syndrome

1. Introduction

The Fontan operation is a palliative procedure in patients with functionally univentricular hearts, which surgically redirects systemic venous blood return to the pulmonary circulation in the absence of a subpulmonary ventricle [1]. Multiple factors are contributing to an increased risk of thromboembolic events in patients with Fontan circulation which are related to Virchow's triad of thrombogenesis comprising altered blood flow, endothelial injury, and hypercoagulability [2,3]. First of all, the loss of pulsatility and subsequent elevated systemic venous pressure predisposes to thrombus formation through stasis of blood [3]. Additionally, a diminished cardiac output in Fontan patients was reported to increase the risk for thrombosis [4]. Finally, artificial intravascular material, chronic hypoxia, and surgical manipulation are thought to be involved in endothelial injury [5,6]. Hemodynamic changes and endothelial dysfunction were shown to increase levels of von Willebrand factor (VWF), platelet reactivity, and thrombin generation in the Fontan circulation [7,8]. However, these aforementioned defects could also be associated with

VWF degradation leading to acquired von Willebrand syndrome (AVWS), but data on VWF function in Fontan patients is lacking.

In addition to coagulation abnormalities, the increased venous pressure in the Fontan circulation is also leading to a chronic state of hepatic congestion. The non-inflammatory structural and functional hepatic changes associated with hemodynamic alterations of the Fontan circulation are summarized as Fontan-associated liver disease (FALD) [9,10]. As FALD progresses, sinusoidal fibrosis becomes inevitable [9]. Intrahepatic coagulation was shown to foster fibrosis in Fontan patients via thrombin generation and intraparenchymal fibrin deposition [11]. Subsequent platelet activation was proven to promote liver fibrosis by the activation of hepatic stellate cells in a mouse model [12]. Additionally, mechanistic and clinical observations in other hepatopathies suggest a link between changes in VWF and liver injury [13]. Taken together, intrahepatic coagulation processes play a detrimental role in the progression of FALD. However, the actual hemostatic trigger for these processes is unknown.

Elevated bile acid (BA) levels are hypothesized to play a key role in the decryption of human tissue factor (TF), which in complex with activated coagulation factor VII (FVIIa) serves as a hemostatic trigger [14]. In a previous study, we could demonstrate increased hepatic TF activity upon incubating hepatocytes with certain BA in vitro [14]. As Fontan patients tend to exhibit mild cholestasis by hepatic congestion, elevated BA levels may subsequently increase TF activity as the principal trigger of plasmatic coagulation. Hence, we hypothesized an interplay between cholestasis and a hemodynamically induced procoagulant state fostering FALD in patients with Fontan circulation.

2. Material and Methods

Study design and patients' characteristics: We conducted an observational study at the Division of Pediatric Cardiology and the GUCH (grown-up with congenital heart disease) Unit of the Medical University of Graz. We included 34 Fontan patients (14 females, 20 males) aged 5 to 38 years from whom we collected blood samples between May 2020 and May 2021. Non-fasting serum samples were taken for BA measurements from all study participants ($n = 34$). A total BA (tBA) cut-off value of ≥ 10 µM was set to determine cholestasis within the study cohort. Citrate plasma was available in 33/34 Fontan patients (14 females, 19 males) for coagulation analysis. From the 33 available plasma samples, 2 patients were not subjected to any anticoagulant medication during sample collection. The remaining subcohorts comprised 15 patients, receiving vitamin K antagonist Phenprocoumon (PhC), and 16 patients medicated with platelet aggregation inhibitor acetylsalicylic acid (ASA) (Supplementary Figure S1).

Blood samples: Blood samples from children and adolescent Fontan patients were collected via venipuncture at the Division of Pediatric Cardiology of the Medical University of Graz during routine diagnostic workup. Blood samples from adult Fontan patients were obtained by venipuncture at the GUCH Unit of the Medical University of Graz. Serum samples ($n = 34$) were collected in serum tubes (1.4 mL) which were centrifuged at $2000\times g$ for 10 min within 3 h before storage at $-80\ °C$ until analysis. Citrate plasma samples ($n = 33$) were collected using a single citrate tube (3 mL), which were processed to platelet-poor plasma by centrifugation at $2598\times g$ for 10 min within 3 h and stored at $-80\ °C$ until analysis.

BA analysis: BA levels including unconjugated, taurine-, and glycine-conjugated BA species (Supplementary Table S1) were measured by high-performance liquid chromatography (HPLC) combined with tandem mass spectrometry (MS/MS) as described previously [15]. Briefly, plasma samples were prepared after the protocol of Humbert et al. [16]. After the addition of internal standards d4-DCA, d4-LCA, d4-GLCA, d4-GCDCA, and d4-TDCA, 0.2 nmol each, plasma samples (10 µL) were vortexed for one minute. Then, 400 µL of acetonitrile (80% v/v; Sigma Aldrich, Taufkirchen, Germany) was added for deproteination. After vortexing, the precipitate was removed by centrifugation at $3200\times g$ for 12 min. The supernatant was dried under a stream of nitrogen (40 °C). The samples were re-dissolved in 100 µL of mobile phase B (methanol with 1.2% v/v formic acid and 0.38% w/v ammonium acetate) and transferred to an autosampler. Individual BA were separated by HPLC using a reversed-phase C18 column (Macherey-Nagel, Düren, Germany) and a kinetex pentafluorophenyl column (Phenomenex, Aschaffenburg, Germany). Quantification and characterization were achieved using a Q Exactive™ mass spectrometer (Thermo Fisher Scientific, Waltham, MA, USA) and a high-performance quadrupole precursor selection with high-resolution and accurate-mass (HR/AM) Orbitrap™ detection [16]. In our Fontan patients, cholestasis was defined by a cut-off value of tBA $\geq$ 10 µM. The cut-off was established during validation of the HPLC-MS method in our laboratory with a broad range of samples from patients that were externally diagnosed with varying degrees or absence of cholestasis.

TF activity analysis: The procoagulant activity of human TF in plasma samples was determined through a commercial chromogenic microplate assay (BioMedica Diagnostics, Windsor, CA, USA). The assay, which is based on the conversion of factor X to factor Xa followed by the enzymatic cleavage of a chromogenic substrate, was performed according to the manufacturer's instructions.

Von Willebrand factor analysis: VWF antigen (VWF:Ag) and VWF collagen binding capacity (VWF:CB) were determined, as described previously [17]. Briefly, VWF:Ag was measured in sodium citrate plasma using an in-house ELISA (Sutor Semin Thromb Haemost 2001). Collagen type I was immobilized on a microtiter plate, and VWF:CB in plasma was measured photometrically via the ELISA technique. Ratios of VWF:CB/VWF:Ag were calculated reflecting the biological capacity of the available VWF to bind to collagen. Ratios < 0.7 were considered pathological and indicative of acquired von Willebrand syndrome (AVWS). VWF was determined using appropriate primary and secondary antibodies and 3.30-diaminobenzidine/cobalt chloride. Standard human plasma was used as control. AVWS was diagnosed if the VWF:CB/VWF:Ag-ratio was reduced.

Endothelial damage analysis: The tissue-type plasminogen activator (tPA) antigen level in plasma was assayed using a commercial in vitro ELISA kit (Hyphen BioMed, Neuville-sur-Oise, France). A commercial in vitro ELISA kit (Hyphen BioMed) was performed to measure the plasminogen activator inhibitor-1 (PAI-1) antigen concentration. The thrombomodulin ™ levels in patient plasma were determined using a commercial ELISA test kit (Abcam, Cambridge, UK). The test procedures were conducted according to the provided protocol.

Clinical data: We collected clinical data and routine laboratory data of the included Fontan patients which comprised current medication, serum bilirubin, gamma-glutamyl transferase (GGT), as well as prothrombin time (PT), and platelet count, amongst others.

Ethics: This clinical study has been approved by the Austrian ethics committee (EK-Nr.32-376ex19/20) and was performed in accordance with the ethics standards as laid down in the 1964 Declaration of Helsinki and its later amendments or comparable ethical standards. Informed parental consent/informed consent was obtained for each included subject.

Statistical analysis: The statistical analysis was performed in IBM SPSS Statistics 28.0.0.0 and GraphPad Prism software. The changes in the examined parameters were visualized using GraphPad Prism Software. After testing for normal distribution, comparison of data from cholestatic and non-cholestatic Fontan patients was made via a Man-n–Whitney U-test. Spearman's correlation coefficient and corresponding p-values were used to investigate the relationships between the examined parameters. The statistical analysis regarding PT was limited to the patient subcohort receiving PhC.

3. Results

3.1. Demographic Data and Clinical Characteristics

Based on a tBA cut-off value of $\geq$10 µM, cholestasis was identified in 6/34 Fontan patients, equaling 17.7% of all patients included in the study. Concerning standard laboratory markers indicating hepatic injury, cholestatic Fontan patients had significantly higher bilirubin and GGT levels compared to non-cholestatic Fontan patients (Table 1).

Table 1. Characteristics of cholestatic and non-cholestatic pediatric and adult Fontan patients.

	Non-Cholestatic FP (n = 28)	Cholestatic FP (n = 6)	p-Value
Baseline demographic data			
Age at Fontan Procedure (y)	3.6 (2.6–6.5)	3.4 (3.0–4.0)	0.973
Gender, female (n,%)	13 (46.4)	1 (16.7)	0.179
Dominant ventricle: (n)			0.383
Left	11	4	
Right	13	1	
Both	4	1	
Type of Fontan:			0.724
TCPC (lateral tunnel)	8	1	
ECFO	19	5	
Other (Kawashima)	1	0	
Last follow-up			
Age at follow-up (y)	23.5 (16.0–32.3)	12.4 (9.3–28.0)	0.183
Time since Fontan (y)	18.0 (13.5–28.5)	9.5 (6.3–24.7)	0.191
Ejection fraction: (n)			0.638
>50%	27 (96.5%)	6 (100%)	
<50%	1 (3.5%)	0	
AV-valve incompetence: (n)			0.401
Mild/moderate	25 (89.3%)	6 (100%)	
Severe	3 (10.7%)	0	
Erythrocytes ($\times 10^6/\mu L$)	5.2 (4.7–5.6)	5.5 (5.3–5.7)	0.175
Hemoglobin (g/dL)	15.0 (13.4–15.4)	16.4 (15.7–17.0)	0.066
Hematocrit (%)	43.5 (40.0–45.0)	46.5 (45.0–48.7)	**0.044**
Platelet count ($\times 10^3/\mu L$)	196.0 (152.0–242.0)	116.0 (70.3–217.0)	**0.013**
ALT (U/L)	25.5 (19.0–30.0)	26.0 (21.8–43.0)	0.428
AST (U/L)	28.5 (22.0–36.0)	30.5 (25.8–42.3)	0.485
GGT (U/L)	46.5 (36.5–73.8)	99.5 (60.8–198.5)	**0.032**
Cholinesterase (U/L)	7241 (6263–8537)	6187 (5814–7687)	0.243
Lactate dehydrogenase (U/L)	227.5 (175.0–255.8)	216.5 (167.5–278.8)	0.935
Bilirubin (mg/dL)	0.8 (0.6–1.2)	1.9 (1.2–2.9)	**0.003**
Creatinine (mg/dL)	0.6 (0.5–0.8)	0.8 (0.7–0.9)	0.219
Total protein (g/dL)	7.5 (6.9–7.6)	7.4 (7.2–7.7)	0.785
Albumin (g/dL)	4.7 (4.5–4.9)	4.7 (4.3–4.8)	0.629
NT-ProBNP (ng/mL)	149.5 (73.8–269.3)	338.0 (103.8–396.3)	0.179
Antithrombin III (%)	101.0 (94.0–106.5)	85.0 (80.5–91.0)	**0.002**
Medication: (n)			0.204
Acetylsalicylic acid (ASA)	16	1	
Phenprocoumone (PhC)	11	4	
ACE inhibitor	15	2	
Antiarrhythmic	5	3	
PH medication	2	2	

Significant differences are shown in bold. Abbreviations: ALT, alanine aminotransferase; AST, aspartate aminotransferase; AV, atrioventricular; ECFO, extracardiac Fontan operation; FP, Fontan patients; GGT, gamma-glutamyl transferase; NTproBNP, N-terminal pro-B-type natriuretic peptide; PH, pulmonary hypertension; TCPC, total cavopulmonary connection; y, years.

3.2. Bile Acids

The tBA concentrations of the cholestatic Fontan subcohort ranged from 10.85 to 59.01 µM (median: 48.38 µM, IQR: 28.42–53.49), whereas the tBA levels of non-cholestatic Fontan patients ranged from 0.72 to 7.86 µM (median: 3.31 µM, IQR: 2.17–5.10). The tBA levels were significantly higher in Fontan patients ≥18- than in patients <18 years of age ($p = 0.033$) (Figure 1A). BA profiles of the cholestatic and non-cholestatic Fontan groups were established by determining the mean of the relative fraction for each of the 15 common human BA (Figure 1B). The relative fractions of glycocholic acid (GCA), taurocholic acid (TCA), taurolitocholic acid (TLCA), and tauroursodeoxycholic acid (TUDCA) were significantly higher, whereas the relative fraction of ursodeoxycholic acid (UDCA) was significantly lower in cholestatic Fontan patients compared to non-cholestatic patients (Supplementary Table S2).

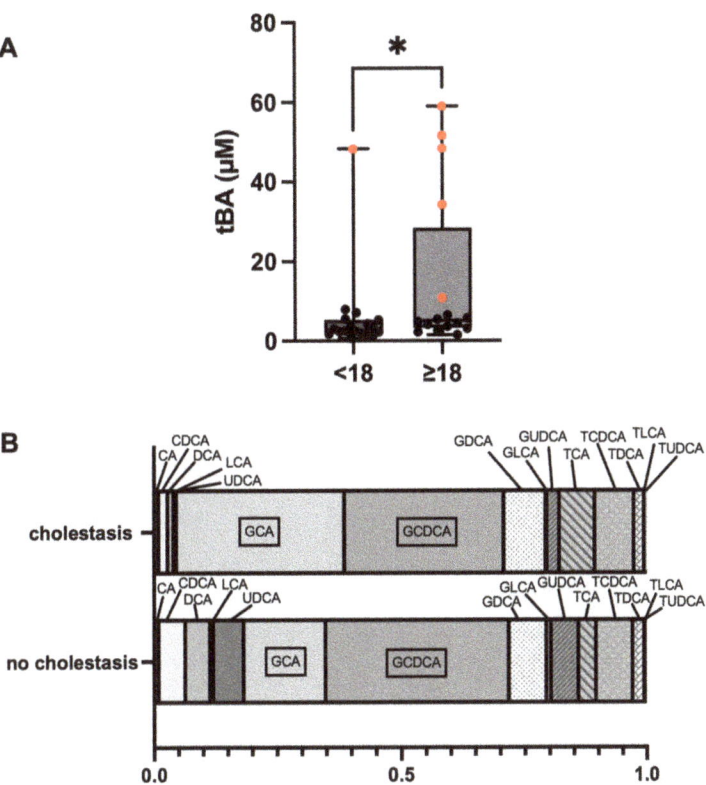

Figure 1. Comparison of the distribution of total bile acid (tBA) concentrations between Fontan patients <18 and ≥18 years of age. Cholestatic patients are highlighted by the red dots (**A**). BA profiles of cholestatic and non-cholestatic Fontan patients (**B**). * $p \leq 0.05$. **Abbreviations:** See Supplementary Table S1.

3.3. Laboratory Parameters and Clinical Data

In PhC-treated Fontan patients with cholestasis, the PT was significantly lower (median: 25.0, IQR: 21.8–28.3) compared to PhC-treated study participants without cholestasis (median: 33.0, IQR: 30.0–41.5, $p = 0.013$). Most cholestatic Fontan patients (5/6) were not treated with ASA (Supplementary Figure S1) and showed significantly lower platelet counts than non-cholestatic study participants ($p = 0.013$) (Table 1). In non-cholestatic individuals, platelet counts ($\times 10^3/\mu L$) were not affected by the type of antithrombotic treatment, as they were comparable between ASA- (median: 167.0, IQR: 132.5–215.8) and PhC-treated (median: 152.0, IQR: 113.0–222.0) patients ($p = 0.677$).

3.4. Tissue Factor Activity Analysis

The TF activity was not significantly higher in cholestatic Fontan patients (median: 6.88 pM, IQR: 3.25–13.71) compared to non-cholestatic patients (median: 7.73 pM, IQR: 2.65–16.43, $p = 1.000$).

3.5. Markers of Endothelial Damage

The endothelial damage was further evaluated by comparison of the TM levels (ng/mL) of cholestatic (median: 4.119, IQR: 2.977–5.836) and non-cholestatic Fontan patients (median: 5.416, IQR: 3.762–6.597) but without a statistically significant difference ($p = 0.276$). Likewise, both endothelial markers tPA and PAI-1 (ng/mL) showed no statistically significant differences between the subcohorts (tPA cholestasis median: 2.78, IQR: 2.63–5.10; tPA no cholestasis median: 2.76, IQR: 2.21–4.29, $p = 0.633$; PAI-1 cholestasis median: 9.51, IQR: 7.47–12.81; PAI-1 no cholestasis median: 10.47, IQR: 5.66–22.50 *p* = 0.760).

3.6. VWF Analysis

The VWF:Ag levels were compared between cholestatic and non-cholestatic Fontan patients. In both groups, VWF:Ag levels were generally elevated (cholestatic median 146.7%, IQR: 125.1–164.7; non-cholestatic median: 138.8%, IQR: 119.6–176.4), however without a statistically significant difference between the groups (*p* = 0.701) (Figure 2A). Interestingly, VWF:Ag levels were significantly lower in Fontan patients receiving ASA (median: 109.0%, IQR: 95.0–122.5) than in Fontan patients without ASA treatment (median 125.0%; IQR: 111.5–171.5, *p* = 0.0436) (Figure 2B). VWF:CB was comparable in cholestatic (median: 84.0%, IQR: 65.3–144.0) compared to non-cholestatic Fontan patients (median 92.5%, IQR: 77.0–144.0, *p* = 0.938) (Figure 2A).

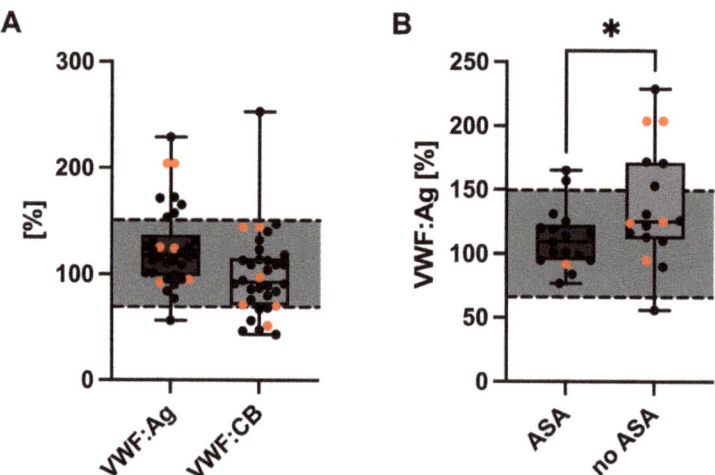

Figure 2. VWF:Ag and VWF:CB (**A**) values in cholestatic (**red dots**) and non-cholestatic Fontan patients. Comparison of VWF:Ag levels between Fontan patients with and without acetylsalicylic acid (ASA) treatment. Cholestatic patients are highlighted by the red dots (**B**). * $p \leq 0.05$. **Abbreviations:** VWF, von Willebrand factor; VWF:Ag, VWF antigen; VWF:CB, VWF collagen binding activity.

However, the VWF:CB/VWF:Ag ratio was pathologically low, indicating AVWS in 10/34 Fontan patients (29.4%). Although the VWF:CB/VWF:Ag ratio did not differ statistically significantly between cholestatic (median: 0.70, IQR: 0.56–0.78) and non-cholestatic Fontan patients (median: 0.77, IQR: 0.73–0.92, *p* = 0.112) (Figure 3), ratios below the pathological threshold were significantly more frequent in cholestatic (4/6) than in non-cholestatic Fontan patients (6/28) (*p* = 0.048) (Figure 3).

Fontan patients with decreased VWF:CB/VWF:Ag ratio ≤ 0.7 were compared with Fontan patients with VWF:CB/VWF:Ag ratio > 0.7 concerning invasively measured hemodynamic parameters and NTproBNP levels. We found no statistically significant differences for the mean Fontan pathway pressure (ratio ≤ 0.7 median: 12.5 mmHg, IQR 10.2–14.5, ratio > 0.7 median: 11.0 mmHg, IQR: 10.0–12.0, *p* = 0.111), pulmonary capillary wedge pressure (ratio ≤ 0.7 median: 7.0 mmHg, IQR 5.0–9.0; ratio > 0.7 median: 6.0 mmHg, IQR: 5.0–8.0, *p* = 0.419) or transpulmonary pressure gradient (ratio ≤ 0.7 median: 5.0 mmHg, IQR 4.0–6.8; ratio > 0.7 median: 5.0 mmHg, IQR: 4.0–6.0, *p* = 0.592). Moreover, there was no statistically significant difference in NTproBNP levels (ratio ≤ 0.7 median: 200 ng/mL, IQR 83–338; ratio > 0.7 median: 148 ng/mL, IQR: 82–310, *p* = 0.655).

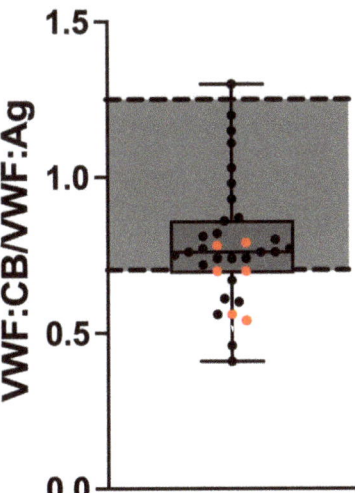

Figure 3. VWF:CB/VWF:Ag ratio in cholestatic (**red dots**) and non-cholestatic Fontan patients. **Abbreviations:** VWF:Ag, von Willebrand factor antigen; VWF:CB, von Willebrand factor collagen binding activity.

3.7. Correlation Analysis

A Spearman's rank correlation was performed to determine a potential relationship between BA parameters and TF activity and endothelial damage parameters. No significant correlation was determined between the analyzed BA variables and TF activity ($p \geq 0.05$). Furthermore, the BA parameters did not correlate with the endothelial damage markers TM, tPA, PAI-1, VWF:Ag, and VWF:CB ($p \geq 0.05$).

4. Discussion

FALD is defined as a hepatic disorder comprising structural and functional alterations which are arising from hemodynamic changes and chronic systemic venous congestion following Fontan surgery [9]. Albeit liver fibrosis seems to be universally present in Fontan patients, hepatic laboratory markers are usually not reflecting histopathological findings [18–21]. In advance of assessing the tBA values within our study cohort, a high incidence rate of cholestasis was hypothesized. However, the HPLC-MS/MS analysis revealed elevated tBA levels (≥ 10 µM) only in six out of 34 Fontan patients. Upon comparing the BA pools of the cholestatic and non-cholestatic Fontan subcohorts, the cholestatic subjects showed a statistically significant increase in GCA, TCA, TLCA and TUDCA. In contrast to the aforementioned, UDCA was significantly decreased in Fontan patients with cholestasis. Out of six cholestatic Fontan patients, five were ≥ 18 years of age, which is in accordance with previous research findings describing the time since Fontan completion as the main risk factor for FALD development [9,22]. In accordance with mild elevations of biochemical hepatic parameters being a common secondary sequela in Fontan patients, serum bilirubin and GGT values were compared in the study cohort. As a result, increased serum bilirubin and GGT levels were discovered in the cholestatic subcohort, suggesting that hepatic congestion serves as a potential confounder of the heightened BA and hepatic function markers bilirubin and GGT.

Even though the exact pathophysiology is not completely understood, a relationship between the advance of FALD and intrahepatic thrombosis has been assumed [8,9,23]. As increased hepatic TF activity was observed in the setting of elevated bile acids, we analyzed the TF activity as the principal trigger of plasmatic coagulation in Fontan patients [14]. In our study population, however, the plasmatic analysis of TF activity in cholestatic and non-cholestatic Fontan patients revealed no significant difference between both groups. Additionally, no correlation was found between the BA and TF activity of the examined patients, arguing against a BA-mediated decryption of hepatic TF in cholestatic patients with Fontan circulation. This mechanism is most likely relevant in primary obstructive liver diseases where bile acid accumulation precedes the activation of coagulation. However, patients with Fontan circulation show coagulatory abnormalities from the beginning due to altered hemodynamics, and only a fraction of patients develop cholestasis years after Fontan completion. Hence, intrahepatic coagulation activation most likely fosters liver fibrosis and precedes the obstruction of bile flow.

Nevertheless, multiple factors are contributing to an increased risk for thromboembolic events in the Fontan circulation including disturbed blood flow, endothelial injury, and coagulopathy [3]. However, controversies exist regarding optimal thromboprophylaxis in Fontan patients [24]. To date, the superiority of either anticoagulation or antiplatelet therapy (ASA) has not been proven. Therefore, treatment recommendation for each patient was based on subjective thromboembolic risk assessment of the treating physician. In two independent randomized controlled trials comparing vitamin K antagonists (e.g., PhC) and ASA, no significant differences have been demonstrated regarding thromboembolic events in children with Fontan circulation [25,26]. Within all included study participants, 16 patients were treated with ASA (cholestatic n = 1, non-cholestatic n = 15), whereas 15 patients received PhC (cholestatic n = 4, non-cholestatic n = 11). Generally, we are preferring the prescription of ASA for thrombophylaxis in our pediatric patients due to the higher risk of bleeding in case of trauma. At the appearance of clear indications such as atrial arrythmias or thromboembolic events, amongst others, pediatric and adult patients are switched to anticoagulation with PhC. Moreover, life events such as pregnancy and additional surgery of course might require changes to thrombophylaxis strategies. In our study, PhC-treated cholestatic Fontan patients had a significantly shorter PT than non-cholestatic patients with PhC, hinting at an impaired synthetic function of the liver, although a variance in PhC treatment cannot be entirely excluded. Independent of PhC treatment, however, platelet counts were significantly lower in cholestatic Fontan patients whereby five out of six were not treated with ASA. In non-cholestatic Fontan patients, platelet counts were comparable between PhC- and ASA-treated individuals. These observations are either pointing to a decreased platelet biogenesis or an increased platelet activation and consumption in cholestatic Fontan patients. In a mouse model, platelet activation has been shown to promote liver fibrosis by activating hepatic stellate cells [12]. Furthermore, the daily use of aspirin was associated with less severe histologic findings and a lower risk of advanced fibrosis progression over time in non-alcoholic fatty liver disease [27]. In Fontan patients, ASA therapy might reduce the risk for advanced liver fibrosis and therefore the severity of FALD; however, this needs further investigation by larger clinical trials.

Endothelial function and fibrinolysis have been investigated previously as potential contributors to thrombosis in Fontan patients. Binotto et al. reported increased VWF levels, pointing to a dysfunction of the vascular endothelium [6]. This is in accordance with our findings of enhanced VWF:Ag levels in all our Fontan patients indicating either endothelial perturbation or increased platelet activation. However, we could not find a significant difference between cholestatic and non-cholestatic Fontan patients.

AVWS is characterized by the loss of high molecular weight multimers of VWF leading to an impaired VWF function, which can be either shear stress-induced or associated with increased platelet activation [28]. It has been shown that the combined interpretation of VWF:Ag, VWF:CB, and VWF:CB/VWF:Ag ratio increases the sensitivity of diagnosing AVWS [29]. A low VWF:CB/VWF:Ag ratio < 0.7 has been shown to correlate with the loss of high molecular weight multimers [29]. Generally, the VWF:CB/VWF:Ag ratio was decreased in 29.4% of all included Fontan patients. Moreover, the incidence of pathological VWF:CB/VWF:Ag ratio was higher in cholestatic Fontan patients. One explanation for our findings could be an increased release of VWF by the dysfunctional vascular endothelium of Fontan patients leading to generally enhanced levels of detectable VWF:Ag. Alternatively, the altered hemodynamics in the Fontan circulation might change the three-dimensional VWF structure and enhance the proteolysis of VWF by ADAMTS-13. Similarly, a loss of high molecular weight multimers of VWF has been reported in patients after continuous-flow left ventricular assist device implantation [30]. However, it remains unclear why all Fontan patients are not affected by a mild AVWS despite comparable invasively measured hemodynamic parameters.

Lastly, we investigated fibrinolysis via the release of tPA and PAI-1, as the processes are primarily mediated by the vascular endothelium. In our study, the analyzed endothelial parameters did not differ significantly between cholestatic- and non-cholestatic Fontan patients. Likewise, in the study of Binotto et al., tPA and PAI-1 levels and activity did not deviate significantly from the control group, showing that not all endothelial functions are impaired following the Fontan procedure [6].

We acknowledge that the representativeness of our results may be limited due to the small number of analyzed patients per study group. Statistical evaluation was constrained by the low incidence rate of cholestasis within the study cohort. Furthermore, as 4/6 cholestatic Fontan patients received PhC, the hemostatic statistical evaluation was limited to the PhC subcohort. Still, we believe that the results of our study revealed valuable new insights into the pathophysiology of FALD with inherent clinical impact as clinical trials investigating coagulation in Fontan patients are sparse.

5. Conclusions

Firstly, the low incidence rate of cholestasis in Fontan patients represents a novel clinical finding. However, elevated bile acid levels were not associated with increased tissue factor activity or endothelial dysfunction. Secondly, the absence of cholestasis in patients receiving ASA is striking and warrants further investigation. Thirdly, the Fontan circulation is associated with a mild acquired von Willebrand syndrome. However, ongoing clinical trials are required to investigate the risk of bleeding events in Fontan patients with acquired von Willebrand syndrome. Due to the higher incidence and possibly impaired hepatic synthetic function in cholestatic patients, testing for acquired von Willebrand syndrome should be considered prior to surgery to avoid bleeding events.

Supplementary Materials: The following supporting information can be downloaded at: https://www.mdpi.com/article/10.3390/jcm12031240/s1, Figure S1: Overview of groups and subcohorts investigated in this study. Table S1. Unconjugated bile acids (BA) and their glycine (G) or taurine (T) conjugates analyzed in this study design. Table S2: Descriptive data and results of the Mann-Whitney U tests, comparing the relative bile acid (BA) values between cholestatic and non-cholestatic Fontan patients.

Author Contributions: K.M. and A.S. conceived the initial idea and wrote the manuscript with the support of M.K. and H.S. Collection of blood samples was performed by K.M., D.B. and A.B., A.S., F.K., M.D., T.S. and B.Z. planned and performed the measurements. F.K., A.S. and K.M. analyzed the data and constructed figures and tables. All authors provided critical feedback and helped shape the manuscript. All authors have read and agreed to the published version of the manuscript.

Funding: This research received no external funding.

Institutional Review Board Statement: This clinical study has been approved by the Austrian ethics committee (EK-Nr.32-376ex19/20) and was performed in accordance with the ethics standards as laid down in the 1964 Declaration of Helsinki and its later amendments or comparable ethical standards.

Informed Consent Statement: Informed parental consent/informed consent was obtained for each included subject.

Data Availability Statement: The data presented in this study are available on request from the corresponding author. The data are not publicly available due to ethical reasons.

Conflicts of Interest: The authors declare no conflict of interest.

References

1. Mazza, G.A.; Gribaudo, E.; Agnoletti, G. The pathophysiology and complications of Fontan circulation. *Acta Biomed.* **2021**, *92*, e2021260. [CrossRef] [PubMed]
2. Odegard, K.C.; McGowan, F.X.; DiNardo, J.A.; Castro, R.A.; Zurakowski, D.; Connor, C.M.; Hansen, D.D.; Neufeld, E.J.; Del Nido, P.J.; Laussen, P.C. Coagulation abnormalities in patients with single-ventricle physiology precede the Fontan procedure. *J. Thorac. Cardiovasc. Surg.* **2002**, *123*, 459–465. [CrossRef] [PubMed]
3. Heidendael, J.F.; Engele, L.J.; Bouma, B.J.; Dipchand, A.I.; Thorne, S.A.; McCrindle, B.W.; Mulder, B.J.M. Coagulation and Anticoagulation in Fontan Patients. *Can. J. Cardiol.* **2022**, *38*, 1024–1035. [CrossRef]
4. Ohuchi, H.; Yasuda, K.; Miyazaki, A.; Ono, S.; Hayama, Y.; Negishi, J.; Noritake, K.; Mizuno, M.; Yamada, O. Prevalence and predictors of haemostatic complications in 412 Fontan patients: Their relation to anticoagulation and haemodynamics. *Eur. J. Cardiothorac. Surg.* **2015**, *47*, 511–519. [CrossRef] [PubMed]
5. Mahle, W.T.; Todd, K.; Fyfe, D.A. Endothelial function following the Fontan operation. *Am. J. Cardiol.* **2003**, *91*, 1286–1288 [CrossRef]
6. Binotto, M.A.; Maeda, N.Y.; Lopes, A.A. Altered endothelial function following the Fontan procedure. *Cardiol. Young* **2008**, *18*, 70–74 [CrossRef]
7. Ravn, H.B.; Hjortdal, V.E.; Stenbog, E.V.; Emmertsen, K.; Kromann, O.; Pedersen, J.; Sorensen, K.E. Increased platelet reactivity and significant changes in coagulation markers after cavopulmonary connection. *Heart* **2001**, *85*, 61–65. [CrossRef]
8. Tomkiewicz-Pajak, L.; Hoffman, P.; Trojnarska, O.; Lipczyńska, M.; Podolec, P.; Undas, A. Abnormalities in blood coagulation, fibrinolysis, and platelet activation in adult patients after the Fontan procedure. *J. Thorac. Cardiovasc. Surg.* **2014**, *147*, 1284–1290 [CrossRef]
9. Téllez, L.; Rodríguez-Santiago, E.; Albillos, A. Fontan-Associated Liver Disease: A Review. *Ann. Hepatol.* **2018**, *17*, 192–204 [CrossRef]
10. Asrani, S.K.; Asrani, N.S.; Freese, D.K.; Phillips, S.D.; Warnes, C.A.; Heimbach, J.; Kamath, P.S. Congenital heart disease and the liver. *Hepatology* **2012**, *56*, 1160–1169. [CrossRef]
11. Simonetto, D.A.; Yang, H.Y.; Yin, M.; de Assuncao, T.M.; Kwon, J.H.; Hilscher, M.; Pan, S.; Yang, L.; Bi, Y.; Beyder, A.; et al. Chronic passive venous congestion drives hepatic fibrogenesis via sinusoidal thrombosis and mechanical forces. *Hepatology* **2015**, *61*, 648–659. [CrossRef] [PubMed]
12. Yoshida, S.; Ikenaga, N.; Liu, S.B.; Peng, Z.W.; Chung, J.; Sverdlov, D.Y.; Miyamoto, M.; Kim, Y.O.; Ogawa, S.; Arch, R.H.; et al. Extrahepatic platelet-derived growth factor-β, delivered by platelets, promotes activation of hepatic stellate cells and biliary fibrosis in mice. *Gastroenterology* **2014**, *147*, 1378–1392. [CrossRef] [PubMed]
13. Groeneveld, D.J.; Poole, L.G.; Luyendyk, J.P. Targeting von Willebrand factor in liver diseases: A novel therapeutic strategy? *J. Thromb. Haemost.* **2021**, *19*, 1390–1408. [CrossRef]
14. Greimel, T.; Jahnel, J.; Pohl, S.; Strini, T.; Tischitz, M.; Meier-Allard, N.; Holasek, S.; Meinel, K.; Aguiriano-Moser, V.; Zobel, J.; et al. Bile acid-induced tissue factor activity in hepatocytes correlates with activation of farnesoid X receptor. *Lab. Investig.* **2021**, *101*, 1394–1402. [CrossRef] [PubMed]
15. Amplatz, B.; Zöhrer, E.; Haas, C.; Schäffer, M.; Stojakovic, T.; Jahnel, J.; Fauler, G. Bile acid preparation and comprehensive analysis by high performance liquid chromatography–high-resolution mass spectrometry. *Clin. Chim. Acta* **2017**, *464*, 85–92 [CrossRef]
16. Humbert, L.; Maubert, M.A.; Wolf, C.; Duboc, H.; Mahé, M.; Farabos, D.; Seksik, P.; Mallet, J.M.; Trugnan, G.; Masliah, J.; et al. Bile acid profiling in human biological samples: Comparison of extraction procedures and application to normal and cholestatic patients. *J. Chromatogr. B Anal. Technol. Biomed. Life Sci.* **2012**, *899*, 135–145. [CrossRef]
17. Heilmann, C.; Geisen, U.; Beyersdorf, F.; Nakamura, L.; Benk, C.; Berchtold-Herz, M.; Trummer, G.; Schlensak, C.; Zieger, B. Acquired von Willebrand syndrome in patients with ventricular assist device or total artificial heart. *Thromb. Haemost.* **2010**, *103*, 962–967. [CrossRef]
18. Wu, F.M.; Ukomadu, C.; Odze, R.D.; Valente, A.M.; Mayer, J.E.; Earing, M.G. Liver disease in the patient with fontan circulation. *Congenit. Heart Dis.* **2011**, *6*, 190–201. [CrossRef]
19. Kiesewetter, C.H.; Sheron, N.; Vettukattill, J.J.; Hacking, N.; Stedman, B.; Millward-Sadler, H.; Haw, M.; Cope, R.; Salmon, A.P.; Sivaprakasam, M.C.; et al. Hepatic changes in the failing Fontan circulation. *Heart* **2007**, *93*, 579–584. [CrossRef]
20. Narkewicz, M.R.; Sondheimer, H.M.; Ziegler, J.W.; Otanni, Y.; Lorts, A.; Shaffer, E.M.; Horgan, J.G.; Sokol, R.J. Hepatic dysfunction following the Fontan procedure. *J. Pediatr. Gastroenterol. Nutr.* **2003**, *36*, 352–357. [CrossRef]
21. Camposilvan, S.; Milanesi, O.; Stellin, G.; Pettenazzo, A.; Zancan, L.; D'Antiga, L. Liver and cardiac function in the long term after Fontan operation. *Ann. Thorac. Surg.* **2008**, *86*, 177–182. [CrossRef] [PubMed]
22. Baek, J.S.; Bae, E.J.; Ko, J.S.; Kim, G.B.; Kwon, B.S.; Lee, S.Y.; Noh, C., II; Park, E.A.; Lee, W. Late hepatic complications after Fontan operation; non-invasive markers of hepatic fibrosis and risk factors. *Heart* **2010**, *96*, 1750–1755. [CrossRef]
23. Greuter, T.; Shah, V.H. Hepatic sinusoids in liver injury, inflammation, and fibrosis: New pathophysiological insights. *J. Gastroenterol.* **2016**, *51*, 511–519. [CrossRef] [PubMed]
24. Alsaied, T.; Alsidawi, S.; Allen, C.C.; Faircloth, J.; Palumbo, J.S.; Veldtman, G.R. Strategies for thromboprophylaxis in Fontan circulation: A meta-analysis. *Heart* **2015**, *101*, 1731–1737. [CrossRef] [PubMed]

25. Pessotti, C.F.X.; Jatene, M.B.; Jatene, I.B.; Oliveira, P.M.; Succi, F.M.P.; De Melo Moreira, V.; Lopes, R.W.; Pedra, S.R.F.F. Comparative trial of the use of antiplatelet and oral anticoagulant in thrombosis prophylaxis in patients undergoing total cavopulmonary operation with extracardiac conduit: Echocardiographic, tomographic, scintigraphic, clinical and laboratory analysis. *Rev. Bras. Cir. Cardiovasc.* **2014**, *29*, 595–605. [CrossRef] [PubMed]
26. Monagle, P.; Cochrane, A.; Roberts, R.; Manlhiot, C.; Weintraub, R.; Szechtman, B.; Hughes, M.; Andrew, M.; McCrindle, B.W. A multicenter, randomized trial comparing heparin/warfarin and acetylsalicylic acid as primary thromboprophylaxis for 2 years after the Fontan procedure in children. *J. Am. Coll. Cardiol.* **2011**, *58*, 645–651. [CrossRef]
27. Simon, T.G.; Henson, J.; Osganian, S.; Masia, R.; Chan, A.T.; Chung, R.T.; Corey, K.E. Daily Aspirin Use Associated With Reduced Risk For Fibrosis Progression In Patients With Nonalcoholic Fatty Liver Disease. *Clin. Gastroenterol. Hepatol.* **2019**, *17*, 2776–2784.e4. [CrossRef]
28. James, A.H.; Eikenboom, J.; Federici, A.B. State of the art: Von Willebrand disease. *Haemophilia* **2016**, *22* (Suppl. 5), 54–59. [CrossRef]
29. Muslem, R.; Caliskan, K.; Leebeek, F.W.G. Acquired coagulopathy in patients with left ventricular assist devices. *J. Thromb. Haemost.* **2018**, *16*, 429–440. [CrossRef]
30. Geisen, U.; Heilmann, C.; Beyersdorf, F.; Benk, C.; Berchtold-Herz, M.; Schlensak, C.; Budde, U.; Zieger, B. Non-surgical bleeding in patients with ventricular assist devices could be explained by acquired von Willebrand disease. *Eur. J. Cardiothorac. Surg.* **2008**, *33*, 679–684. [CrossRef]

Disclaimer/Publisher's Note: The statements, opinions and data contained in all publications are solely those of the individual author(s) and contributor(s) and not of MDPI and/or the editor(s). MDPI and/or the editor(s) disclaim responsibility for any injury to people or property resulting from any ideas, methods, instructions or products referred to in the content.

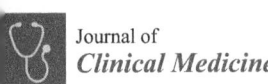

Journal of
Clinical Medicine

Article

Pregnancy Outcomes in Women after the Fontan Procedure

Agnieszka Bartczak-Rutkowska [1,*], Lidia Tomkiewicz-Pająk [2], Katarzyna Kawka-Paciorkowska [3], Natalia Bajorek [4], Aleksandra Ciepłucha [1], Mariola Ropacka-Lesiak [3] and Olga Trojnarska [1]

1. 1st Department of Cardiology, Poznan University of Medical Sciences, 61-848 Poznan, Poland
2. Institute of Cardiology, Jagiellonian University Medical College, 31-202 Krakow, Poland
3. Department of Perinatology and Gynecology, Poznan University of Medical Sciences, 60-535 Poznan, Poland
4. Department of Medical Education, Centre for Innovative Medical Education, Jagiellonian University Medical College, 30-688 Krakow, Poland
* Correspondence: aga.bartczak@gmail.com

Abstract: Women with single ventricle physiology after the Fontan procedure, despite numerous possible complications, can reach adulthood and give birth. Pregnancy poses a hemodynamic burden for distorted physiology of Fontan circulation, but according to the literature, it is usually well tolerated unless the patient is a "failing" Fontan. Our study aimed to assess maternal and fetal outcomes in patients after the Fontan procedure followed up in two tertiary Polish medical centers. We retrospectively evaluated all pregnancies in women after the Fontan procedure who were followed up between 1995–2022. During the study period, 15 women after the Fontan procedure had 26 pregnancies. Among 26 pregnancies, eleven ended with miscarriages, and 15 pregnancies resulted in 16 live births. Fetal complications were observed in 9 (56.3%) live births, with prematurity being the most common complication ($n = 7$, 43.8%). We recorded 3 (18.8%) neonatal deaths. Obstetrical complications were present in 6 (40%) out of 15 completed pregnancies—two (13.3%) cases of abruptio placentae, two (13.3%) pregnancies with premature rupture of membranes, and two (13.3%) patients with antepartum hemorrhage. There was neither maternal death nor heart failure decompensation during pregnancy. In two (13.3%) women, atrial arrhythmia developed. One (6.7%) patient in the second trimester developed ventricular arrhythmia. None of the patients suffered from systemic thromboembolism during pregnancy. Pregnancy in women after the Fontan procedure is well tolerated. However, it is burdened by a high risk of miscarriage and multiple obstetrical complications. These women require specialized care provided by both experienced cardiologists and obstetricians.

Keywords: congenital heart disease; Fontan procedure; single ventricle; miscarriage; pregnancy; prematurity

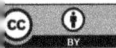

1. Introduction

The Fontan procedure is one of the most inventive cardiosurgical concepts. It enables patients with complex congenital heart defects unsuitable for biventricular repair to reach adulthood. Fontan palliation through the complete separation of pulmonary and systemic circulation alleviates cyanosis but creates a challenge for the cardiovascular system [1]. Lack of the subpulmonary ventricle leads to nonpulsatile pulmonary blood flow that depends on low pulmonary vascular resistance and high systemic venous pressures. This solution tremendously improves the survival of these patients but also leads to numerous complications. Single ventricular dysfunction, refractory arrhythmia, Fontan-associated liver dysfunction, thromboembolic events, plastic bronchitis, protein-losing enteropathy, and cognitive disorders are examples of Fontan circulation failure. [2,3]. However, women who reach childbearing age desire to have children. Pregnancy is a hemodynamic burden to the normal cardiovascular system. At a six-week pregnancy, both heart rate and stroke volume start to increase, leading to a 30–50% rise in cardiac output [4]. As a result of progesterone, nitric oxide, and prostaglandin actions, there is a decrease in systemic and pulmonary vascular resistance. Volume loading results in hemodilution and physiologic anemia. Additionally, there is a rise in prothrombotic factors during pregnancy. All these changes challenge the distorted univentricular heart after the Fontan procedure [5]. Moreover, high systemic venous pressures and limited reserve to increase cardiac output may impact placental perfusion [6].

As per European Society of Cardiology (ESC) guidelines for the management of cardiovascular diseases during pregnancy, uncomplicated Fontan patients belong to modified World Health Organization (WHO) class III, which means a significantly increased risk of maternal mortality or severe morbidity [7]. However, patients called failing Fontans who demonstrate the above-mentioned complications of Fontan circulation are classified as a modified WHO class IV and should be counseled against pregnancy.

Our study aimed to assess maternal and fetal outcomes in patients after the Fontan procedure followed up in two tertiary Polish medical centers.

2. Materials and Methods

In this retrospective two-center (First Department of Cardiology, University of Medical Sciences, Poznan, and Institute of Cardiology, Jagiellonian University Medical College Krakow) observational study, we evaluated all pregnancies of women after the Fontan procedure who were followed up between 1995–2022. We did not include ongoing pregnancies. Information from medical records included demographic data, initial heart anatomy, prior surgical procedures, cardiac complications before pregnancy, the latest echocardiography examination, age at first pregnancy, week, and mode of delivery. We also analyzed the number of patients' visits to the outpatient clinic during pregnancy.

Echocardiography (Vivid 9, GE Healthcare, Wauwatosa, WI, USA) was performed by two experienced echocardiographers (ABR and LTP) according to a predetermined study protocol. The echocardiograms included 2D and Doppler imaging to identify the morphology of the single ventricle—dominant left, right, or mixed ventricle and the presence of thrombus. Based on biplane modified Simpson's rule, the ejection fraction (EF) of a single ventricle was calculated. Impaired ventricular function was considered when EF was <50% [8]. Color-mode Doppler determined atrioventricular valve (AVV) regurgitation in a 4-chamber view.

Fetal outcomes were recorded and included: termination of pregnancy before 20 weeks of gestation (WG), miscarriage as spontaneous fetal loss before 24 WG, stillbirth as fetal death after 24 WG [9], premature delivery (delivery before 37 WG), small size for gestational age (SGA) (birth weight below 10th percentile), neonatal death (death within the first month after birth), and diagnosis of congenital malformations.

Maternal complications included: maternal death, heart failure, systemic thromboembolic complication, new cyanosis (SO_2—oxygen saturation drop below 90% at rest), protein-losing enteropathy, and atrial or ventricular arrhythmia. Obstetrical complications were classified as preeclampsia, abruptio placentae, premature rupture of membranes before 37 WG, and antepartum and postpartum hemorrhage. Postpartum hemorrhage was defined as a loss of >1000 mL of blood after cesarean section until 24 h postpartum [10].

We also calculated the risk scores for adverse cardiac complications during pregnancy according to ZAHARA and CARPREG II scores [11,12].

As approved by our institutional Ethics Committee, the study protocol conformed to the ethical guidelines set forth by the 1975 Declaration of Helsinki.

3. Statistics

Data were expressed as means with SD or medians with range (according to normal distribution) for continuous variables and percentages for categorical variables for descriptive analysis. Analysis was performed using PQStat v.1.8.2. (PQStat Software, Poznan/Plewiska, Poland).

4. Results

4.1. Baseline Characteristics

During the study period, 15 women after the Fontan procedure had 26 pregnancies. Among them, three women had two pregnancies, two patients had three pregnancies, and one woman had five pregnancies. The mean age (SD) at first pregnancy was 25.4 (3.5) years. Underlying congenital heart defects and baseline maternal characteristics are presented in Table 1.

Table 1. Pre-conception baseline maternal characteristic.

Population Characteristics	n = 15
Type of congenital heart defect	
Tricuspid atresia	5 (33.3%)
Double inlet left ventricle	4 (26.7%)
Pulmonary atresia	3 (20%)
Double outlet right ventricle	3 (20%)
Type of palliation	
Atrio-pulmonary connection	1 (6.7%)
Total cavo-pulmonary connection	14 (93.3%)
Fenestration	6 (40%)
Functional state	
NYHA I/II/III/IV	3/12/0/0
Hypoxemia (<90%)	1 (6.7%)
Past medical history	
Sick sinus syndrome	4 (26.7%)
Atrial arrhythmia	4 (26.7%)
Ventricular arrhythmia	2 (13.3%)
Permanent pacemaker	2 (13.3%)
Thromboembolic complications	2 (13.3%)
Age at first pregnancy (years) mean (SD)	25.4 (3.5)
Incidence of patient's visits median (range)	3 (2–6)
Echocardiography	
SV morphology	RV—3 (20%), LV—12 (80%)
SV function normal/impaired	14 (93.3%)/1 (6.7%)
Atrio-ventricular regurgitation mild/moderate/severe	10 (66.7%)/5 (33.3%)/0
Thrombus	1 (6.7%)

LV—left ventricle; NYHA—New York Heart Association scale; RV—right ventricle; SV—single ventricle.

All palliations, except one—atrio-pulmonary connection—were total cavo-pulmonary connections (TCPC) performed at the mean age (SD) of 7.1 (4.4) years. Fenestrated TCPC was performed in six (40%) patients. One fenestration was closed with an Amplatzer device six years after Fontan's completion. Hypoxemia was observed before pregnancy in one (6.7%) patient with patent fenestration (SO_2—87%). All pregnancies were delivered by cesarean section.

4.2. Fetal Outcomes

Among 26 pregnancies, 11 ended in miscarriage at the median gestational age of 9.3 (5–18) WG, and the mean age (SD) of patients was 24.1 (3.1) years. Fifteen pregnancies resulted in sixteen live births at the median gestational age of 35.5 (26–40) WG and the mean age (SD) of patients of 26.3 (3.8) years. The mean birth weight (SD) was 2519 (758) g. Fetal complications were observed in 9 (56.3%) live births, with prematurity being the most common complication (n = 7, 43.8%). Four (25%) children were born before 33 WG. We recorded three (18.8%) neonatal deaths resulting from one twin and one singleton pregnancy. Twin pregnancy was delivered in 26 WG due to premature rupture of membranes, and babies also had morphological abnormalities: hypotrophy, abnormalities of lower and upper limbs, and calcification around the stomach (probably due to a genetic disorder which was not specified). They died one month after delivery. The third neonatal death occurred in a patient with placental hematoma and ablation. Cesarean section was performed at 27 WG, and the child died due to complications of extreme prematurity. Two (12.5%) other children were diagnosed with congenital malformations—one child presented with patent ductus arteriosus, and the other was born with a diaphragmatic hernia (Table 2).

Table 2. Fetal/neonatal complications—n = 16 (one twin pregnancy).

Birth Weight (g) Mean (SD)	2519 (758)
Termination of pregnancy <20 WG	0
Stillbirth	0
Neonatal death	3 (18.8%)
Small for gestational age	1 (6.25%)
Congenital malformations	2 (12.5%)
Prematurity	7 (43.8%)
33–36 + 6 WG	3
28–32 + 6 WG	1
22–27 + 6 WG	3

WG—week of gestation.

4.3. Obstetrical Status

Obstetrical complications were present in 6 (40%) out of 15 completed pregnancies, among which 1 was multiparous. Two (13.3%) pregnancies were complicated with abruptio placentae. In another two (13.3%), premature rupture of membranes occurred. Antepartum hemorrhage complicated two (13.3%) pregnancies and both patients were followed up using prophylactic anticoagulation. Preeclampsia was not observed in our study group. All the above-mentioned complications resulted in premature delivery before 37 WG (Table 3).

Table 3. Maternal cardiovascular and obstetrical complications.

Pt	Age at Fontan (Years)	Age at First P (Years)	CARPREG II	ZAHARA	P	M	L	Anticoag	NYHA	Arrhythmia before 1st Pregnancy	Complications during Pregnancy
1	1	29	5	4	1	0	1	Prophyl	II	AA	None
2	4	24	3	6.25	1	0	1	Prophyl	II	AA	PD, AH
3	5	27	8	4.75	1	1	0	Therap	II	SSS, VA	VB
4	7	26	3	4.75	1	0	1	Prophyl	II	SSS	PD; AP; Takotsubo syndrome
5	14	23	3	4.75	3	2	1	Therap	II	SSS	1- Miscarriage 2- Miscarriage 3- AFl
6	4	24	2	2.5	2	1	1	ASA	II	-	1- Miscarriage 2- None
7	5	17	2	2.5	5	3	2	None -1st Therap -2nd -5th pregnancy	II	-	1- None 2- Miscarriage- AF, hypoxemia 3- Miscarriage 4- Miscarriage 5- PD, AP
8	12	24	5	4.75	2	1	1	None	II	AA, VA	1- Miscarriage 2- None
9	5	22	3	2.5	1	0	1	None	I	AA	VA
10	13	28	2	2.5	1	0	1	None	II	-	None
11	5	28	0	1	1	0	1	None	I	-	None
12	7	28	5	5.5	3	2	1	None -1st -2nd Prophyl -3rd pregnancy	II	SSS	1- Miscarriage 2- Miscarriage 3- PD, AH
13	8	23	2	0	2	1	1	None	I	-	1- PD, PROM 2- Miscarriage
14	15	30	2	1.75	1	0	1	Prophyl	II	-	PD, PROM
15	2	29	0	1	1	0	1	Prophyl	I	-	None

AA—atrial arrhythmia; AF—atrial fibrillation; AFl—atrial flutter; AH—antepartum hemorrhage; Anticoag—anticoagulation; AP—abruptio placentae; ASA—aspirin; L—live birth; CARPREG II—the risk score of primary maternal cardiac event, calculated for the first pregnancy, was 5% with a score of 1, 10% for a score of 2, 15% with a score of 3, 22% for a score of 4, and 41% if the score was greater than 4 points; M—miscarriage; NYHA—New York Heart Association; P—pregnancy; PD—preterm delivery; PROM—premature rupture of membranes; Prophyl—prophylactic anticoagulation; SSS—sick sinus syndrome; SV—single ventricle; Therap—therapeutic anticoagulation; VA—ventricular arrhythmia; VB—vaginal bleeding; ZAHARA—the risk score of maternal cardiovascular complications calculated for first pregnancy is 2.9% with <0.5 points, 7.5% with 0.5–1.5 points, 17.5% with 1.51–2.50 points, 43.1% with 2.51–3.5 points, and 70% with >3.5 points.

4.4. Maternal Cardiovascular Complications

There was neither maternal death nor heart failure decompensation during pregnancy. However, episodes of new-onset arrhythmia occurred. In two (13.3%) women, atrial arrhythmia developed. One patient presented with atrial flutter in the second trimester and required anticoagulation and beta-blocker therapy. The other who had five pregnancies presented with atrial fibrillation during the second pregnancy (this woman suffered three miscarriages and died five years after her last pregnancy because of heart failure). One (6.7%) patient in the second trimester developed ventricular arrhythmia (premature ventricular contractions), which resolved after delivery. She did not require medications. New onset of hypoxemia was observed in one patient with classic (atrio-pulmonary) Fontan palliation (SO_2—89%) when atrial fibrillation occurred and complicated her second pregnancy. As late maternal complications, we observed Takotsubo syndrome in relation to abruptio placentae and premature delivery of a baby who died subsequently. Four years after delivery, one (6.7%) patient suffered from a pulmonary embolism (Table 4).

Table 4. Maternal cardiovascular complications during pregnancy and after delivery.

Type of Complication	n = 15	Trimester
Atrial arrhythmia	2 (13.3%)	2nd
Ventricular arrhythmia	1 (6.7%)	2nd
Hypoxemia ($SO_2 < 90\%$)	1 (6.7%)	2nd
Systemic thromboembolism	0	-
Heart failure	0	-
Takotsubo syndrome	1 (6.7%)	After delivery
Protein-losing enteropathy	0	-
Maternal death	0	-

4.5. Anticoagulation Regimen during Pregnancy

There were three different types of anticoagulation used in our population. Twelve (46.2%) pregnancies were followed without anticoagulation therapy. One of them was treated with aspirin 75mg/d. Prophylactic anticoagulation was administered during six (23%) pregnancies due to abnormal (accelerated in comparison to previous examinations) flow in the TCPC tunnel as well as patent fenestration with a right to left shunt. Therapeutic anticoagulation was used in eight (30.8%) pregnancies due to atrial arrhythmia or thromboembolic complications, diagnosed by abnormal perfusion in pulmonary scintigraphy examination or presence of thrombus in the echocardiographic examination (Table 3).

5. Discussion

Our analysis confirmed that pregnancy in Fontan survivors is possible and may also be successful [1,5,7,13]. However, a woman considering pregnancy must be aware of potential risks and complications for herself and the baby. The earliest is a miscarriage, which happened in the analyzed population in 11 (42%) pregnancies, all but one in the first trimester. These observations were the same as described by Bonner et al. [14] and were similar to the incidence of 27–69% published in previous reports [1,5,7,13,15,16]. These numbers are much higher than the spontaneous miscarriage rates of 10–15% observed in the general European population [17]. The reason for this fatal condition is not completely clear, but it may result from abdominal venous congestion, increased venous pressure, and inability to increase cardiac output [1,5,6,18].

As we already know from published data, pregnancies that prevail into the second trimester should be eventually completed [13,14,16,19]. Therefore, it is reasonable to assume that well-functioning Fontan patients are more likely to achieve pregnancy. This was confirmed by Arif et al. based on an analysis of 55 pregnancies in women after the Fontan procedure [16]. These authors proposed a novel three-step risk stratification model based on patients' functional class and the presence of complications typical for Fontan circulation. They observed a high (93.3%) miscarriage rate among women with poor cardiovascular status. Our data showed similar results. Eleven patients who suffered miscarriage had worse cardiovascular status than women who completed their pregnancies.

5.1. Maternal Cardiovascular Complications

What is worth underlining, fortunately, and consistently with published data, is that we did not observe any maternal deaths in our study [1,5,14,16,20].

Our study's most frequent Fontan-related complication was atrial and ventricular arrhythmia, which occurred in three (20%) patients and responded well to pharmacotherapy.

In the reported literature, supraventricular arrhythmia is the most common cardiovascular adverse event in these pregnant women [1]. According to the published data, an arrhythmia occurs, similarly to our observations, in 8.1–31.5% of patients [16,20,21]. Women after the Fontan procedure are prone to arrhythmia development not only due to the atrial surgical scars, sinus node disease, or altered and injured atrial tissue organization but also as a result of typical changes in the pregnant state, i.e., hyperdynamic circulation, myocardial stretch, or hormonal changes (progesterone increase) [1,13,16,22,23].

None of our patients suffered from heart failure during pregnancy, unlike the published series, where 9.5–15.7% of pregnancies were complicated by heart failure. [16,20,21]. These observations result from our patients' good clinical and hemodynamical status. This is consistent with the conception made by Arif et al., which states that successful pregnancy is strictly related to the preconceptional clinical state of women after the Fontan procedure [16]. Heart failure was the second most common cardiovascular complication in their studied population. Hence, hyperdynamic circulation typical for pregnancy and resulting from increased cardiac output and dilation of vascular bed impairs the functioning of fragile Fontan circulation. A single ventricle must create such energy to enable blood flow into pulmonary circulation against decreased preload and gravity [18].

Furthermore, obstetrical complications, such as gestational hypertension, preeclampsia, or anemia, may result in heart failure development.

In the analyzed group, in accordance with other published series, we did not observe any new systemic thromboembolism during pregnancy [16,21]. Considering the presence of both thromboembolic risk in women after the Fontan procedure and the hypercoagulable state of pregnancy, patients at risk of thromboembolic complications (presence of arrhythmia, right to left shunt) received anticoagulation in our study. Cauldwell et al demonstrated only one (out of 50 pregnant women) venous thromboembolism case in the postpartum period [23]. In the series from Gouton et al. as well as Ropero et al., only isolated cases of antepartum pulmonary embolism and cerebral ischemic events were reported [1,20]. In relation to the presented thromboembolic risk, these results require validation in more extensive studies. Initiation of anticoagulation in the studied group must balance the potential risk of bleeding, which is present even in nonpregnant patients [24].

In our study group, all women were of NYHA $\leq$ II class, and none of the patients had a mechanical valve or pulmonary hypertension. In this setting, the identification of women at risk of primary cardiovascular events using ZAHARA or CARPREG II scores was not particularly discriminative [11,12]. Additionally, the low incidence of cardiovascular complications in our study group could not prove the strength of these risk scores.

5.2. Obstetrical Status

Although European guidelines do not give explicit recommendations regarding the delivery mode, all our patients were delivered by semi-elective cesarean section [7]. Almost in half of the patients (6 out of 15), deliveries were conducted before the 37 WG, which significantly increased the risk of potential peri-delivery complications. Similar decisions were made by Arif et al. [16]. Organization of cardiological and obstetrical care in our unit was an additional factor in favor of cesarean section. In the centers participating in our study, obstetrical departments are located in the other part of the city, rendering hours-long high-specialty cardiological and obstetrical care impossible.

As noted in our analysis and described in previous studies, such obstetrical complications as abruptio placentae, premature rupture of membranes, and antepartum hemorrhage are observed significantly more often in pregnancies with Fontan circulation than in the general population [1,20,21,25]. In our study, we had two (13.3%) cases of each complication. In other series, the rate of premature rupture of membranes amounted to 15.3–28.2% vs. 1.25% found in the general population [23,25]. The main reason for this high incidence of complications is hypoperfusion of the fetoplacental unit and vascular dysfunction resulting from the existing Fontan hemodynamic inability to increase stroke volume together with systemic venous hypertension [5]. Antepartum hemorrhage was described to complicate 5.7–21% of pregnancies of women after the Fontan procedure [20,21,23]. We did not observe postpartum hemorrhage, but others reported that complication in 2.8–42.8% of pregnancies in Fontan survivors [20,21,23]. Vascular malformations, liver disease due to abdominal venous congestion, or thrombotic disorders typical for Fontan circulation could be responsible for this observation [24,26]. Not without meaning when postpartum hemorrhage is considered is a mode of delivery, and its protocol, i.e., common use of oxytocin to avoid uterus atony—a potential cause for hemorrhagic complications [27]. In addition, anticoagulation treatment during pregnancy may play a role [21]; however, not all authors support this finding [15,25]. Although current European guidelines suggest consideration of anticoagulation treatment during pregnancy, patients analyzed in our retrospective study were anticoagulated only when additional indications for anticoagulation, i.e., atrial arrhythmia, right to left shunt, or previous thromboembolic events occurred [7]. As was already mentioned, and what needs to be considered while planning pregnancy, anticoagulation can entail miscarriage in these patients.

5.3. Neonatal Complications

In our study group, we observed three (18.8%) neonatal deaths, prematurity amounted to 40% of live births, and the birth weight was smaller than in the general population. These results are comparable to other published reports of neonatal deaths at 2.7–25% [20,23,25]. In the other series, prematurity rates in Fontan patients amounted to 60–82% [14,21,23,28] and were six–eight-fold more frequent than in the general population [25]. Presented neonatal complications arise from the above-mentioned adverse hemodynamics regarding Fontan circulation physiology [18,28]. Another predisposing factor for neonatal outcomes could be desaturation due to fenestration, which was present in 40% of patients [20], although Caudwell et al. do not support this thinking [23]. Certainly, maternal medications also play a role, i.e., beta-blockers or diuretics decreasing placental perfusion [1,28].

5.4. Management of Pregnant Patients in Our Center

When a patient reaches adulthood and is transferred to our outpatient clinic for adults with congenital heart defects, we analyze previous medical history and talk about reproductive plans. If a patient is considered as "failing" Fontan according to medical records, we discourage her from pregnancy. At preconception evaluation, we perform the echocardiographic examination, laboratory tests (i.e., morphology, NTproBNP, liver function), and cardiopulmonary exercise test. Once a patient gets pregnant, she is asked to come for a visit. Usually, we invite patients once in every trimester for a clinical visit comprising ECG, oxygen saturation, blood pressure, and echocardiographic examination. If additional problems occur (arrhythmia, heart failure symptoms, obstetrical complications), we schedule further visits or hospitalize the patient. Between 20–22 weeks gestation, we advise obtaining a fetal echocardiographic examination. Our patients are comanaged by obstetricians whom we sensify to careful placental and uterus perfusion assessment and thorough evaluation of fetal growth. Usually, we recommend delivery between 37–39 weeks gestation, but its timing depends on the advancement of fetal growth and the presence of potential obstetrical complications. Within three months after delivery, we ask the patient to schedule a clinical visit.

5.5. Study Limitations

Single ventricle anatomy and physiology encompasses a spectrum of various defects that may alter Fontan hemodynamics and outcomes. Therefore, the heterogeneity of the studied population makes any comparisons difficult. In addition, this study is limited by the retrospective nature of data collection. Finally, the small sample size is another limitation of this study.

6. Conclusions

Pregnancy in women after the Fontan procedure, although it increases the risk of morbidity, is well tolerated. However, it is burdened by a high risk of miscarriage and multiple obstetrical complications, including losing a child, which a young woman and her family should be counseled about. These women require specialized care provided by both experienced cardiologists and obstetricians.

Author Contributions: Conceptualization, A.B.-R. and O.T.; methodology, A.B.-R. and O.T.; validation, O.T., L.T.-P. and M.R.-L.; formal analysis, A.B.-R. and O.T.; investigation, A.B.-R., O.T., L.T.-P., A.C., N.B. and K.K.-P.; resources, O.T. and L.T.-P.; data curation, A.B.-R. and O.T.; writing—original draft preparation, A.B.-R.; writing—review and editing, O.T.; visualization, A.B.-R. and O.T.; supervision, O.T.; project administration, A.B.-R. All authors have read and agreed to the published version of the manuscript.

Funding: This research received no external funding.

Institutional Review Board Statement: The study was conducted in accordance with the Declaration of Helsinki and approved by the Institutional Review Board (or Ethics Committee) of Poznan University of Medical Sciences (Protocol code 475/19, date of approval 11 April 2019).

Informed Consent Statement: Not applicable.

Data Availability Statement: The data presented in this study are available on request from the corresponding author.

Acknowledgments: The authors thank Jacek Bil (JO Medical Solutions) for providing medical writing support.

Conflicts of Interest: The authors declare no conflict of interest.

References

1. Garcia Ropero, A.; Baskar, S.; Roos Hesselink, J.W.; Girnius, A.; Zentner, D.; Swan, L.; Ladouceur, M.; Brown, N.; Veldtman, G.R. Pregnancy in women with a Fontan circulation: A systematic review of the literature. *Circ. Cardiovasc. Qual. Outcomes* **2018**, *11*, e004575. [CrossRef]
2. Kramer, P.; Schleiger, A.; Schafstedde, M.; Danne, F.; Nordmeyer, J.; Berger, F.; Ovroutski, S. A Multimodal Score Accurately Classifies Fontan Failure and Late Mortality in Adult Fontan Patients. *Front. Cardiovasc. Med.* **2022**, *9*, 767503. [CrossRef] [PubMed]
3. Alsaied, T.; Possner, M.; Lubert, A.M.; Trout, A.T.; Gandhi, J.P.; Garr, B.; Palumbo, J.S.; Palermo, J.J.; Lorts, A.; Veldtman, G.R.; et al. Thromboembolic Events Are Independently Associated with Liver Stiffness in Patients with Fontan Circulation. *J. Clin. Med.* **2020**, *9*, 418. [CrossRef] [PubMed]
4. Monga, M.; Mastrobattista, J.M. Maternal cardiovascular, respiratory, and renal adaptation to pregnancy. In *Creasy and Resnik's Maternal-Fetal Medicine: Principles and Practice*, 8th ed.; Resnik, R., Lockwood, C.J., Moore, T., Greene, M.F., Copel, J., Silver, R.M., Eds.; Elsevier Saunders: Philadelphia, PA, USA, 2018; pp. 141–147.
5. Ordonez, M.V.; Trinder, J.; Curtis, S.L. Success in a Fontan pregnancy: How important is ventricular function? *Cardiol Young* **2019**, *29*, 225–227. [CrossRef] [PubMed]
6. Ordoñez, M.V.; Biglino, G.; Caputo, M.; Kelly, B.; Mohan, A.; Trinder, J.; Curtis, S.L. Case of placental insufficiency and premature delivery in a Fontan pregnancy: Physiological insights and considerations on risk stratification. *Open Heart* **2021**, *8*, e001211. [CrossRef]
7. Regitz-Zagrosek, V.; Roos-Hesselink, J.W.; Bauersachs, J.; Blomstrom-Lundqvist, C.; Cifkova, R.; De Bonis, M.; Iung, B.; Johnson, M.R.; Kintscher, U.; Kranke, P.; et al. ESC Guidelines for the management of cardiovascular diseases during pregnancy. *Eur. Heart J.* **2018**, *39*, 3165–3241. [CrossRef]
8. Chowdhury, S.M.; Graham, E.M.; Taylor, C.L.; Savage, A.; McHugh, K.E.; Gaydos, S.; Nutting, A.C.; Zile, M.R.; Atz, A.M. Diastolic Dysfunction with Preserved Ejection Fraction After the Fontan Procedure. *J. Am. Heart Assoc.* **2022**, *11*, e024095. [CrossRef]

9. Vause, S.; Clarke, B.; Tower, C.L.; Hay, C.; Knight, M. Pregnancy outcomes in women with mechanical prosthetic heart valves: A prospective descriptive population based study using the United Kingdom Obstetric Surveillance System (UKOSS) data collection system. *BJOG* **2017**, *124*, 1411–1419. [CrossRef]
10. van Hagen, I.M.; Roos-Hesselink, J.W.; Ruys, T.P.; Merz, W.M.; Goland, S.; Gabriel, H.; Lelonek, M.; Trojnarska, O.; Al Mahmeed, W.A.; Balint, H.O.; et al. Pregnancy in women with a mechanical heart valve: Data of the European Society of Cardiology Registry of Pregnancy and Cardiac Disease (ROPAC). *Circulation* **2015**, *132*, 132–142. [CrossRef]
11. Silversides, C.K.; Grewal, J.; Mason, J.; Sermer, M.; Kiess, M.; Rychel, V.; Wald, R.M.; Colman, J.M.; Siu, S.C. Pregnancy Outcomes in Women with Heart Disease: The CARPREG II Study. *J. Am. Coll. Cardiol.* **2018**, *71*, 2419–2430. [CrossRef]
12. Drenthen, W.; Boersma, E.; Balci, A.; Moons, P.; Roos-Hesselink, J.W.; Mulder, B.J.; Vliegen, H.W.; van Dijk, A.P.; Voors, A.A.; Yap, S.C.; et al. Predictors of pregnancy complications in women with congenital heart disease. *Eur. Heart J.* **2010**, *31*, 2124–2132. [CrossRef] [PubMed]
13. Wolfe, N.K.; Sabol, B.A.; Kelly, J.C.; Dombrowski, M.; Benhardt, A.C.; Fleckenstein, J.; Stout, M.J.; Lindley, K.J. Management of Fontan circulation in pregnancy: A multidisciplinary approach to care. *Am. J. Obstet. Gynecol. MFM* **2021**, *3*, 100257. [CrossRef] [PubMed]
14. Bonner, S.J.; Asghar, O.; Roberts, A.; Vause, S.; Clarke, B.; Keavney, B. Cardiovascular, obstetric and neonatal outcomes in women with previous fontan repair. *Eur. J. Obstet. Gynecol. Reprod. Biol.* **2017**, *219*, 53–56. [CrossRef] [PubMed]
15. Cauldwell, M.; Von Klemperer, K.; Uebing, A.; Swan, L.; Steer, P.J.; Babu-Narayan, S.V.; Gatzoulis, M.A.; Johnson, M.R. A cohort study of women with a Fontan circulation undergoing preconception counselling. *Heart* **2016**, *102*, 534–540. [CrossRef] [PubMed]
16. Arif, S.; Chaudhary, A.; Clift, P.F.; Morris, R.K.; Selman, T.J.; Bowater, S.E.; Hudsmith, L.E.; Thompson, P.J.; Thorne, S.A. Pregnancy outcomes in patients with a fontan circulation and proposal for a risk-scoring system: Single centre experience. *J. Congenit. Heart. Dis.* **2017**, *1*, 10. [CrossRef]
17. Ford, H.B.; Schust, D.J. Recurrent pregnancy loss: Etiology, diagnosis, and therapy. *Rev. Obstet. Gynecol.* **2009**, *2*, 76–83. [PubMed]
18. Gewillig, M. The Fontan circulation. *Heart* **2005**, *91*, 839–846. [CrossRef]
19. Walker, F. Pregnancy and the various forms of the Fontan circulation. *Heart* **2007**, *93*, 152–154. [CrossRef]
20. Gouton, M.; Nizard, J.; Patel, M.; Sassolas, F.; Jimenez, M.; Radojevic, J.; Mathiron, A.; Amedro, P.; Barre, E.; Labombarda, F.; et al. Maternal and fetal outcomes of pregnancy with Fontan circulation: A multicentric observational study. *Int. J. Cardiol.* **2015**, *187*, 84–89. [CrossRef]
21. Pundi, K.N.; Pundi, K.; Johnson, J.N.; Dearani, J.A.; Bonnichsen, C.R.; Phillips, S.D.; Canobbio, M.C.; Driscoll, D.J.; Cetta, F. Contraception practices and pregnancy outcome in patients after fontan operation. *Congenit Heart Dis.* **2016**, *11*, 63–70. [CrossRef]
22. Pujol, C.; Hessling, G.; Telishevska, M.; Schiele, S.; Deisenhofer, I.; Ewert, P.; Tutarel, O. Prevalence and Treatment Outcomes of Arrhythmias in Patients with Single Ventricle Physiology over the Age of 40 Years. *J. Clin. Med.* **2022**, *11*, 6568. [CrossRef] [PubMed]
23. Cauldwell, M.; Steer, P.J.; Bonner, S.; Asghar, O.; Swan, L.; Hodson, K.; Head, C.E.G.; Jakes, A.D.; Walker, N.; Simpson, M.; et al. Retrospective UK multicentre study of the pregnancy outcomes of women with a Fontan repair. *Heart* **2018**, *104*, 401–406. [CrossRef] [PubMed]
24. Monagle, P.; Cochrane, A.; Roberts, R.; Manlhiot, C.; Weintraub, R.; Szechtman, B.; Hughes, M.; Andrew, M.; McCrindle, B.W. Fontan Anticoagulation Study Group. A multicenter, randomized trial comparing heparin/warfarin and acetylsalicylic acid as primary thromboprophylaxis for 2 years after the Fontan procedure in children. *J. Am. Coll Cardiol.* **2011**, *58*, 645–651. [CrossRef] [PubMed]
25. Drenthen, W.; Pieper, P.G.; Roos-Hesselink, J.W.; van Lottum, W.A.; Voors, A.A.; Mulder, B.J.; van Dijk, A.P.; Vliegen, H.W.; Sollie, K.M.; Moons, P.; et al. Pregnancy and delivery in women after Fontan palliation. *Heart* **2006**, *92*, 1290–1294. [CrossRef]
26. McCrindle, B.W.; Manlhiot, C.; Cochrane, A.; Roberts, R.; Hughes, M.; Szechtman, B.; Weintraub, R.; Andrew, M.; Monagle, P. Fontan Anticoagulation Study Group. Factors associated with thrombotic complications after the Fontan procedure: A secondary analysis of a multicenter, randomized trial of primary thromboprophylaxis for 2 years after the Fontan procedure. *J. Am. Coll. Cardiol.* **2013**, *61*, 346–353. [CrossRef]
27. Cauldwell, M.; Swan, L.; Uebing, A.; Gatzoulis, M.; Patel, R.; Steer, P.J.; Johnson, M.R. The management of third stage of labour in women with heart disease needs more attention. *Int. J. Cardiol.* **2016**, *223*, 23–24. [CrossRef]
28. Afshar, Y.; Tan, W.; Jones, W.M.; Canobbio, M.; Lin, J.; Reardon, L.; Lluri, G.; Aboulhosn, J.; Koos, B.J. Maternal Fontan procedure is a predictor of a small-for gestational-age neonate: A 10-year retrospective study. *Am. J. Obstet Gynecol. MFM* **2019**, *1*, 100036. [CrossRef]

Disclaimer/Publisher's Note: The statements, opinions and data contained in all publications are solely those of the individual author(s) and contributor(s) and not of MDPI and/or the editor(s). MDPI and/or the editor(s) disclaim responsibility for any injury to people or property resulting from any ideas, methods, instructions or products referred to in the content.

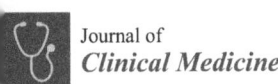

Article

Interventional Occlusion of Large Patent Ductus Arteriosus in Adults with Severe Pulmonary Hypertension

Zeming Zhou [1,2,†], Yuanrui Gu [3,†], Hong Zheng [1,*], Chaowu Yan [1], Qiong Liu [1], Shiguo Li [1], Huijun Song [1], Zhongying Xu [1], Jinglin Jin [1], Haibo Hu [1] and Jianhua Lv [1]

[1] Department of Structural Heart Disease, Fuwai Hospital, State Key Laboratory of Cardiovascular Disease, National Center for Cardiovascular Diseases, Chinese Academy of Medical Sciences, Peking Union Medical College, Beijing 100037, China

[2] Department of Cardiology, Fuwai Hospital, State Key Laboratory of Cardiovascular Disease, National Center for Cardiovascular Diseases, Chinese Academy of Medical Sciences, Peking Union Medical College, Beijing 100037, China

[3] Department of Vascular Surgery, Fuwai Hospital, State Key Laboratory of Cardiovascular Disease, National Center for Cardiovascular Disease, Chinese Academy of Medical Sciences, Peking Union Medical College, Beijing 100037, China

* Correspondence: zheng_hung@126.com
† These authors contributed equally to this work.

Abstract: (1) Background: the indications for transcatheter closure of large patent ductus arteriosus (PDA) with severe pulmonary hypertension (PH) are still unclear, and scholars have not fully elucidated the factors that affect PH prognosis. (2) Methods: we retrospectively enrolled 134 consecutive patients with a PDA diameter $\geq$10 mm or a ratio of PDA and aortic >0.5. We collected clinical data to explore the factors affecting follow-up PH. (3) Results: 134 patients (mean age 35.04 ± 10.23 years; 98 women) successfully underwent a transcatheter closure, and all patients had a mean pulmonary artery pressure (mPAP) >50 mmHg. Five procedures were deemed to have failed because their mPAP did not decrease, and the patients experienced uncomfortable symptoms after the trial occlusion. The average occluder (pulmonary end) size was almost twice the PDA diameter (22.33 ± 4.81 mm vs. 11.69 ± 2.18 mm). Left ventricular end-diastolic dimension (LVEDD), mPAP, and left ventricular ejection fraction (LVEF) significantly reduced after the occlusion, and LVEF recovered during the follow-up period. In total, 42 of the 78 patients with total pulmonary resistance >4 Wood Units experienced clinical outcomes, and all of them had PH in the follow-up, while 10 of them had heart failure, and 4 were hospitalized again because of PH. The results of a logistic regression analysis revealed that the postoperative mPAP had an independent risk factor (odds ratio = 1.069, 95% confidence interval: 1.003 to 1.140, $p = 0.040$) with a receiver operating characteristic curve cut-off value of 35.5 mmHg ($p < 0.001$). (4) Conclusions: performing a transcatheter closure of large patent ductus arteriosus is feasible, and postoperative mPAP was a risk factor that affected the follow-up PH. Patients with a postoperative mPAP >35.5 mmHg should be considered for targeted medical therapy or should undergo right heart catheterization again after the occlusion.

Keywords: patent ductus arteriosus; pulmonary hypertension; transcatheter closure; risk factor; prognosis

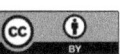

1. Introduction

Patent ductus arteriosus (PDA) is one of the most common congenital heart diseases (CHD) as it accounts for 10–16% of CHDs [1,2]. Since 1967, when Porstmann conducted the first transcatheter closure to treat PDA [3], scientists have enhanced the device and delivery systems that physicians use when performing transcatheter closures tremendously. Currently, factors that determine whether a physician should perform a transcatheter closure to treat an individual with a normal-size PDA are clear and definite, and transcatheter closure is the first treatment choice of cardiologists. However, challenges still exist when closing large PDAs, especially those >10 mm. Various difficulties, including insufficient device sizes and pulmonary hypertension (PH), considerably decrease the success rate of the procedure. The invention of an oversized device larger than the 18/16 mm mushroom PDA occluder made it possible for physicians to close large PDAs. However, a large PDA is always accompanied by severe PH, and the mean pulmonary artery pressure (mPAP) is usually >50 mmHg. Thus, the irreversible pulmonary vascular change caused by severe PH results in persistent PH during the follow-up period which elevates the poor prognosis risk.

Right heart catheterization (RHC) is the method most commonly used to assess hemodynamics. Qp/Qs are less accurate at predicting the prognosis; nevertheless, scholars regard pulmonary vascular resistance (PVR) as a useful index [4–11]. However, the samples used in previous studies were small or the PDAs of the enrolled patients were not large enough. The indicators that predict follow-up PH after the occlusion of large PDAs with severe PH remain unclear. Thus, we retrospectively examined patients with large PDAs who underwent interventional treatment from 2010 to 2020, analyzed the feasibility of interventional treatments for large PDAs, and found a clear predictor regarding the postoperative persistence of PH.

2. Materials and Methods

2.1. Patients

We recruited patients who were diagnosed with large PDAs and underwent interventional treatment from 2010 to 2020. All the patients underwent an X-ray, electrocardiography, and transthoracic echocardiography (TTE). Some patients underwent multislice computed tomography before surgery. Researchers at the Structural Heart Disease Department at Fuwai Hospital conducted this retrospective study. The procedures of this study followed the ethical guidelines of the Declaration of Helsinki, and the Ethics Committee of Fuwai Hospital approved this study. Additionally, we obtained informed consent from all the participants (2021-1452).

2.2. Inclusion and Exclusion Criteria

Currently, the classification of PDA according to diameter is unclear. We defined a PDA diameter $\geq$10 mm or a ratio of PDA and aortic >0.5 as a large PDA. We defined indications that a transcatheter closure should be performed as follows: (1) large PDA; (2) pulmonary hypertension; and (3) an audible cardiac murmur attributable to the PDA. The exclusion criteria were as follows: (1) endocarditis; (2) resistant pulmonary hypertension; and (3) accompanied by other heart diseases requiring surgical repair [12].

2.3. Right Heart Catheterization and Transcatheter Closure

All patients underwent fluoroscopy-guided procedures under local anesthesia. We punctured the right femoral artery and vein and inserted puncture sheaths. We performed routine right heart catheterization, and we inserted a 5 or 6 Fr MPA2 catheter into the pulmonary artery and right ventricle to measure the pulmonary arterial pressure. We calculated total pulmonary resistance (TPR) based on blood oxygen saturation. If the TPR was >4 Wood Units, the patient inhaled oxygen for 10 min, and we repeated the procedure to calculate the TPR. Then, we inserted a 5 Fr pigtail catheter into the aorta (AO) and performed an aortography. We observed and measured the shape and diameter of the ducts using an aortography. The device deployment procedure was as follows: we passed a 5 or 6 Fr MPA2 catheter across the PDA into the aorta, exchanged the extra-stiff wire, and passed the delivery sheath. We passed the delivery sheath into the aorta via the PDA from the femoral vein. We deployed the device using fluoroscopy and angiographic guidance. The size of the pulmonary end of the PDA occluder used was larger than 16 mm and was produced by Lifetech Scientific Co., Ltd. (Shenzhen, China) or Starway Medical Tec Co., Ltd. (Beijing, China). We repeated the aortography and measured the continuous pressure. Finally, we released the device under X-ray and TTE guidance after confirming the correct position. We measured the pressure when the patient was stable after we released the device.

2.4. Postoperative and Follow-Up Outcomes

All patients underwent TTE, X-ray, and ECG again at 1, 3, 6, and 12 months. We detected the position and residual shunt of the occluder using TTE. We performed an X-ray to measure the cardiothoracic ratio after the procedure. We evaluated the PAP and predicted the PH in all the patients using TTE. The PH diagnostic criteria that we used to evaluate the TTE were based on the 2022 ESC guidelines [13]. We recommended that the patients repeat the RHC at 6 months after closure if doing so was deemed possible based on their TTE results. We defined the follow-up outcome according to the PH assessed with TTE or RHC after the occlusion. We conducted a telephone follow-up with all the patients before we analyzed the data. The follow-up time was the length from the discharge to the time of the last follow-up result that we could collect. We defined clinical outcomes as the follow-up PH, heart failure (NYHA III or IV), and/or hospitalization caused by PH.

2.5. Statistical Analysis

We used SPSS version 26.0 (IBM), R version 4.2.0 software, and GraphPad Prism version 8.0 (GraphPad Software Inc., La Jolla, CA, USA) to calculate and illustrate the data. The continuous variables in this study are expressed as the mean ± standard deviation (SD) or as the median (IQR), and the categorical variables are expressed as numbers and percentages. We compared the continuous variables using the independent sample t-test or the Wilcoxon rank-sum test. We performed a risk factor estimation of the outcomes using a combination of the least absolute shrinkage selection operator (LASSO) and univariate or multivariate logistic regression to determine the association measures. We used the receiver operating characteristic curve to define the cut-off value. We set statistical significance at $p < 0.05$.

3. Results

3.1. Patient Characteristics

A total of 152 patients underwent transcatheter therapy. We excluded 11 patients with other congenital heart diseases that required surgical repair or staged operation and 2 patients with severe residual shunts. The procedure failed in 5 patients whose PAP did not decrease and who also experienced uncomfortable symptoms after the trial occlusion; because of this, we pulled the device back. Thus, we recruited 134 patients for this study. A total of 88 patients underwent RHC, and 78 had a TPR >4 Wood Units.

Table 1 presents the baseline characteristics of the patients. The results of the preoperative TTE indicated a large PDA with an accompanying left-sided heart enlargement in all the patients. The results of the X-ray suggested heart enlargement with an increased cardiothoracic ratio. Five patients had a trivial pericardiac effusion before the operation which may have been caused by heart failure and disappeared after closure. Nine patients had other congenital heart diseases, including three with patent foramen ovale, four with a small atrial septal defect (7, 5, 5, and 4 mm), and two with small ventricular septal defects (3 and 2 mm). Twelve patients participated in targeted medical therapy before and after closure.

Table 1. Baseline characteristics of patients.

Variables	N
Patients, n	134
Female, n (%)	98 (73.1)
Age, y	35.04 ± 10.23
BMI, kg/m^2	20.43 ± 3.60

Table 1. Cont.

Variables	N
Heart function (NYHA)	
I, II	115
III, IV	19
Cardiothoracic ratio	0.60 ± 0.07
PDA diameter, mm	11.69 ± 2.18
Occluder size, mm	22.33 ± 4.81
Presence of other heart diseases, n	
PFO	3
Small ASD	4
Small VSD	2
Trivial pericardiac effusion, n	5
Complications, n	
Residual shunt	7
Femoral arteriovenous fistula	1
Systolic Pp/Ps ratio, %	82.93 ± 18.47
Targeted medical therapy, n	12
Endothelin receptor antagonists, n	7
Phosphodiesterase 5 inhibitors and guanylate cyclase stimulators, n	8
Prostacyclin analogues and prostacyclin receptor agonists, n	1

NYHA: New York Heart Association; ASD: atrial septal defect; BMI: body mass index; PDA: patent ductus arteriosus; PFO: patent foramen ovale; Pp/Ps: pulmonary pressure, systemic pressure.

3.2. Transcatheter Closure and Postoperative PAP

We measured PAP and aortic pressure (AP) at baseline in all the patients using a catheter. The average size of the occluder (pulmonary end) was 22.33 ± 4.81 mm and was almost twice the size of the PDA diameter (β = 1.88; 95% confidence interval [CI] 1.682–2.081; R^2 = 0.73; $p < 0.001$). The left ventricular end-diastolic dimension (LVEDD) showed significant shrinkage accompanied with a decrease in the left ventricular ejection fraction (LVEF) below the normal level (Table 2). After closure, the mPAP of all 134 patients for whom the procedure was successful decreased (40.99 ± 12.34 mmHg), and the mean AP increased (14.52 ± 10.40 mmHg) (Table 2). Although the LVEF decreased after the occlusion, the clinical symptoms were not significant without pericardial effusion or heart failure. All the patients were able to walk out of the hospital one or two days after the occlusion.

Table 2. Pre- and postoperative variable comparison.

Variables	Preoperative	Postoperative	p
mPAP	76.79 ± 14.96	35.31 ± 12.05	<0.001
mAP	89.17 ± 12.23	103.70 ± 13.39	<0.001
RVEDD	24.22 ± 5.37	23.83 ± 4.86	>0.05
LVEDD	63.75 ± 10.05	58.53 ± 9.35	<0.001
LVEF	59.60 ± 8.11	52.94 ± 9.90	<0.001

mPAP: mean pulmonary artery pressure; mAP: mean arterial pressure; LVEDD: left ventricular end-diastolic dimension; LVEF: left ventricular ejection fraction; RVEDD: right ventricular end-diastolic dimension.

The preoperative mPAP (76.0 [67.0,83.0] mmHg vs. 86.0 [70.5,94.0] mmHg; $p > 0.05$) in women aged <45 years was similar to that of men, but the postoperative mPAP (32.0 [24.0,41.0] mmHg vs. 41.0 [32.0, 52.5] mmHg; $p = 0.015$) was lower in women aged <45 than in men. The average difference between the pre- and postoperative mPAP in women and men was 5.53 mmHg and 8.59 mmHg, respectively, and they were not significant ($p > 0.05$). Both the preoperative (22.68 ± 4.84 mm vs. 27.24 ± 5.30 mm, $p < 0.001$) and postoperative (22.38 ± 4.26 mm vs. 27.21 ± 5.38 mm; $p < 0.001$) RVEDD were smaller in women.

3.3. Follow-Up Data

The average follow-up period for the 134 patients was 17.56 months. We conducted a follow-up TTE to assess the PAP, ventricle diameter, and LVEF. The follow-up LVEDD was normal and statistically different from the postoperative LVEDD ($p < 0.001$), and the RVEDD measured during the follow up was similar to the postoperative RVEDD ($p > 0.05$). However, the LVEF at the follow up was elevated compared with the postoperative LVEF ($p < 0.001$), and it gradually recovered to a normal level ($p > 0.05$) (Figure 1). Twelve patients who received targeted medical therapy stopped taking drugs and continued to have PH, but they were still alive at the final follow up.

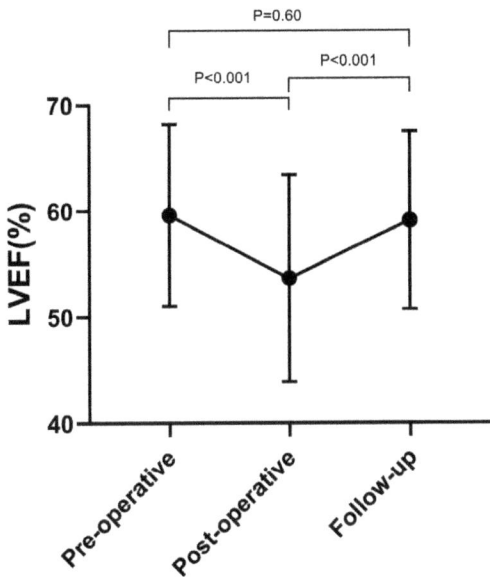

Figure 1. The postoperative LVEF was significantly reduced after occlusion and recovered to a normal level during the follow-up period. LVEF: left ventricular ejection fraction.

3.4. Baseline of the Five Failed Patients

Although we did not include data from five failed patients, we compared them to the 78 successful patients who had a TPR >4 Wood Units. These five failed patients had a higher postoperative mPAP (62.20 ± 25.08 vs. 37.38 ± 11.23), a lower mPAP decrease (18.60 ± 22.50 vs. 41.94 ± 12.41), a lower Qp/Qs (1.58 ± 0.28 vs. 2.13 ± 1.04), a smaller LV diameter (52.60 ± 8.05 vs. 61.76 ± 9.27), and a higher LVEF (70.70 ± 7.05 vs. 61.16 ± 8.05). We created a logistic regression model based on these 83 patients and found that the mPAP after the occlusion was the only risk factor for closure failure (odds ratio [OR] = 1.115; 95% CI: 1.020–1.217; $p = 0.016$). The cut-off value of the mPAP was 49.5 mmHg, and the area under the curve (AUC) was 88.5% ($p = 0.004$).

3.5. Prognostic Value of the Post-Operative PAP after Occlusion

We assessed the PAP using TTE of 78 successful closure patients with a TPR >4 Wood Units, and only 5 patients repeated the RHC 6 months later. Forty-two patients had experienced clinical outcomes during the 12.00 (IQR:3.00-29.25, only 4 patients <3 months) months follow-up, and all of them were detected during the follow-up PH. Ten of them experienced heart failure, and four were hospitalized again because of PH. During follow-up, 42 patients (Group 1) still had PH, and 36 patients' (Group 2) PAP had returned to normal. Group 1 had a higher postoperative mPAP and larger RVEDD during all periods

(Table 3). Group 1 had a larger TPR and systolic Pp/Ps ratio than Group 2 before the occlusion (Table 3).

Table 3. Comparison of variables between patients with and without follow-up PH.

Variables	With Follow-Up PH (n = 42)	Without Follow-Up PH (n = 36)	p
Female, n (%)	32 (76.2)	25 (69.2)	0.61
Age, y	35.48 ± 9.97	33.81 ± 10.80	
Heart function (NYHA), n			0.21
I, II	34	33	
III, IV	8	3	
PDA diameter, mm	12.17 ± 2.52	12.14 ± 1.85	0.95
Occluder size, mm	23.29 ± 4.90	23.00 ± 4.67	0.79
Before occlusion at baseline			
Baseline TPR, Wood Units	12.95 ± 5.87	10.47 ± 4.77	0.047
Systolic Pp/Ps ratio, %	88.03 ± 17.40	81.40 ± 19.74	0.11
Qp/Qs	2.00 ± 1.18	2.29 ± 0.84	0.22
mPAP, mmHg	81.29 ± 11.32	78.14 ± 13.24	0.26
LVEDD, mm	58.95 ± 8.00	65.03 ± 9.67	0.003
RVEDD, mm	25.57 ± 5.61	22.89 ± 5.13	0.03
LVEF, %	61.40 ± 7.55	60.88 ± 8.70	0.78
Femoral artery SaO$_2$, %	93.91 ± 3.52	94.42 ± 2.38	0.045
After occlusion at devices released			
Systolic Pp/Ps ratio, %	43.95 ± 11.99	35.39 ± 9.50	<0.001
mPAP, mmHg	41.69 ± 10.45	32.36 ± 10.07	<0.001
LVEDD, mm	54.81 ± 7.59	65.03 ± 9.67	0.023
RVEDD, mm	25.12 ± 5.26	22.53 ± 4.16	0.020
LVEF, %	55.28 ± 8.98	53.09 ± 8.70	0.28
mPAP difference before and after occlusion, mmHg	41.69 ± 10.45	32.36 ± 10.07	0.072

PH: pulmonary hypertension; PDA: patent ductus arteriosus; TPR: total pulmonary resistance; Pp/Ps: pulmonary pressure, systemic pressure.

Table 3 shows the potential risk factors for follow-up PH which we selected using the LASSO method (Figure 2). Table 4 shows the logistic regression analysis results. The postoperative mPAP was a risk factor that significantly affected the follow-up PH ($p = 0.040$, as shown in Table 4). We used the receiver operating characteristic (ROC) curve to determine the postoperative mPAP cut-off value to predict the PH, and we found that the cut-off value was 35.5 mmHg with an AUC of 74.4% (Figure 3A). The results of the logistic regression analysis showed that those with a higher PAP (>35.5 mmHg) had a higher risk of experiencing follow-up PH than those with a lower PAP (<35.5 mmHg) (OR = 5.682; 95% CI: 2.143–15.067; $p < 0.001$).

The LVEDD had no significant effect according to the multivariable regression model. However, when the regression model only included the preoperative factors, such as the baseline LVEDD, RVEDD, age, and sex, LVEDD was the only detected risk factor. Thus, we built an ROC curve, and the cut-off value was 56.5 mm with an AUC of 67.6% (Figure 3B). The results of the logistic regression analysis showed that those with a large LVEDD (>56.5 mm) had a lower risk of experiencing follow-up PH than those with a small LVEDD (<56.5 mm) (OR = 0.242; 95% CI: 0.083–0.703; $p = 0.009$).

Table 4. Univariable and multivariable logistic regression of persistent PH at follow-up.

Variables	Univariable (OR, 95% CI)	p	Multivariable (OR, 95% CI)	p
Postoperative mPAP	1.097 (1.040–1.158)	0.001	1.069 (1.003–1.140)	0.040
Preoperative LVEDD	0.921 (0.869–0.977)	0.006	0.958 (0.897–1.022)	0.195
Postoperative systolic Pp/Ps	1.083 (1.028–1.141)	0.003	1.027 (0.961–1.098)	0.428

PH: pulmonary hypertension; mPAP: mean pulmonary artery pressure; LVEDD: left ventricular end-diastolic dimension.

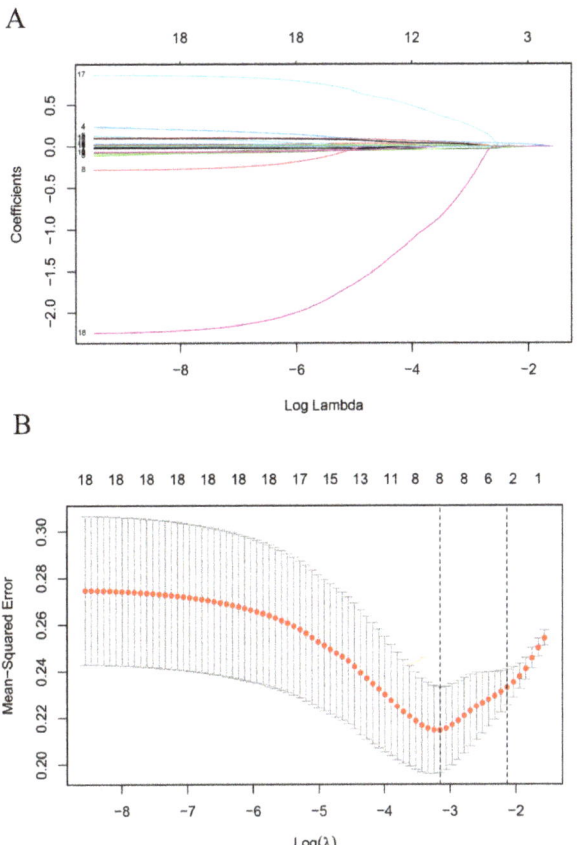

Figure 2. Least absolute shrinkage and selection operator (LASSO) analysis (**A**). We used LASSO regression to screen the prognostic factors. Coefficients of the determined characteristics are exhibited via lambda parameters (**B**). Cross validation indicated that three factors (postoperative mPAP, preoperative LVEDD, and postoperative systolic Pp/Ps) could be used in logistic regression. mPAP: mean pulmonary artery pressure; LVEDD: left ventricular end-diastolic dimension; Pp/Ps: pulmonary pressure, systemic pressure.

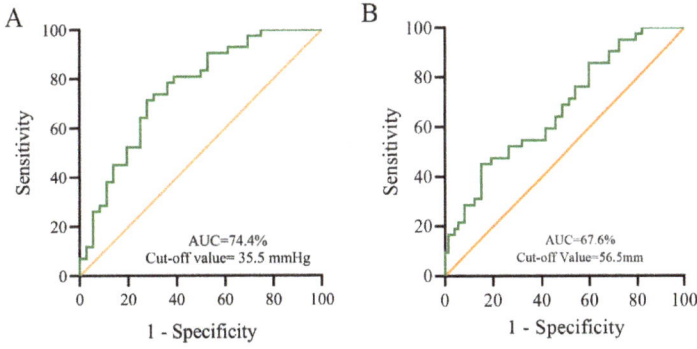

Figure 3. Receiver operating characteristic curve of postoperative mPAP (**A**) and LVEDD (**B**) for follow-up PH. AUC: area under the curve; mPAP: mean pulmonary artery pressure; LVEDD: left ventricular end-diastolic dimension.

4. Discussion

Presently, physicians still face difficulties when closing large PDAs, especially when treating patients with severe PH. Although there are different recommended closure strategies for different PVR grades, the ability to recognize the feasibility of closure and the postoperative persistence of PH is inconsistent across institutions. We analyzed and summarized the feasibility of large PDA interventional closures and found a clear predictor of PH postoperative persistence.

In small- or medium-sized PDAs, a device that is <16 mm can usually satisfy the clinical requirements. However, the PDA diameter in this study was ≥9 mm in all cases, and the size of the mushroom occluder was almost twice the PDA diameter. Thus, the size of the PDA occluder was larger than 16 mm. The normal-sized PDA could not provide sufficient support, and thus, the device was unstable and easily transposed under the large differential pressure of the AO and PA after implantation. Moreover, accurately measuring the diameters of the large PDAs was difficult, even with aortic angiography. After we implanted the device, the left disc of the device bulged into the aorta. Thus, the risk of obstructing the aorta still existed. Performing aortic angiography and measuring the continuous pressure from the aortic arch to the descending aorta below the device is necessary. The aorta and expanding pulmonary artery in adults can provide enough space for an oversized device; however, physicians still need to perform TTE and catheter examination with caution. We still do not recommend a transcatheter closure for a large PDA in children because of the higher risk of obstructing the descending aorta.

Many institutions are proficient with PDA transcatheter closure technology, but some questions still need special attention.

The first question concerns transcatheter closure criteria. The 2020 ESC Guidelines recommend that physicians should consider shunt closures for PDA patients with a PVR of 3–5 Wood Units and Qp/Qs >1.5 (IIa, C) and that physicians may consider a shunt closure after careful evaluation in a specialized center for patients with a PVR >5 Wood Units and Qp/Qs >1.5 (IIb, C) [14]. Compared with the 2015 ESC/ERS guidelines [15], this guideline attempts to make shunt closures more accessible for patients with over 5 Wood Units. This may benefit some patients with a higher PVR. Physicians in some clinical centers have adopted a trial occlusion strategy where some patients with >4 Wood Units undergo treatment. In this study, we adopted TPR, which is different from the recommended guidelines. Thus, when we set the inclusion criteria, we set the TPR dividing line to 4 Wood Units to control the PVR of patients at 3 Wood Units. In total, 78 patients with >4 Wood Units successfully implanted the PDA occluders, while their mPAP significantly decreased, and their heart function recovered. However, the closure eventually failed in five patients because of an increase in their pulmonary artery pressure and the accompanying uncomfortable symptoms after the occlusion. We could easily decide whether the occluder was suitable for release after observing clinical symptoms and analyzing the hemodynamics after the trial occlusion. One cannot deny that trial occlusions provide opportunities for patients with severe PH.

The second question focuses on the LVEF change after the occlusion. In this study, we found that the LVEF in several patients was reduced to <30%, and no clinical symptoms were present according to the patients' self-description. The LVEF reduced significantly after the closure, but it recovered after several months. LVEF is an index influenced by the preload and afterload. The preload decreases and the afterload increases after PDA treatment; therefore, the LVEF decreases after treatment. After several months, the cardiac reserve was gradually restored, and the LVEF and LV gradually recovered to a normal level. Therefore, the patient could return to daily life and perform physical labor several months after the operation. Ruth et al. reported the same result in children [16]. In practice, we observed that the change in the LVEF mostly happened in patients with a large PDA and LVEDD, and we predicted a significant reduction in the LVEF during the LV remodeling. A European study with a large sample revealed that the PDA diameter correlates well with postoperative LV dysfunction [17]. However, this was not significant in our study because we did not recruit patients with a normal PDA diameter.

The final question we should ask concerns PH prognosis after occlusion, especially in patients with TPR >4 Wood Units. For these patients, factors that affected follow-up PH were still unclear. Predicting follow-up PH could help physicians determine the subsequent treatment strategy, namely whether they should subsequently perform targeted medical treatment. Barst et al. suggested that Pp/Ps is appropriate to define PH, and Zhang et al. revealed that the postoperation systolic Pp/Ps ratio is a sensitive and specific parameter to identify postoperative PH [18,19]. However, the systolic Pp/Ps in our study was not significant in the multivariable regression model. The reasons may include the following. (1) The proportion of PH patients was different. Only 17 (12.6%) patients who participated in the previous study had PH during the follow up, whereas 42 (54%) patients who participated in our study had PH during the follow up. (2) Although the results of our study and the previous study showed that the systolic pulmonary pressure was similar in the baseline (115 ± 16 vs. 119 ± 18 mmHg), the postoperative systolic pulmonary pressure of the 42 follow-up PH patients who participated in this study was less than that of the participants who participated in the previous study (62 ± 15 vs. 85 ± 13 mmHg), and the mean pulmonary pressure decreased more significantly in the patients who participated our study. Thus, the average systolic Pp/Ps that we found was less than what the authors of the previous study found (44 ± 12% vs. 68 ± 15%). Therefore, postoperative systolic Pp/Ps was not significant in our study. However, the systolic Pp/Ps values between the patients with and without PH who participated in our study were also significantly different (43.95 ± 11.99% vs. 35.39 ± 9.50%; $p < 0.001$). This finding also indicates that the follow-up PH patients had a higher postoperative PAP.

We found that postoperative mPAP and mPAP differences were higher in the patients who had PH at follow-up than in those who did not have PH at follow-up. Postoperative mPAP was the only significant factor that affected the follow-up PH in patients with a TPR >4 Wood units. Using a logistic regression model, we found that those with a higher postoperative mPAP had a higher risk of having follow-up PH. The cut-off value suggested that a postoperative mPAP <35.5 mmHg was preferable. If the postoperative mPAP was greater than 35.5 mmHg, the patient was required to undergo targeted medical therapy or repeat the RHC 6 months later. As for the 12 patients who received targeted medical therapy, stopped taking the drugs, and were unwilling to undergo RHC again due to the economic burden, their prognosis may be relatively pessimistic. Many of these individuals were from developing countries and low-income populations. Cost efficiency is thus the largest concern when implementing RHC. Undergoing RHC is important regardless of whether patients with mild postoperative PH need to undergo targeted medical therapy. Thus, we are still recruiting a large sample population, and the pulmonary-pressure-based targeted medical therapy strategy is still under observation.

Although the LVEDD was not significant in the multivariable regression model, it was significant when we included only the preoperative factors in the model. This result was consistent with our clinical experience. The cut-off value of the LVEDD was similar to that found during clinical practice. Two reasons may explain this phenomenon: one is that a large RV compresses the LV and thus causes it to present a "D" shape on the TTE, and another is that the increased PAP changed the pre- and afterload of the left ventricle. A small LV may cause a patient to have a severe prognosis at follow-up. Physicians could even directly conduct targeted medical therapy without RHC in some circumstances. Therefore, patients with small LVEDD might need to have a further evaluation when undergoing this invasive operation.

As for the 5 failed patients, we compared their clinical data to the data of the 78 successful patients, and the differences were statistically significant. In clinical practice, a postoperative mPAP >49.5 mmHg is always combined with occlusion failure, which was consistent with our findings. Although the sample was too small to have enough power to draw firm conclusions, the patients reported clinical symptoms of chest pain and dyspnea after the trial occlusion. This demonstrates that a trial occlusion is necessary and important when closing a large PDA.

This study has some limitations. First, it was a single-center retrospective study with inescapable referral bias. Second, we only recorded the terminal status of the patients over the telephone. Some early patients were missing local hospital TTE results or were absent from the examination for many years. Thus, collecting the exact time when the PAP returned to normal was difficult. Third, the patients who received targeted medicine therapy may have withdrawn from the therapy or only participated in half of it. Thus, evaluating the drug therapy efficiency was difficult. Fourth, over half of the patients did not declare whether they used diuretics and vasodilators in their medication records. Thus, we may have underestimated the PAP before closure. Fifth, 46 patients did not undergo the RHC. These patients' PAP were similar to those of the patients with RHC, and the proportion of patients with >35.5 mmHg was not significantly different between these two populations (all $p > 0.05$). However, this finding was based on the experiences of our center and has certain limitations. Sixth, we measured the TPR in the past 10 years, which is different from what the guidelines recommend. Thus, when setting the inclusion criteria, we set the TPR dividing line as 4 Wood Units to control the PVR of patients at 3 Wood Units. Adopting the PVR would have been more appropriate. Finally, the TTE results obtained by the researchers at local clinical centers and our institution may have been inconsistent, and thus, the detected PH may have not been accurate.

5. Conclusions

The closure of large PDA with severe PH is feasible with 96.4% success (5 out of 139 patients failed). However, mPAP over 35.5 mmHg after closure predicts follow-up PH and clinical outcomes that are likely worse. These patients should probably be treated with target therapy, and repeated RHC should be performed after PDA closure, optimally with PVR assessment. PVR (not TPR) should also be calculated before PDA closure. Patients with smaller LV before closure (less than 56.5 mm LVEDD) should be observed more carefully.

Unfortunately, the importance of PVR assessment before the closure and evaluation of an upper value of PVR that is safe for PDA closure cannot be derived from this study.

Author Contributions: Conceptualization, Z.Z. and Y.G.; methodology, Z.Z.; software, Z.Z.; validation, Z.Z., Y.G. and H.Z.; formal analysis, Z.Z.; investigation, Z.Z. and Y.G.; resources, H.Z., C.Y., Q.L., S.L., H.S., Z.X., J.J., H.H. and J.L.; data curation, Z.Z. and H.Z.; writing—original draft preparation, Z.Z.; writing—review and editing, Y.G. and H.Z.; visualization, H.Z.; supervision, H.Z.; project administration, H.Z.; funding acquisition, H.Z. All authors have read and agreed to the published version of the manuscript.

Funding: This research was funded by the National Key Research and Development Program of China (grant number 2018YFB1107100), and the APC was funded by 2018YFB1107100.

Institutional Review Board Statement: The study was conducted in accordance with the Declaration of Helsinki and approved by the Institutional Ethics Committee of Fuwai Hospital (protocol code 2021-1452).

Informed Consent Statement: Informed consent was obtained from all subjects involved in the study.

Data Availability Statement: Not applicable.

Conflicts of Interest: The authors declare no conflict of interest.

References

1. Schneider, D.J.; Moore, J.W. Patent ductus arteriosus. *Circulation* **2006**, *114*, 1873–1882. [CrossRef] [PubMed]
2. Hammerman, C. Patent ductus arteriosus. Clinical relevance of prostaglandins and prostaglandin inhibitors in PDA pathophysiology and treatment. *Clin. Perinatol.* **1995**, *22*, 457–479. [CrossRef] [PubMed]
3. Porstmann, W.; Wierny, L.; Warnke, H. Closure of persistent ductus arteriosus without thoracotomy. *Ger. Med. Mon.* **1967**, *12*, 259–261. [PubMed]

6. Yamaki, S.; Mohri, H.; Haneda, K.; Endo, M.; Akimoto, H. Indications for surgery based on lung biopsy in cases of ventricular septal defect and/or patent ductus arteriosus with severe pulmonary hypertension. *Chest* **1989**, *96*, 31–39. [CrossRef] [PubMed]
7. Kannan, B.R.; Sivasankaran, S.; Tharakan, J.A.; Titus, T.; Kumar, V.K.A.; Francis, B.; Krishnamoorthy, K.M.; Harikrishnan, S.; Padmakumar, R.; Nair, K. Long-term outcome of patients operated for large ventricular septal defects with increased pulmonary vascular resistance. *Indian Heart J.* **2003**, *55*, 161–166. [PubMed]
8. Sinha, S.K.; Razi, M.; Pandey, R.N.; Kumar, P.; Krishna, V.; Jha, M.J.; Mishra, V.; Asif, M.; Abdali, N.; Tewari, P.; et al. Prospective evaluation of the feasibility, safety, and efficacy of Cocoon Duct Occluder for transcatheter closure of large patent ductus arteriosus: A single-center study with short- and medium-term follow-up results. *Anatol. J. Cardiol.* **2017**, *18*, 321–327. [CrossRef] [PubMed]
9. Kanabar, K.; Bootla, D.; Kaur, N.; Pruthvi, C.; Krishnappa, D.; Santosh, K.; Guleria, V.; Rohit, M.K. Outcomes of transcatheter closure of patent ductus arteriosus with the off-label use of large occluders (≥16 mm). *Indian Heart J.* **2020**, *72*, 107–112. [CrossRef] [PubMed]
10. Rohit, M.K.; Gupta, A. Transcatheter closure of large patent ductus arteriosus using custom made devices. *Catheter. Cardiovasc. Interv.* **2017**, *89*, E194–E199. [CrossRef] [PubMed]
11. Lehner, A.; Ulrich, S.; Happel, C.M.; Fischer, M.; Kantzis, M.; Schulze-Neick, I.; Haas, N.A. Closure of very large PDA with pulmonary hypertension: Initial clinical case-series with the new Occlutech® PDA occluder. *Catheter. Cardiovasc. Interv.* **2017**, *89*, 718–725. [CrossRef] [PubMed]
12. Yan, C.; Zhao, S.; Jiang, S.; Xu, Z.; Huang, L.; Zheng, H.; Ling, J.; Wang, C.; Wu, W.; Hu, H.; et al. Transcatheter closure of patent ductus arteriosus with severe pulmonary arterial hypertension in adults. *Heart* **2007**, *93*, 514–518. [CrossRef] [PubMed]
13. Konagai, N.; Fukui, S.; Kitano, M.; Fujimoto, K.; Nishii, T.; Ogo, T.; Yasuda, S. Very Large Patent Ductus Arteriosus With Severe Pulmonary Arterial Hypertension. *Circ. J.* **2019**, *83*, 2325. [CrossRef] [PubMed]
14. Stout, K.K.; Daniels, C.J.; Aboulhosn, J.A.; Bozkurt, B.; Broberg, C.S.; Colman, J.M.; Crumb, S.R.; Dearani, J.A.; Fuller, S.; Gurvitz, M.; et al. 2018 AHA/ACC Guideline for the Management of Adults With Congenital Heart Disease: Executive Summary: A Report of the American College of Cardiology/American Heart Association Task Force on Clinical Practice Guidelines. *J. Am. Coll. Cardiol.* **2019**, *73*, 1494–1563. [CrossRef] [PubMed]
15. Humbert, M.; Kovacs, G.; Hoeper, M.M.; Badagliacca, R.; Berger, R.M.F.; Brida, M.; Carlsen, J.; Coats, A.J.S.; Escribano-Subias, P.; Ferrari, P.; et al. 2022 ESC/ERS Guidelines for the diagnosis and treatment of pulmonary hypertension. *Eur. Heart J.* **2022**, *43*, 3618–3731. [CrossRef] [PubMed]
16. Baumgartner, H.; De Backer, J.; Babu-Narayan, S.V.; Budts, W.; Chessa, M.; Diller, G.-P.; Lung, B.; Kluin, J.; Lang, I.M.; Meijboom, F.; et al. 2020 ESC Guidelines for the management of adult congenital heart disease. *Eur. Heart J.* **2021**, *42*, 563–645. [CrossRef] [PubMed]
17. Galiè, N.; Humbert, M.; Vachiery, J.; Gibbs, S.; Lang, I.; Torbicki, A.; Simmonneau, G.; Peacock, A.; Vonk Noordegraaf, A.; Beghetti, M.; et al. 2015 ESC/ERS Guidelines for the diagnosis and treatment of pulmonary hypertension: The Joint Task Force for the Diagnosis and Treatment of Pulmonary Hypertension of the European Society of Cardiology (ESC) and the European Respiratory Society (ERS): Endorsed by: Association for European Paediatric and Congenital Cardiology (AEPC), International Society for Heart and Lung Transplantation (ISHLT). *Eur. Heart J.* **2016**, *37*, 67–119. [CrossRef] [PubMed]
18. Rafaeli Rabin, R.; Rosin, I.; Matitiau, A.; Simpson, Y.; Flidel-Rimon, O. Assessing Patent Ductus Arteriosus (PDA) Significance on Cardiac Output by Whole-Body Bio-impedance. *Pediatr. Cardiol.* **2020**, *41*, 1386–1390. [CrossRef] [PubMed]
19. Kiran, V.S.; Tiwari, A. Prediction of left ventricular dysfunction after device closure of patent ductus arteriosus: Proposal for a new functional classification. *EuroIntervention* **2018**, *13*, e2124–e2129. [CrossRef] [PubMed]
20. Zhang, D.-Z.; Zhu, X.-Y.; Lv, B.; Cui, C.-S.; Han, X.-M.; Sheng, X.-T.; Wang, Q.-G.; Zhang, P. Trial occlusion to assess the risk of persistent pulmonary arterial hypertension after closure of a large patent ductus arteriosus in adolescents and adults with elevated pulmonary artery pressure. *Circ. Cardiovasc. Interv.* **2014**, *7*, 473–481. [CrossRef] [PubMed]
21. Hester, J.; Ventetuolo, C.; Lahm, T. Sex, Gender, and Sex Hormones in Pulmonary Hypertension and Right Ventricular Failure. *Compr. Physiol.* **2019**, *10*, 125–170. [CrossRef] [PubMed]

Disclaimer/Publisher's Note: The statements, opinions and data contained in all publications are solely those of the individual author(s) and contributor(s) and not of MDPI and/or the editor(s). MDPI and/or the editor(s) disclaim responsibility for any injury to people or property resulting from any ideas, methods, instructions or products referred to in the content.

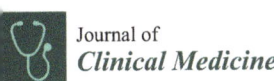

Case Report

CT Detection of an Anomalous Left Circumflex Coronary Artery from Pulmonary Artery (ALXCAPA) in 81-Year-Old Female Patient

Marian Pop [1,2], Zsófia Kakucs [3,*] and Simona Coman [2]

1. ME1 Department, George Emil Palade University of Medicine, Pharmacy, Science and Technology of Targu Mures, 540142 Târgu Mureș, Romania
2. Emergency Institute for Cardiovascular Disease and Transplant of Targu Mures, 540136 Târgu Mureș, Romania
3. Mures County Clinical Emergency Hospital, 540136 Târgu Mureș, Romania
* Correspondence: kakucs_zsofia@yahoo.com

Abstract: Background: The left circumflex coronary artery from the pulmonary artery is a very rare congenital anomaly with few cases described, so far, worldwide. Case report: An 81-year-old female presented complaining of dyspnea. The transthoracic echocardiogram revealed severe degenerative aortic stenosis in addition to a hypertrophied left ventricle with normal function and no wall motion abnormalities. As part of the pre-TAVI planning, she underwent a CT examination, which revealed an anomalous left circumflex artery originating from the right pulmonary artery. The case is currently being managed conservatively. Conclusion: The presented congenital coronary anomaly is, to our knowledge, the first to be described in the literature in this age group (80+).

Keywords: coronary vessels anomalies; anomalous origin of the left circumflex coronary artery from the pulmonary artery; ALXCAPA; coronary CT angiography

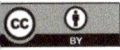

1. Introduction

The classic configuration of coronary tree anatomy consists of the left main coronary artery (LMCA) and the right coronary artery (RCA), arising from the left and right coronary sinuses, respectively, in the aortic root. Typically, the LMCA is a short common stem, which bifurcates into the left anterior descending (LAD) artery and the left circumflex (LCX) artery [1].

The prevalence of coronary artery anomalies (CAAs) shows a wide variation between 0.3% and 2% in the general population [2]. CAAs are typically found incidentally during coronary angiography or autopsy studies. Considering that many hemodynamically insignificant cases remain undiagnosed, the actual prevalence rate is probably higher. Anomalous origins of the coronary arteries from the pulmonary trunk are relatively rare [3]. The left coronary artery from the pulmonary artery (ALCAPA), also known as Bland-White-Garland syndrome, is a well-recognized cardiovascular malformation affecting 1 in 300,000 births and constitutes 0.25–0.5% of total congenital heart defects [4–7].

The anomalous LCX coronary artery from the pulmonary artery (ALXCAPA) can be considered an extremely rare variant of the ALCAPA, with the first adult case documented in 1992 [8] and only 47 cases reported worldwide by 2021 [9]. The presence of an ALXCAPA in adult patients without congenital heart disease is extremely uncommon. Since 1992, only few cases have been described, with stable angina being the most frequent presenting symptom. While the ALCAPA is frequently identified in infancy due to ischemic symptoms related to flow changes consecutive to pulmonary artery pressure decrease [10,11], the ALXCAPA is usually discovered in adults [9,12], appearing concomitantly with other congenital symptomatic or life-threatening cardiac defects. It is often accompanied by aortic coarctation, patent ductus arteriosus, and subaortic or pulmonary valve stenosis [13].

The ALXCAPA identification in the more senior population has asked [14,15] for a reconsideration of its impact on the patient's prognosis.

2. Case Description

We reported a case of an 81-year-old female patient, diagnosed five years before with aortic stenosis and arterial hypertension. She was in good health, with two adult children and minor non-cardiovascular complaints (lumbar disc herniation) at the time.

Three months before a CT examination, she was referred again to the cardiology outpatient clinic due to a worsening of the clinical status with palpitations and fatigability.

At the time of the examination, the patient's clinical condition was stable, with a heart rate of 52 beats per minute and a blood pressure of 180/100 mmHg. A systolic murmur of grade 3/6 was found during the clinical examination, but there was no pulmonary or systemic congestion.

Her ECG showed a sinus rhythm with pressure overload changes, large R-waves, and end-phase diffuse ischemic changes.

The echocardiography showed concentric left ventricular hypertrophy with no cardiac wall motion abnormalities and an ejection fraction of 58%. The right ventricle function was normal, and there were no signs of pulmonary arterial hypertension. The aortic valve was intensely hyperechoic, with a maximum gradient of 100 mmHg and an average of 23 mmHg, and the diagnosis of severe degenerative aortic stenosis was set. The patient was referred to the cardiovascular radiology department for a CT evaluation prior to the trans-catheter aortic valve implantation (TAVI).

In accordance with the local pre-TAVI protocol, the examination included a native coronary calcium score assessment, an ECG-gated thoracic Angio CT examination with multiphasic contrast agent administration, and a non-ECG-gated Angio CT examination of the abdomen and pelvis. Minor breathing artifacts were noted.

Extensive coronary artery calcifications were discovered in systemically supplied coronary arteries, but they were very mild in the circumflex coronary artery, which originated from the pulmonary artery (Supplementary Video S1). The total Agatston score was 4322.72, placing her in the 99th percentile according to age, gender, and ethnicity; however, the LCX calcification represented only 6.56 of those.

A normal left main coronary artery was found to arise from the left coronary sinus, giving rise only to a dilated left anterior descending (LAD) artery (5.9 mm). The dilation of the LAD was evident at the level of the diagonals (4 mm) and septal perforator branches (2 mm) as well.

The enlarged left circumflex coronary artery (LCX; 3.5 mm) arose from the inferior aspect of the right pulmonary artery (Figures 1 and 2 and Supplementary Video S2) and gave two thin branches (retroatrial and lateroatrial). It was enlarged up to 8 mm, with a large obtuse marginal, and ended as a posterolateral branch.

The right coronary artery (RCA) was codominant, originated in the typical location, and ended as the posterior descending artery with a serpiginous course.

While the overall coronary circulation was dilated, no definite RCA–LCA collaterals were observed; however, the presence of atypical LCX branches and the enlarged intramyocardial branches was indicative of an established network of collaterals draining eventually into the RPA.

The left ventricle appeared with a normal volume (75.6 mL, 508.5 mL/m^2), with thickened walls up to 17.8 mL in the septum and 14.6 mm in the lateral wall.

No congenital malformations have been identified.

The main pulmonary artery was in normal size (26 mm), but both branches were enlarged, with the right pulmonary artery displaying a fusiform aneurysmal aspect reaching 29 mm in the region of the LCX ostium. The normal right-to-left ventricle diameter ratio and the normal arterio-bronchial ratio also implied the lack of pulmonary hypertension.

A general thoraco-abdominal assessment showed minor TB sequelae, diffuse atheromatous plaques, and diffuse bone demineralization, but no further lesions.

The TAVI procedure has been reconsidered, with the patient currently undergoing medical treatment, with mild improvement of the symptoms at the last clinical re-evaluation.

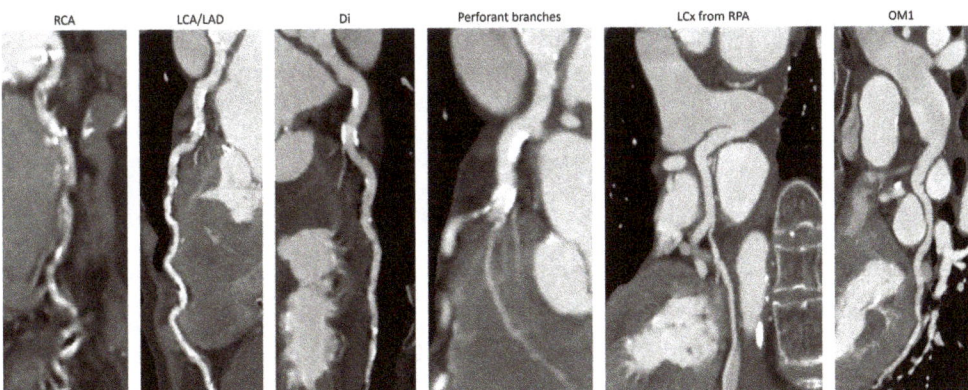

Figure 1. Curved reformat of the coronary arteries from their ostia. There were extensive calcification on the branches, starting from the systemic circulation (RCA, LCA/LAD, and diagonals), and only trivial calcification spots in the left circumflex coronary artery and in the obtuse marginal branch. The coronary arteries are enlarged, with perforant branches from the LAD reaching 2 mm in diameter. RCA—right coronary artery; LCA—left coronary artery; LAD—left anterior descending coronary artery; Di—diagonal branch; LCx—left circumflex coronary artery; OM1—first obtuse marginal.

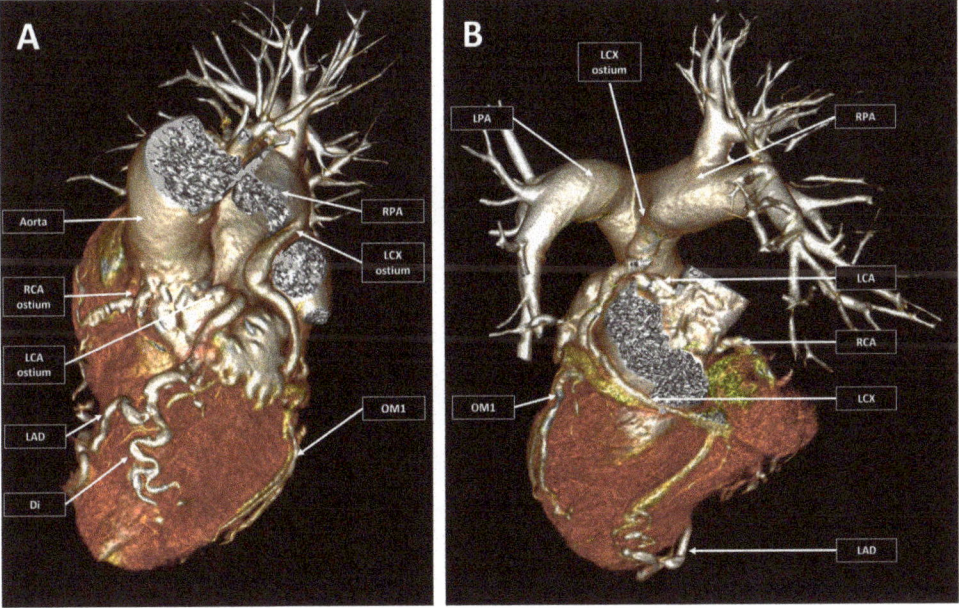

Figure 2. 3D virtual rendering technique reconstruction of the heart, main vessels, and coronary arteries. Pannel (**A**) (left) Left/cranial double oblique anterior reconstruction with the main pulmonary artery and the left pulmonary artery removed from the image. Pannel (**B**) (right) Right/cranial double oblique posterior reconstruction with the removal of the atria, ascending aorta, aortic arch, and descending aorta. The coronary arteries are enlarged and had a tortuous course. There were both left and right coronary arteries emerging from the corresponding coronary sinuses, and a circumflex coronary artery emerged from the right pulmonary artery. RCA—right coronary artery; LCA—left coronary artery; LAD—left anterior descending coronary artery; Di—diagonal branch; LCx—left circumflex coronary artery; OM1—first obtuse marginal; LPA—left pulmonary artery; RPA—right pulmonary artery.

3. Discussion

We reported the case of an 81-year-old female patient who was diagnosed with ALX CAPA following an Angio CT examination.

This type of anomaly may cause hemodynamic impairment. In case of the ALXCAPA the posterolateral wall of the left ventricle (LV) is perfused by the abnormally arising coronary artery providing relatively low perfusion pressure and deoxygenated blood. In case of well-developed collateral circulation and decreased pulmonary vascular resistance steal of blood flow will occur, a retrograde filling of the LCX from LAD artery and the RCA circulation (left-to-right shunt). Additionally, due to volume overload via left-to-right shunt pulmonary hypertension may occur. Pulmonary hypertension can minimize the shunt from the LCX to pulmonary arteries and maintain the myocardial perfusion at a sufficient level. The hypoperfusion of myocardium will be prevented by a well-collateralized and pressured system, enabling survival to adulthood. However, the left-to-right shunt will induce a chronic increase in the LV preload, which will cause progressive dilatation of the LV and deterioration of the LV function [16].

Clinical presentation and survival depend upon the degree of collateralization from the two other coronary arteries. Adult patients may initially present with new-onset stable angina, palpitation, dyspnea, abnormal ischemic changes on electrocardiogram, or wall motion abnormalities observed on echocardiography [13]. Sudden cardiac death can occur after myocardial ischemia during physical activity, stress, or ventricular arrhythmias triggered by a previously developed scar tissue [17]. The symptoms of the ALXCAPA may present in different periods of life; however, some patients remain asymptomatic with the anomaly being identified incidentally during diagnostic procedures [18]. We hypothesize that our patient remained asymptomatic throughout her life and reached the age of 81 due to the development of adequate coronary collateralization and the relatively small area of myocardium supplied by the LCX artery.

Invasive coronary angiography (ICA), which is widely available and considered the gold standard diagnostic method, provides visualization of collateral vessels and enables assessing the amount of retrograde flow from collateral vessels [14]. Moreover, in case of CAAs, ICA should be performed to exclude additional stenosis. The coronary computed tomography angiography (CCTA) has been shown to be a promising substitute for cardiac catheterization as a non-invasive imaging method of identifying abnormal coronary origin and course [19]. In some cases, the precise origin of aberrant coronary vessels could not be identified by ICA. In such cases, CCTA and cardiac magnetic resonance imaging are recommended, which allow unambiguous identification of coronary origins [13].

CT allows for the quantification of calcified plaques, which we found to be extensive for systemic-supplied coronaries and only trivial in the branch connected to pulmonary circulation. In previously reported ALXCAPA cases [12], we found no mention of such extensive calcification and we believe that their asymmetrical distribution may be attributable to the variations in the local pulse pressure; however, since survival in untreated ALCAPA patients is uncommon beyond the age of 50, there are little data on the amount of calcified plaques in very elderly patients with coronary anomalies.

In diagnosing the ischemic effects of anomalous coronary arteries, stress testing (echocardiogram, magnetic resonance imaging, or CT stress perfusion) has proven useful [20], demonstrating perfusion deficit in the territory affected. Our CT examination, conducted with the patient at rest, did not reveal any structural changes in the myocardium that might indicate perfusion deficit or long-term ischemic damage.

There are no consensus defining the standard management and operative techniques for patients with the ALXCAPA [15]. Although the latest guidelines recommend surgical treatment for asymptomatic ALCAPA, there is no specific guidance on variants such as the ALXCAPA. The clinical course of the ALXCAPA may not always be favorable, and some patients need surgical treatment in early infancy. In the ALCAPA, the surgical correction is mandatory, when symptoms are attributed to ischemia [14]. Surgical treatment options include reimplantation of the anomalous vessel into the aorta [17,21], ligation, or ligation with aorto-coronary bypass. Even if in many previous cases the surgical technique of choice was ligation followed by bypass [5], the current surgical techniques focus, whenever possible, on the anatomical reimplantation, regardless of the patient age [12], with overall good results [22]. Although cardiovascular surgery has been mostly used, the conservative approach may be an option in some circumstances. Although cardiovascular surgery has been mostly used, the conservative approach may be an option in some circumstances [15].

There is limited experience on the management of concurrent ALCAPA and aortic valve disfunction [23], with surgical correction in such an age group being uncertain to provide a survival benefit. Transcatheter replacement of the aortic valve might improve aortic stenosis symptoms; however, in a patient that has been balancing such conditions for a long time, a change in the hemodynamic status can provide unpredictable results.

4. Conclusions

We described a rare case of the isolated left circumflex coronary artery from the right pulmonary artery. This is the first case report of a patient with ALXCAPA in the age group of 80+, and it shows extensive calcification in systemic-supplied coronary arteries and trivial calcification spots in pulmonary-connected coronary arteries.

Supplementary Materials: The following supporting information can be downloaded at: https://www.mdpi.com/article/10.3390/jcm12010226/s1, Video S1: Calcium score examination; Video S2: 3D virtual rendering technique reconstruction of the heart, main vessels, and coronary arteries.

Author Contributions: Conceptualization, M.P.; methodology, M.P.; software, M.P.; validation, M.P.; formal analysis, M.P.; investigation, M.P. and Z.K.; resources, M.P.; data curation, M.P.; writing—original draft preparation, M.P. and Z.K.; writing—review and editing, M.P. and Z.K.; visualization, M.P. and Z.K.; supervision, S.C.; project administration, M.P.; funding acquisition, M.P. All authors have read and agreed to the published version of the manuscript.

Funding: This research received no external funding.

Institutional Review Board Statement: The study was conducted in accordance with the Declaration of Helsinki and approved by the Ethics Committee of The Targu Mures Emergency Institute for Cardiovascular Diseases and Heart Transplant (8596/2022).

Informed Consent Statement: Written informed consent has been obtained from the patient to publish this paper.

Data Availability Statement: Not applicable.

Conflicts of Interest: The authors declare no conflict of interest.

References

1. Angelini, P. Curicculum in Cardlology Normal and Anomalous Coronary Arterys: Definitions and Classification.
2. Namgung, J.; Kim, J.A. The Prevalence of Coronary Anomalies in a Single Center of Korea: Origination, Course, and Termination Anomalies of Aberrant Coronary Arteries Detected by ECG-Gated Cardiac MDCT. *BMC Cardiovasc. Disord.* **2014**, *14*, 48. [CrossRef]
3. Gentile, F.; Castiglione, V.; de Caterina, R. Coronary Artery Anomalies. *Circulation* **2021**, *144*, 983–996. [CrossRef]
4. Sadoma, D.; Valente, C.; Sigal, A. Anomalous Left Coronary Artery From The Pulmonary Artery (ALCAPA) as a Cause of Heart Failure. *Am. J. Case Rep.* **2019**, *20*, 1797. [CrossRef]
5. Liu, B.; Fursevich, D.; O'dell, M.C.; Flores, M.; Feranec, N. Anomalous Left Circumflex Coronary Artery Arising from the Right Pulmonary Artery: A Rare Cause of Aborted Sudden Cardiac Death. *Cureus* **2016**, *8*, e499. [CrossRef]
6. Hauser, M. Congenital Anomalies of the Coronary Arteries. *Heart* **2005**, *91*, 1240. [CrossRef]
7. Angelini, P. Coronary artery anomalies: An entity in search of an identity. *Circulation* **2007**, *115*, 1296–1305. [CrossRef]
8. Garcia, C.M.; Chandler, J.; Russell, R. Anomalous Left Circumflex Coronary Artery from the Right Pulmonary Artery: First Adult Case Report. *Am. Heart J.* **1992**, *123*, 526–528. [CrossRef]
9. Ziermann, F.K. Fehlkonnektierte Koronararterien Zur Pulmonalarterie—Primäre Befunde Und Anatomische Besonderheiten. Ph.D. Thesis, Technische Universität München, München, Germany, 2021.
10. Walsh, M.A.; Duff, D.; Oslizlok, P.; Redmond, M.; Walsh, K.P.; Wood, A.E.; Coleman, D.M. A Review of 15-Year Experience with Anomalous Origin of the Left Coronary Artery. *Ir. J. Med. Sci.* **2008**, *177*, 127–130. [CrossRef]
11. Peña, E.; Nguyen, E.T.; Merchant, N.; Dennie, C. ALCAPA Syndrome: Not Just a Pediatric Disease. *Radiographics* **2009**, *29*, 553–565. [CrossRef]

12. Guenther, T.M.; Sherazee, E.A.; Gustafson, J.D.; Wozniak, C.J.; Brothers, J.; Raff, G. Anomalous Origin of the Circumflex or Left Anterior Descending Artery From the Pulmonary Artery. *World J. Pediatr. Congenit. Heart Surg.* **2020**, *11*, 765–775. [CrossRef]
13. Korosoglou, G.; Ringwald, G.; Giannitsis, E.; Katus, H.A. Anomalous Origin of the Left Circumflex Coronary Artery from the Pulmonary Artery. A Very Rare Congenital Anomaly in an Adult Patient Diagnosed by Cardiovascular Magnetic Resonance. *J. Cardiovasc. Magn. Reson.* **2008**, *10*, 4. [CrossRef]
14. Cabrera-Huerta, S.P.; Martín-Lores, I.; Cabeza, B.; Gómez de Diego, J.J.; Pérez de Isla, L.; Vilacosta, I.; Pozo-Osinalde, E. Circumflex Artery Arising From the Pulmonary Artery: Always a Malignant Coronary Anomaly? *JACC Case Rep.* **2020**, *2*, 1702–1707. [CrossRef]
15. Separham, A.; Aliakbarzadeh, P. Anomalous Left Coronary Artery from the Pulmonary Artery Presenting with Aborted Sudden Death in an Octogenarian: A Case Report. *J. Med. Case Rep.* **2012**, *6*, 12. [CrossRef]
16. Cambronero-Cortinas, E.; Moratalla-Haro, P.; González-García, A.E.; Oliver-Ruiz, J.M. Case Report of Asymptomatic Very Late Presentation of ALCAPA Syndrome: Review of the Literature since Pathophysiology until Treatment. *Eur. Heart J. Case Rep.* **2020**, *4*, 1. [CrossRef]
17. Vergara-Uzcategui, C.E.; Urquiza, R.V.; Salinas, P.; Nunez-Gil, I.J. Anomalous Origin of Left Circumflex Artery from the Right Pulmonary Artery of an Adult. *REC Interv. Cardiol.* **2021**, *3*, 65–72. [CrossRef]
18. Al-Muhaya, M.A.; Syed, A.; Najjar, A.H.A.; Mofeed, M.; Al-Mutairi, M. Anomalous Origin of Circumflex Coronary Artery from Right Pulmonary Artery Associated with Atrial Septal Defect. *J. Saudi Heart Assoc.* **2017**, *29*, 219–222. [CrossRef]
19. Kakucs, Z.; Heidenhoffer, E.; Pop, M. Detection of Coronary Artery and Aortic Arch Anomalies in Patients with Tetralogy of Fallot Using CT Angiography. *J. Clin. Med.* **2022**, *11*, 5500. [CrossRef]
20. Laflamme, E.; Alonso-Gonzalez, R.; Roche, S.L.; Wald, R.M.; Swan, L.; Silversides, C.K.; Thorne, S.A.; Horlick, E.M.; Benson, L.N.; Osten, M.; et al. Anomalous Origin of a Coronary Artery from the Pulmonary Artery Presenting in Adulthood: Experience from a Tertiary Center. *Int. J. Cardiol. Congenit. Heart Dis.* **2021**, *4*, 100169. [CrossRef]
21. Bolognesi, R.; Alfieri, O.; Tsialtas, D.; Manca, C. Surgical Treatment of the Left Circumflex Coronary Artery from the Pulmonary Artery in an Adult Patient. *Ann. Thorac. Surg.* **2003**, *75*, 1642–1643. [CrossRef]
22. Fudulu, D.P.; Dorobantu, D.M.; Taghavi, M.; Sharabiani, A.; Angelini, G.D.; Caputo, M.; Parry, A.J.; Stoica, S.C. Outcomes Following Repair of Anomalous Coronary Artery from the Pulmonary Artery in Infants: Results from a Procedure-Based National Database. *Open Heart* **2015**, *2*, 277. [CrossRef]
23. Yong, L. Asymptomatic Adult Type ALCAPA Syndrome Coexisting with Bicuspid Aortic Valve- A Case Report. *J. Cardiol. Cardiovasc. Res.* **2021**, *2*. [CrossRef] [PubMed]

Disclaimer/Publisher's Note: The statements, opinions and data contained in all publications are solely those of the individual author(s) and contributor(s) and not of MDPI and/or the editor(s). MDPI and/or the editor(s) disclaim responsibility for any injury to people or property resulting from any ideas, methods, instructions or products referred to in the content.

Becoming a Teenager after Early Surgical Ventricular Septal Defect (VSD) Repair: Longitudinal Biopsychological Data on Mental Health and Maternal Involvement

Laura Lang [1,†], Jennifer Gerlach [1,†], Anne-Christine Plank [1], Ariawan Purbojo [2], Robert A. Cesnjevar [2,3], Oliver Kratz [1], Gunther H. Moll [1] and Anna Eichler [1,*]

[1] Department of Child and Adolescent Mental Health, University Hospital Erlangen, Friedrich-Alexander-Universität Erlangen-Nürnberg (FAU), 91054 Erlangen, Germany
[2] Department of Pediatric Cardiac Surgery, University Hospital Erlangen, Friedrich-Alexander-Universität Erlangen-Nürnberg (FAU), 91054 Erlangen, Germany
[3] Department of Pediatric Cardiovascular Surgery, Pediatric Heart Center, University Children's Hospital Zürich, 8032 Zürich, Switzerland
* Correspondence: anna.eichler@uk-erlangen.de
† These authors contributed equally to this work.

Abstract: Beside somatic strains of congenital heart diseases (CHD), affected children often show developmental impairments in the long term. Ventricular septal defect (VSD) is the most common congenital heart defect and early surgical repair is associated with positive somatic outcomes. However, psychological adjustment is of lifelong relevance. We investigated 24 children with a surgically-corrected isolated VSD and their mothers from primary school (6–9 years) to adolescence (10–14 years) and compared them to controls. Both times, mothers reported child internalizing/externalizing problems, mothers and children rated child quality of life, and children performed neurodevelopmental tests. Adolescents also rated internalizing/externalizing problems themselves, and their hair cortisol levels were analyzed. Maternal anxiety and proactive parenting behavior were considered as moderators. Results revealed no group differences in child neurodevelopment (language, cognition), externalizing problems, and cortisol levels at any time. In reports from mothers, internalizing problems (depression, anxiety) were elevated in children with a VSD at both times—when mothers reported anxiety symptoms themselves. In adolescent reports, VSD patients' quality of life was increased and internalizing problems were decreased—proactive parenting behavior went along with decreased symptoms in VSD-affected adolescents and with increased symptoms in controls. The findings pronounce the crucial role of parenting behavior and the influence of maternal anxieties on child mental health after surgical VSD repair and might highlight the need for parent-centered interventions.

Keywords: congenital heart disease; ventricular septal defect; child development; psychological adjustment; quality of life; stress; adolescence; longitudinal study; mental health; cortisol

1. Introduction

Congenital heart disease (CHD) is the most frequent birth malformation, with isolated ventricular septal defect (VSD) representing the largest sub-category in children (approximately 37%) [1–4]. Most isolated VSDs close spontaneously during the first 12 months of life. As a result of modern cardiological and cardiac surgical management, children who require surgery have an excellent long-term outcome regarding their physical abilities [1,5–7]. Therefore, the recent research focus has shifted towards examining psychological adjustments in children with CHD. Most of these studies find affected children to be developmentally impaired. especially those with more severe CHD conditions [8,9]. In particular, studies concentrating on neurodevelopmental outcomes showed reduced cognitive development in children with CHD compared to non-affected controls [10–13] and found that these deficits remain into young adulthood [14,15]. It is also widely understood that children and adolescents with CHD are at an increased risk of internalizing and externalizing problems [12,16,17]. In clinical classification systems such as the DSM-IV internalizing problems are described as emotional problems that can include disorders such as anxiety and depression, while externalizing or behavior problems comprise disorders such as ADHD or antisocial behavior [18]. In addition, children with CHD are reported to have a higher lifetime prevalence of psychiatric disorders, such as attention deficit/hyperactivity disorder (ADHD) or anxiety disorders [19–21]. Still, a recent review found most of these dysfunctions to be high in prevalence but mild [8], which accounts specifically for less severe conditions, as with VSD [22]. Moreover, most of them seem to be more relevant in younger children [23] and might decrease over the individual's lifetime [24]. The limitations in neurodevelopmental, internalizing, and externalizing function could lead to reduced health-related quality of life (HRQOL) in children with CHD [25,26]. Nevertheless, results on the perceived HRQOL of children with CHD are still inconsistent. Some studies reported satisfactory overall HRQOL with no differences or even better scores compared to non-affected controls [19,27–29], whereas other studies found these children to be at a greater risk of impaired HRQOL [30–32]. These differences could be attributed to variability in method designs, such as the age of the children at the time of assessment [33] or the severity of CHD [32]. One long-term study exclusively including children with surgically corrected VSDs found increased HRQOL three months after cardiac surgery and even higher scores after at the one-year follow-up [34]. To fully understand psychological development in children with CHD, it seems important to investigate these adjustments on a physiological level, in additional to self-reporting and proxy reports. Some studies found that early stressful life events such as cardiac surgery could lead to alterations to the hypothalamic–pituitary–adrenal (HPA) axis, the key system of stress response, and thus to different patterns of cortisol release [35–37]. This dysregulation of the HPA axis could be one mechanism underlying impaired neurodevelopmental and psychopathological outcomes in children [35–37]. However, after using a homogeneous sample of children who underwent surgery for a VSD, no differences were found regarding the stress system when compared to non-affected controls.

A CHD does not only affect the child. Besides the impacts of CHD on children's physical development and later psychological adjustment, the diagnosis, medical treatments, and surgery have a major influence on parents as well [38,39]. Many parents experience tremendous emotional distress (e.g., shock, sadness, guilt); mothers, who are often the primary caregiver, describe immense suffering and anxiety, as well as the burden of caring for a child with CHD [40–42]. In addition, mothers of children with CHD have been shown to be less involved in interactions with their child [43], and the parent–child relationship seems to encounter difficulties [44]. Moreover, maternal characteristics such as a lower educational level, anxiety symptoms, or parenting stress were found to be risk factors for increased internalizing and externalizing problems [45–47], early delays in cognitive development (e.g., communication difficulties) [10], and lower quality of life (QoL) [28] in children with CHD. Thus, family-related variables (e.g., maternal mental health and parenting style) seem to have an even greater impact on predicting behavioral and cognitive outcomes in children with CHD than disease or surgical factors themselves [48]. In reverse, positive parenting behavior could be a potential protective factor and improve emotional and behavior problems in children with CHD [49]. To summarize, the characteristics of the mother (e.g., parenting behavior, maternal psychopathology) seem to be highly relevant moderators of child development and psychological adjustment and should be considered in studies targeting the longitudinal development of children with CHD.

2. Aims of This Study

Even though there is growing interest in the psychological development of children with CHD [9,12,22], there is still a lack of relevant literature focusing exclusively on children with surgically corrected isolated VSDs. Previously, we compared psychological long-term outcomes between primary school-aged children (t1) who underwent surgery for a VSD in infancy and typically developing children, including assessment of maternal anxiety and proactive parenting behavior as potential moderators [50,51]. The aim of this follow-up study was to reinvestigate these children in adolescence (t2) to reveal potential changes in their psychological adjustments. Specifically, this follow-up study explored the long-term consequences of early surgical VSD correction on children's neurodevelopment (cognitive development and language), internalizing and externalizing problems (depression, anxiety, attention deficit/hyperactivity disorder (ADHD), and antisocial behavior), HRQOL, and cortisol levels and additionally sought to reveal the role of maternal characteristics (proactive parenting behavior and maternal anxiety) in child development from primary school to adolescence. The development of children who underwent surgery for a VSD was compared to non-affected matched controls.

Neurodevelopment. For primary school-aged children, our study team found no differences in cognitive development (IQ scores) between the groups but did observe weaker language skills in children with VSDs [50]. Since intelligence is a psychological construct that is considered to be stable over time [52], it was hypothesized that adolescents with VSDs do not significantly differ in their cognitive development from typically developing adolescents. In line with the findings of Eichler et al. [50], this study assumed significantly poorer language outcomes in adolescents with VSDs than the comparison group at adolescence.

Emotional and behavioral problems. Regarding the development of psychopathological symptoms, the current literature is still inconsistent regarding whether these symptoms increase or decline over time in children with CHD. At primary school age, Eichler et al. [50] found no differences in internalizing and externalizing behavior problems between the VSD group and the non-affected control group. As adolescence is a critical stage in life when many mental health symptoms appear for the first time [53–55], some studies reported adolescents with CHD to have more internalizing and externalizing symptoms and to be at higher risk of a lifetime prevalence of psychiatric disorders compared to non-affected controls [19,21,56]. Moreover, Karsdorp, et al. [57] found that only adolescents with CHD displayed an increased risk of adverse psychological adjustment, which could not be demonstrated in younger children. In contrast, other studies showed that younger children had more internalizing and externalizing problems [23] and that these symptoms might decrease over time [24]. The studies reported above used inhomogeneous samples of children with CHD, including a variety of different disease severities, which could account for the differences in the results. Therefore, this study aimed to investigate whether internalizing and externalizing problems occur in adolescence by using a homogeneous sample of children with an early surgically corrected isolated VSD compared to non-affected controls [51].

HRQOL. Many studies have targeted the HRQOL of children with CHD, but findings are still heterogeneous. Some authors reported higher HRQOL in adolescence for those with CHD [19,28], while others found their HRQOL to be impaired compared to typically developing adolescents [30,31]. In our study of primary school-aged children [50], we found a trend in mothers of children with a VSD: mothers reported higher HRQOL in their children than the control group (child self-rating did not differ between groups). Since ratings on HRQOL seem to depend on the severity of CHD [32], this study hypothesized, in line with our previous findings [50], that mothers report higher child HRQOL scores compared to non-affected controls in adolescence.

Physiological stress regulation. In addition to self-reporting and proxy reports of child psychological adjustment, we were also interested in physiological stress regulation in children with surgically corrected VSDs compared to typically developing children. Therefore, children's cortisol levels were assessed. Studies on the association of children with (surgically corrected) CHD and cortisol levels are rare and inconsistent. One study found differences from normal reference values regarding the diurnal variability of salivary cortisol levels in children with CHD [58], while Stonawski et al. [51]—based on our own data—found no differences in diurnal cortisol release between the VSD and control group at primary school age. In adolescence, instead of salivary cortisol, which rather measures acute cortisol production and is sensitive to diurnal rhythm [59], hair cortisol values were used to enable the investigation of cumulative distress over a one-month time period [60]. Since existing studies were heterogeneous in terms of methods and designs and revealed mixed results, this study aimed to investigate whether children with early surgically corrected isolated VSDs differed in their hair cortisol levels from non-affected children.

Maternal characteristics as moderators of development. As mentioned above, maternal characteristics such as parenting behavior and maternal anxiety symptoms can be considered as important moderators of child development, especially in children with surgically corrected VSDs. In the previous study of primary school-aged children, Eichler et al. [50] found mothers' proactive parenting behavior to be a protective factor that levelled impairments in language development in the VSD group, whereas high maternal anxiety was identified as a risk factor for the development of anxiety symptoms in children with surgically corrected VSDs. Therefore, the final goal of this study was to explore the potential moderating role of maternal parenting behavior and anxiety in children's psychological adjustment in adolescence.

3. Methods

3.1. Study Design and Participants

Between March 2006 and March 2012, 86 children with an isolated VSD underwent surgery in the Department of Cardiac Surgery at the Erlangen University Hospital, Germany. A total of 26 children were excluded because of genetic syndromes, additional congenital malformations, complex heart defects, or non-cardiological death. Finally, 60 children fulfilled the inclusion criteria. Six families were not available, and fifteen families chose not to participate. Finally, $n = 39$ took part and were invited to a first investigation in 2015 at the Department of Child and Adolescent Mental Health at the Erlangen University Hospital, Germany, to assess their psychological adjustment when they were primary school-aged (t1) (see Eichler et al. [50] for further information). When children were in adolescence, families were reinvited between July 2019 and June 2021 to participate in a follow-up assessment (t2). In total, 15 of the original 39 children (38.5% drop out) did not attend the follow-up assessment, either because they were not interested ($n = 7$) or they were not available ($n = 8$). Children who attended the study at t2 did not differ in sex ($\chi^2 = 0.60, p = 0.440$), age ($t = -0.90, df = 37, p = 0.372$), or socioeconomic status ($t = 0.25, df = 37, p = 0.801$) from the 15 non-attending children. A total of 24 children and their mothers participated in the study at both time points, of which 16 came directly to the Department of Child and Adolescent Mental Health, 4 were visited at home, and 4 participated via mail (non-contact attendance due to the coronavirus pandemic). The VSD group was matched with a non-affected control group ($n = 24$) for sex, age, and socioeconomic status (VSD: $M = 11.08, SD = 2.55$; Controls: $M = 11.63, SD = 2.50$; for details see Section 3.2.1). The control group was recruited from the Franconian Cognition and Emotion Studies sample [61]. An overview of the study's design, data assessments, and measurements relevant for this publication can be seen in Figure 1.

Most mothers and fathers had a national origin (87.5–91.7%), with no differences between the VSD group and the controls. Parental education levels were comparable in both groups (VSD group—none/low: mothers 33.4%, fathers 25%; middle: mothers 29.2%, fathers 33.3%; high: mothers 33.3%, fathers 29.2%; 4.1% to 12.5% did not provide any information. Control group— none/low: mothers 25%, fathers 37.5%; middle: mothers 29.2%, fathers 12.5%; high: mothers 45.8%, fathers 50%). Family monthly net income did not differ between the VSD group and the control group (VSD: $M = 4.05, SD = 1.15$; Controls: $M = 4.17, SD = 1.17$).

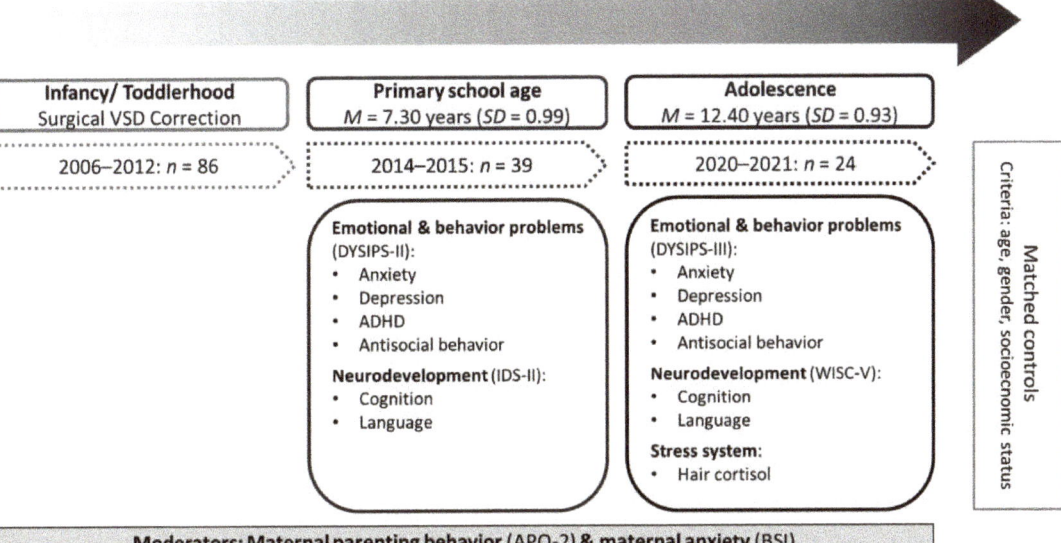

Figure 1. Visual concept model of the study design and variables of interest. *M* = Mean, *SD* = Standard Deviation, *n* = sample size; VSD = ventricular septal defect; DYSIPS = Diagnostic System for Psychiatric Disorders according to ICD-10/DSM-IV [18]; IDS = Intelligence and Development Scales [62]; WISC = Wechsler Intelligence Scale for Children [63]; APQ = Alabama Parenting Questionnaire [64,65]; BSI = Brief Symptom Inventory [66].

Sample characteristics are shown in Table 1. Age in the VSD group ranged from 10 years 9 months to 14 years 7 months (M = 12 years 4 months, SD = 0.93), and age in the comparison group ranged between 12 years 9 months and 13 years 8 months (M = 13 years 2 moths, SD = 0.24). Affected and unaffected children did not differ significantly in sex (VSD: 13 females, 11 males; Controls: 14 females, 10 males; χ^2 = 0.09, p = 0.771) or socioeconomic status (t = −0.74, df = 46, p = 0.461) but differed significantly in age (t = 4.04, df = 46, p = 0.001). Children with VSDs and non-affected controls were tested for differences in corporal diseases (auditory, ocular, cutaneous, respiratory, gastrointestinal, cardiovascular, thyroid, endocrine, kidney), mental health (ADHD, anxiety), and medications (antibiotics, corticosteroids, methylphenidate, ketoconazole). No significant differences between the two groups could be demonstrated (p = 0.074–1.000). Descriptive sample characteristics are summarized in Table 1.

At both times of measurement, mothers answered standardized questionnaires about their child's psychopathology and HRQOL, as well as questions about parenting style and maternal anxiety. Children performed a neurodevelopmental test battery and answered a self-report questionnaire on HRQOL. At t2 (adolescence), children were asked about their own psychopathology using standardized questionnaires and child hair samples were taken. The study protocol was approved by the local ethics committee of the University of Erlangen–Nürnberg and conducted in accordance with the Declaration of Helsinki. Mothers gave written informed consent and assent of the children was obtained.

Table 1. Descriptive Data.

	VSD (n = 24)		Controls (n = 24)		Statistics	
	M/n	SD/%	M/n	SD/%	t/χ^2	d/φ
Mother-related						
Anxiety$_{t1}$	44.48	8.68	46.38	7.87	−0.79	−0.23
Anxiety$_{t2}$	39.88	4.52	46.75	9.49	3.20	0.93 **
Parenting$_{t1}$	3.41	0.62	3.59	0.49	1.05	0.31
Parenting$_{t2}$	3.47	0.67	3.23	0.51	−1.34	0.41
Child-related						
Child's age (y)	12.40	0.93	13.19	0.24	4.04	1.17 **
Sex					0.09	−0.04
Male	11	45.80	10	41.70		
Female	13	54.20	14	58.30		
Physical development						
BMI	20.58	7.29	20.05	3.14	−0.32	−0.09
School level					2.65	0.24
low	9	37.50	4	16.70		
middle	7	29.20	9	37.50		
high	8	33.30	11	45.80		

Note. ** $p < 0.01$. Continuous variables are reported as M (SD) and group differences were tested using a t-test with Cohen's d as the effect size measure; categorical variables are reported with n (%) and group differences were tested using the χ^2 test with the phi-coefficient φ as the effect size measure. Single missing data are demonstrated by reduced degrees of freedom (df): Anxiety df = 45–46, Parenting df = 42–44, Child's age df = 46, Sex df = 1, BMI df = 45, School level df = 2. Anxiety = maternal anxiety: German version of the Brief Symptom Inventory [66]; Parenting = proactive parenting behavior: German version of the Alabama Parenting Questionnaire [64,65]. BMI = body mass index; VSD = ventricular septal defect.

3.2. Measurements

3.2.1. Socioeconomic Status

For assessing families' socioeconomic status, a sum index was created based on maternal and paternal education level (four categories: <9 [1], 9 [2], 10–12 [3], or 13 [4] years of education), maternal and paternal origin (two categories: international [0] or national [1]), and monthly family income (six categories: less than EUR 1000 [1], EUR 1000–2000 [2], EUR 2000–3000 [3], EUR 3000–4000 [4], EUR 4000–5000 [5], more than EUR 5000 [6]) with a theoretical range from 6 to 16 [50].

3.2.2. Neurodevelopment

At t1, the Intelligence and Development Scales (IDS) were applied for measuring children's neurodevelopment [67] (for more details, see Eichler et al. [50]). At t2, adolescents neurodevelopment was assessed using the Wechsler Intelligence Scale for Children—Fifth Edition (WISC-V) [63]. Both procedures represent standardized developmental test batteries for measuring cognitive development and yield IQ ($M = 100$, $SD = 15$) and language competencies (IDS: language score [$M = 10$, $SD = 3$], WISC-V: 'verbal comprehension' subtest [$M = 10$, $SD = 3$]). Z-standardization was used in order to transfer the language scales of the IDS and WISC-V into a common unit for further analyses.

3.2.3. Child Internalizing and Externalizing Outcomes

To measure children's internalizing and externalizing problems, the Diagnostic System for Psychiatric Disorders (DYSIPS-II) according to ICD-10/DSM-IV for children and adolescents was conducted [18]. With this inventory, different symptoms of psychiatric disorders in childhood and adolescence can be assessed in separate questionnaires. On a four-point Likert scale, with values of "not at all" (0), "a little bit" (1), "to a great extent" (2) and "particularly" (3), both children via self-rating at t2 and mothers via external rating at t1 and t2 assessed statements about the child's internalizing and externalizing problems during the last six months. In this study, the symptoms of four psychiatric disorders were investigated: anxiety (44 items, e.g., "shows single intense anxiety states that develop within a few minutes"/"I am suddenly overcome by very strong fear, that develops within a few minutes"), depression (29 items, e.g., "seems sad most of the time; often appears close to tears"/"I am sad most of the time and often close to tears"), ADHD (20 items, e.g., "describes a frequently occurring strong feeling of inner restlessness"/"I often run around or climb permanently when it is inappropriate"), and antisocial behavior (38 items, e.g., "I am often angry or offended/"Is often angry or offended"). In all four questionnaires, the mean raw sum was calculated for a total score with a theoretical range of 0.00 ("not at all") to 3.00 ("particularly").

3.2.4. Health-Related Quality of Life

At t1, the mother and child versions of the Revised Quality of Life Questionnaire were used to assess the child's HRQOL [68] (for more details, see Eichler et al. [50]). Both mothers and children rated the child's HRQOL at t2 using the German version of the Kidscreen-10 questionnaire, which provides a global score [69]. It comprises ten statements about physical, psychological, and social aspects of HRQOL in relation to the previous week (e.g., "Have you been full of energy?/Was your child full of energy?"), which are scored on a 5-point scale: "not at all/never" (1), "a little bit/rarely" (2), "moderate/sometimes" (3), "quite a bit/often" (4), and "very much/always" (5). The mean raw sum scores of both inventories were transformed into percentage scales ranging from 0 to 100%.

3.2.5. Maternal Anxiety

At both measurement time points, the German version of the Brief Symptom Inventory was used to assess maternal anxiety [66]. The inventory contains 53 items that measure psychological distress and from which nine subscales and a global score (Global Severity Index [GSI]) can be formed. In this study, the 6-item "anxiety" subscale was used as a potential moderator to assess maternal anxiety (t-scores, $M = 50$, $SD\ 10$). The statements of the scale refer to physical and psychological symptoms over the last seven days (e.g., "fearfulness") and were rated by the mothers on a 5-point Likert scale: "not at all" (0), "a little bit" (1), "quite a bit" (2), "highly" (3), and "very much" (4).

3.2.6. Maternal Proactive Parenting Behavior

To assess parenting behavior at t1 and t2, the German version of the Alabama Parenting Questionnaire was used as a self-rating inventory for mothers [65,70]. The questionnaire consists of 72 items that form seven subscales. In line with the findings of Eichler et al. [50], this study focused on the subscale "proactive parenting", which comprises 6 items (e.g., "You explain to your child how to behave well in a certain situation") and which was rated on a 5-point Likert scale. The mean raw sum score was calculated, with a theoretical range of 1.00 ("almost never") to 5.00 ("almost ever").

3.2.7. Hair Cortisol

At t2, to measure children's hair cortisol concentration (HCC), an at least 1 cm wide strand of hair was cut off near the hairline of the posterior vertex (as close as possible to the scalp) and stored in paper envelopes at 4 °C until analysis. Mothers answered questions about the chemical treatment of their children's hair, medication intake, infection symptoms, and endocrine diseases over the last six months. In the control group, three children were excluded because of corticosteroid medication and one child was excluded because of chemical hair treatment, resulting in a final sample of 20 controls. From the 24 children with VSDs, 1 child was excluded because their hair sample was missing. There were no relevant medication intake or hair treatment abnormalities in this group. One child had an endocrinological disease but was excluded anyway because no hair cortisol could be extracted (information is listed below). Child body mass index (BMI) was measured as a confounder and one child had an obesity score $>30\ kg/m^2$ but was still included in the study.

For HCC quantification, the first proximal centimeter of each sample was cut (1 cm of hair corresponds to about one month of growth) and processed according to the protocol published by Frisch, et al. [71]. Briefly, each sample was subjected to a repeated washing procedure with 2.5 mL isopropanol [72], air-dried, and minced with grinding balls in a ball mill. To calculate the weight of the hair sample, the tar weight (vial and grinding balls) was subtracted from the gross weight (vial, grinding balls, and hair sample). For cortisol extraction, a 4-step method [72,73] with alternating methanol and acetone extraction steps was applied as described by Frisch et al. [71]. The accumulated methanol–acetone supernatants were evaporated at 50 °C and the resulting pellets were stored at −20 °C until analysis.

To quantify cortisol concentrations, pellets were dissolved in 250 µL of phosphate-buffered saline and cortisol concentrations were determined using a salivary ELISA assay kit (RE52611; IBL International, Hamburg, Germany; intra-assay coefficient of variation (CV): 6.7%) according to the manufacturer's instructions. Each sample was assayed in duplicate; the mean value and CV of each duplicate were calculated and used for statistical analysis. The cortisol-to-weight ratio was calculated (pg/mg) as follows:

$$\text{Cortisol-to-weight ratio (pg/mg)} = \frac{\text{HCC}\left[\frac{\text{ng}}{\text{mL}}\right] \times 0.25 \text{ mL}}{\text{hair sample weight [mg]}} \times 1000.$$

In the VSD group, four samples had to be excluded because the CV for the duplicate measurement exceeded 30%. Two samples had CV values between 20% and 30% and were not excluded in view of the small sample size, since their inclusion did not lead to significantly different results. Another five samples were excluded as no cortisol could be extracted ($n = 4$) or because the cortisol-to-weight ratio (pg/mg) was too high (outlier value exceeded mean + 3 SD; $n = 1$), resulting in $n = 14$ valid samples for the VSD group. Since the Shapiro–Wilk test revealed that neither HCC mean values nor cortisol-to-weight ratios were normally distributed, both were ln-transformed. Testing sex, age, menarche, and BMI as potential covariates via t-tests/Pearson correlations did not reveal any significant association with cortisol concentrations, which is why no covariates were taken into account. Descriptive statistics of children's hair cortisol are presented in Table 2. For further information see Frisch et al. [71] and Grimm, et al. [74].

Table 2. Hair Analysis Results: Descriptive Data.

	VSD				Controls				Statistics (df = 32)		
	n	M (SD)	Min	Max	n	M (SD)	Min	Max	t	p	d
HCC, ng/mL	14	0.11 (0.08)	0.02	0.31	20	0.19 (0.13)	0.04	0.51	2.04	0.050	0.71
Hair sample weight, mg	14	19.34 (5.71)	9.80	29.60	20	21.97 (10.57)	3.06	56.90	0.85	0.404	0.30
Cortisol-to-weight-ratio, pg/mg	14	1.41 (0.87)	0.33	3.45	20	2.33 (1.51)	0.60	7.20	2.04	0.050	0.71

Variables are reported as M (SD) and group differences were tested using a t-test with Cohen's d as the effect size measure. HCC = hair cortisol concentration; VSD = ventricular septal defect.

4. Statistical Analyses

Statistical analyses were performed using the statistical software IBM SPSS Statistics version 28.0 (IBM Corporation, Armonk, NY, USA). All tests were chosen according to individual requirements. In case of non-fulfilment of the specific requirements of single variables, additional non-parametric analyses were conducted. Results of non-parametric analyses showed no differences in statistical significance; therefore, only results of parametric tests are reported in the manuscript. At the beginning of data analyses, potential confounders (age, sex, menarche, BMI, and socioeconomic status) were initially detected by significant Pearson correlations (r) (age, BMI, socioeconomic status) or independent t-tests (sex, menarche) with regard to child outcomes. Group differences in mother-rated psychological adjustment (depression, anxiety, ADHD, and antisocial behavior, as well as HRQOL) and child neurodevelopment between the VSD group and control group over both periods of measurement were analyzed using repeated measures analysis of covariance (rm ANCOVAs), which were conducted separately for each outcome. Potential moderators were separately entered as covariates (Model A: maternal anxiety moderator; Model B: maternal parenting moderator) into separate t1 (Model A_{t1}/B_{t1}) and t2 (Model A_{t2}/B_{t2}) moderator models. As a main time effect was not of interest in the present study, only group effects and group x time interactions are presented in the results. For conducting group comparisons of children's self-reported problems and HCC, which were only available at t2, ANCOVAs with maternal characteristics as covariates were conducted. All analyses were two-tailed and the level of significance was defined as $p \leq 0.05$. As our sample size was small, results with a level of significance of $p \leq 0.10$ were interpreted as trends and partial eta-squared (η_p^2) values were reported as the measure for effect sizes in (rm) ANCOVAs, with $0.01 \leq \eta_p^2 \geq 0.05$ representing small, $0.06 \leq \eta_p^2 \geq 0.13$ medium, and $\eta_p^2 > 0.13$ large effects [75].

5. Results
5.1. Preliminary Analyses

Potential effects of sex, age, and socioeconomic status on the dependent variables (cognitive development, language, internalizing and externalizing problems, HRQOL, and hair cortisol) and moderators were tested. Additionally, BMI and menarche were tested as potential covariates with regard to hair cortisol analyses. No significant effects for age, sex, socioeconomic status, BMI, and menarche were observed on the outcome variables and moderators (p = 0.052–0.979). However, there was a significant correlation between age and maternal anxiety at t2 (r = 0.291, p = 0.045) and between socioeconomic status and language at t1 and t2 (t1: r = 0.331, p = 0.024; t2: r = 0.385, p = 0.010), cognitive development at t1 (r = 0.538, p < 0.001), and ADHD symptoms at t1 (r = −0.322, p = 0.026). The VSD group and non-affected controls did not differ significantly by socioeconomic status. However, as socioeconomic status is frequently related to child neurodevelopment, it was still considered as a confounder when analyzing cognitive development and language scores.

Maternal anxiety (Table 3) and proactive parenting behavior (Table 4) were considered as potential moderators. In the VSD group, the self-reported maternal anxiety of mothers at t1 did not differ from mothers' reports of typically developing children (VSD_{t1}: M = 44.48, SD = 8.68; $Controls_{t1}$: M = 46.38, SD = 7.87; $t(45)$ = 0.79, p = 0.436). However, mothers of children with VSD showed significantly lower maternal anxiety scores at t2 than mothers of non-affected controls (VSD_{t2}: M = 39.88, SD = 4.52; $Controls_{t2}$: M = 46.75, SD = 9.49; $t(46)$ = 3.20, p = 0.002). The two groups showed no differences in maternal proactive parenting behavior at both time points (VSD_{t1}: M = 3.41, SD = 0.62; $Controls_{t1}$: M = 3.59, SD = 0.49; $t(44)$ = 1.05, p = 0.298; VSD_{t2}: M = 3.47, SD = 0.67; $Controls_{t2}$: M = 3.23, SD = 0.51; $t(42)$ = −1.34, p = 0.187).

Table 3. Repeated Measures ANCOVA-Tested Differences between the VSD Group and Controls. Covariate: Maternal Anxiety t1 (Model A_{t1}).

	VSD		Controls		Statistics F (η^2_p)							
	M	SD	M	SD	Group		Group × Time		Group × Anxiety t1		Group × Anxiety t1 × Time	
Neurodevelopment												
Cognitive$_{t1}$	97.11	12.19	105.17	11.34	0.08	(0.00)	0.13	(0.00)	0.59	(0.02)	0.12	(0.00)
Cognitive$_{t2}$	99.72	11.42	107.83	10.04								

Table 3. Cont.

	VSD		Controls		Statistics $F\ (\eta^2_p)$							
	M	SD	M	SD	Group		Group × Time		Group × Anxiety t1		Group × Anxiety t1 × Time	
Language$_{t1}$	−0.42	1.06	0.46	0.78	0.44	(0.01)	2.93 +	(0.07)	0.02	(0.00)	4.04 +	(0.10)
Language$_{t2}$	−0.26	1.12	0.18	0.67								
Maternal psychopathology rating												
Depression$_{t1}$	0.17	0.20	0.10	0.16	4.01 +	(0.09)	0.07	(0.00)	5.40 *	(0.12)	0.13	(0.00)
Depression$_{t2}$	0.15	0.21	0.10	0.12								
Anxiety$_{t1}$	0.30	0.32	0.20	0.17	4.71 *	(0.11)	0.28	(0.01)	6.84 *	(0.15)	0.39	(0.01)
Anxiety$_{t2}$	0.18	0.27	0.09	0.14								
ADHD$_{t1}$	0.62	0.47	0.60	0.45	1.04	(0.02)	0.29	(0.01)	1.15	(0.03)	0.19	(0.00)
ADHD$_{t2}$	0.38	0.39	0.42	0.40								
Antisocial$_{t1}$	0.17	0.14	0.20	0.17	0.54	(0.01)	0.00	(0.00)	0.52	(0.01)	0.01	(0.00)
Antisocial$_{t2}$	0.11	0.10	0.11	0.09								
Quality of life												
Mother$_{t1}$	86.35	7.11	80.30	9.06	2.06	(0.05)	1.11	(0.03)	1.55	(0.04)	2.12	(0.05)
Mother$_{t2}$	64.60	9.86	64.00	7.89								
Child$_{t1}$	74.15	12.96	74.24	9.29	0.31	(0.01)	0.48	(0.01)	0.27	(0.01)	0.62	(0.02)
Child$_{t2}$	63.25	9.77	62.00	8.94								

Note. + $p < 0.10$, * $p < 0.05$. VSD = ventricular septal defect. Neurodevelopment: t1, Intelligence and Development Scales, IDS [67]; t2, Wechsler Intelligence Scale for Children—Fifth Edition, WISC-V [63]; Cognitive = cognitive development: $M = 100$, $SD = 15$; Language: z-standardization was used in order to transfer the IDS and WISC-V values into a common unit, $M = 0$, $SD = 1$. Maternal psychopathology ratings at t1 and t2: Diagnostic System for Psychiatric Disorders according to ICD-10/DSM-IV, DYSIPS [18]—0, 'not at all'; 1, 'a little bit'; 2, 'to a great extent'; 3, 'particularly'. ADHD = attention deficit/hyperactivity disorder, Antisocial = antisocial behavior. Quality of life: t1, Revised Quality of Life Questionnaire [68]; t2, German version of the Kidscreen-10 questionnaire [69] (0 to 100% quality of life). Sample size (n): VSD: Cognitive/Language $n = 18$; maternal psychopathology ratings, Depression/Anxiety/Antisocial $n = 20$, ADHD $n = 23$; quality of life, Mother $n = 20$, Child $n = 16$. Controls: Cognitive/Language $n = 24$; maternal psychopathology ratings, Depression/ADHD/Antisocial $n = 24$, Anxiety $n = 23$; quality of life, Mother/Child $n = 24$. Covariates—Cognitive/Language: socioeconomic status. Degrees of freedom in rm ANCOVAs (df_F): Cognitive/Language $df_F = 37$, Depression $df_F = 40$, Anxiety $df_F = 39$, ADHD $df_F = 43$, Antisocial $df_F = 40$, Quality of life Mother $df_F = 40$, Quality of life Child $df_F = 36$. $df_H = 1$. η^2_p, partial eta-squared, effect size measure: ≥0.01 small effect, ≥0.06 medium effect, ≥0.14 large effect.

Table 4. Repeated Measures ANCOVA-Tested Differences between the VSD Group and Controls. Covariate: Maternal Parenting t1 (Model B $_{t1}$).

	VSD		Controls		Statistics $F\ (\eta^2_p)$							
	M	SD	M	SD	Group		Group × Time		Group × Parenting t1		Group × Parenting t1 × Time	
Neurodevelopment												
Cognitive$_{t1}$	97.11	12.19	104.38	11.46	1.60	(0.04)	1.41	(0.04)	0.82	(0.02)	1.37	(0.04)
Cognitive$_{t2}$	99.72	11.42	107.39	10.02								
Language$_{t1}$	−0.42	1.06	0.50	0.78	3.22 +	(0.08)	3.23 +	(0.08)	1.89	(0.05)	2.51	(0.07)
Language$_{t2}$	−0.26	1.12	0.20	0.68								
Maternal psychopathology rating												
Depression$_{t1}$	0.17	0.20	0.10	0.16	2.83	(0.07)	0.24	(0.01)	2.30	(0.06)	0.17	(0.00)
Depression$_{t2}$	0.15	0.21	0.10	0.12								
Anxiety$_{t1}$	0.30	0.32	0.20	0.17	3.12 +	(0.08)	0.34	(0.01)	2.42	(0.06)	0.30	(0.01)
Anxiety$_{t2}$	0.18	0.27	0.10	0.14								
ADHD$_{t1}$	0.62	0.47	0.60	0.46	0.74	(0.02)	3.01 +	(0.07)	0.75	(0.02)	2.89	(0.06)
ADHD$_{t2}$	0.38	0.39	0.41	0.40								
Antisocial$_{t1}$	0.17	0.14	0.19	0.18	0.56	(0.01)	0.06	(0.00)	0.59	(0.02)	0.10	(0.00)
Antisocial$_{t2}$	0.11	0.10	0.11	0.09								

Table 4. Cont.

	VSD		Controls		Statistics $F\ (\eta^2_p)$							
	M	SD	M	SD	Group		Group × Time		Group × Parenting t1		Group × Parenting t1 × Time	
Quality of life												
Mother$_{t1}$	86.35	7.11	80.07	9.20	2.94 +	(0.07)	2.50	(0.06)	3.82 +	(0.10)	3.90 +	(0.09)
Mother$_{t2}$	64.60	9.86	64.17	8.02								
Child$_{t1}$	74.15	12.96	74.44	9.45	4.52 *	(0.11)	0.83	(0.02)	4.60 *	(0.12)	0.77	(0.02)
Child$_{t2}$	63.25	9.77	62.26	9.05								

Note. + $p < 0.10$, * $p < 0.05$. VSD = ventricular septal defect. Neurodevelopment: t1, Intelligence and Development Scales, IDS [67]; t2, Wechsler Intelligence Scale for Children—Fifth Edition, WISC-V [63]; Cognitive = cognitive development: $M = 100$, $SD = 15$; language: z-standardization was used in order to transfer the IDS and WISC-V values into a common unit, $M = 0$, $SD = 1$. Maternal psychopathology ratings at t1 and t2: Diagnostic System for Psychiatric Disorders according to ICD-10/DSM-IV, DYSIPS [18]—0, 'not at all'; 1, 'a little bit'; 2, 'to a great extent'; 3, 'particularly'. ADHD = attention deficit/hyperactivity disorder, Antisocial = antisocial behavior. Quality of life: t1, Revised Quality of Life Questionnaire [68]; t2: German version of the Kidscreen-10 questionnaire [69] (0 to 100% quality of life). Sample size (n): VSD: Cognitive/Language $n = 18$; maternal psychopathology ratings, Depression/Anxiety/Antisocial $n = 20$, ADHD $n = 23$; quality of life, Mother $n = 20$, Child $n = 16$. Controls: Cognitive/Language $n = 23$; maternal psychopathology ratings, Depression/ADHD/Antisocial $n = 23$, Anxiety $n = 22$; quality of life, Mother/Child $n = 23$. Covariates—Cognitive/Language: socioeconomic status. Degrees of freedom in rm ANCOVAs (df_F): Cognitive/Language $df_F = 36$, Depression $df_F = 39$, Anxiety $df_F = 38$, ADHD $df_F = 42$, Antisocial $df_F = 39$, Quality of life Mother $df_F = 39$, Quality of life Child $df_F = 35$. $dfH = 1$. η^2_p, partial eta-squared, effect size measure: ≥ 0.01 small effect, ≥ 0.06 medium effect, ≥ 0.14 large effect.

5.2. Longitudinal Outcomes

As t2 moderator models did not prove to be significant ($p = 0.108$–0.988), only the results with maternal anxiety (Model A$_{t1}$, Table 3) and proactive parenting behavior (Model B$_{t1}$, Table 4) at t1 are presented below.

5.2.1. Children's Neurodevelopment

Cognitive development. There were no significant main group effects or interaction effects. Affected children's intelligence did not significantly differ from controls at any time point and was not moderated by any maternal characteristic.

Language development. A marginal significant main effect occurred, in which children with VSDs demonstrated lower language scores compared to non-affected controls (Model B$_{t1}$: $F(1,36) = 3.22$, $p = 0.081$, $\eta_p^2 = 0.08$). There was a marginally significant interaction effect (group x time: Model A$_{t1}$: $F(1,37) = 2.93$, $p = 0.095$, $\eta_p^2 = 0.07$; Model B$_{t1}$: $F(1,36) = 3.23$, $p = 0.081$, $\eta_p^2 = 0.08$) at t1, with the VSD group exhibiting weaker language skills than the comparison group (Model A$_{t1}$/B$_{t1}$: $p = 0.002/0.003$). In addition, there was a marginally significant three-way interaction (Model A$_{t1}$: group x maternal anxiety t1 × time: $F(1,37) = 4.04$, $p = 0.052$, $\eta_p^2 = 0.10$). However, post-hoc analyses revealed no significant associations.

5.2.2. Internalizing and Externalizing Behavior Outcomes—Maternal Reports

Depressive Symptoms. Regarding internalizing problems, there was a marginally significant main group effect, demonstrating that children with VSDs had higher depression symptoms compared to non-affected controls (Model A$_{t1}$: $F(1,40) = 4.02$, $p = 0.052$, $\eta_p^2 = 0.09$). Additionally, a significant interaction effect between group and maternal anxiety at t1 (Model A$_{t1}$: $F(1,40) = 5.40$, $p = 0.025$, $\eta_p^2 = 0.12$) showed that higher maternal anxiety at t1 was associated with higher depression symptoms in the VSD group, both at t1 and t2 (t1: $r = 0.607$, $p = 0.002$, t2: $r = 0.645$, $p = 0.002$). This interaction remained equally strong over both points of time and was not found in the control group.

Anxiety. There was a significant main group effect: children with VSDs had higher anxiety symptoms than non-affected controls (Model A$_{t1}$: $F(1,39) = 4.71$, $p = 0.036$, $\eta_p^2 = 0.11$). Furthermore, a significant interaction effect between group and maternal anxiety at t1 (Model A$_{t1}$: $F(1,39) = 6.84$, $p = 0.013$, $\eta_p^2 = 0.15$) was found. Post-hoc analyses showed higher maternal anxiety at t1 was associated with higher anxiety symptoms in children in the VSD group, both at t1 and t2 (t1: $r = 0.673$, $p < 0.001$; t2: $r = 0.475$, $p = 0.034$). Conversely, the relationship between children's anxiety scores and maternal anxiety symptoms at t1 was not significant in the control group.

ADHD. Regarding ADHD symptoms, there was no significant main group effect. A marginally significant interaction effect between group and time (Model B$_{t1}$: $F(1,42) = 3.01$, $p = 0.090$, $\eta_p^2 = 0.07$) demonstrated that ADHD symptoms decreased over time and that the difference in ADHD symptoms between t1 and t2 was larger in the VSD group ($p < 0.001$) than in the control group ($p = 0.003$). Additionally, there was a marginally significant three-way interaction (Model B$_{t1}$: group x proactive parenting behavior t1 × time: $F(1,42) = 2.89$, $p = 0.096$, $\eta_p^2 = 0.06$). However, post-hoc analyses revealed no significant associations.

Antisocial behavior. There were no significant main group or interaction effects.

5.2.3. Health-Related Quality of Life (HRQOL)

Maternal ratings. A marginally significant main effect for groups could be demonstrated: children with VSDs showed higher HRQOL scores than typically developing children (Model B$_{t1}$: $F(1,39) = 2.94$, $p = 0.095$, $\eta_p^2 = 0.07$). A slightly significant interaction effect (Model B$_{t1}$: group × proactive parenting behavior t1: $F(1,39) = 3.82$, $p = 0.058$, $\eta_p^2 = 0.09$) and a slightly significant three-way interaction effect (Model B$_{t1}$: group x proactive parenting behavior t1 × time: $F(1,39) = 3.90$, $p = 0.055$, $\eta_p^2 = 0.09$) were found. Post-hoc analyses revealed that children with VSDs showed significantly higher HRQOL scores at t1 ($p = 0.015$) but not at t2. Further, it was demonstrated that, in the control group, more pronounced proactive parenting behavior at t1 was significantly associated with lower scores in HRQOL at t1 ($r = -0.443$, $p = 0.034$). This association was no longer significant at t2. No significant correlations between proactive parenting behavior and HRQOL occurred in the VSD group.

Child ratings. A significant main group effect could be demonstrated: children with VSDs reported higher HRQOL compared to non-affected controls (Model B$_{t1}$: $F(1,35) = 4.52$, $p = 0.041$, $\eta_p^2 = 0.11$). Additionally, there was a significant interaction effect (Model B$_{t1}$: group x proactive parenting behavior t1: $F(1,35) = 4.60$, $p = 0.039$, $\eta_p^2 = 0.12$), with post-hoc analyses demonstrating that, in the control group, more pronounced proactive parenting behavior at t1 was related to significantly lower child self-reports in HRQOL at t1 ($r = -0.455$, $p = 0.029$) and marginally lower HRQOL scores at t2 ($r = -0.361$, $p = 0.091$). In the VSD group, no significant associations between proactive parenting behavior at t1 and self-reported HRQOL could be found at both times of measurement.

5.3. Cross-Sectional Outcomes

5.3.1. Internalizing and Externalizing Behavior Outcomes—Children's Reports

Depressive symptoms. A significant main effect occurred, showing that children with VSDs reported less depressive symptoms than their non-affected peers (Model B$_{t1}$: $F(1,38) = 6.56$, $p = 0.015$, $\eta_p^2 = 0.15$). Furthermore a significant interaction effect between group and maternal proactive parenting behavior at t1 was found (Model B$_{t1}$: $F(1,38) = 6.87$, $p = 0.013$, $\eta_p^2 = 0.15$). In the control group, more pronounced maternal proactive parenting behavior was significantly correlated with higher reported depressive symptoms ($r = 0.424$, $p = 0.044$). No significant association between maternal proactive parenting behavior and depressive symptoms was found in the VSD group.

Anxiety. A slightly significant main group effect (Model B$_{t1}$: $F(1,37) = 3.98$, $p = 0.053$, $\eta_p^2 = 0.10$) was detected: children with VSDs reported marginally lower anxiety symptoms than typically developing children. Additionally, a significant interaction effect (Model B$_{t1}$: group × proactive parenting behavior t1: $F(1,37) = 4.42$, $p = 0.042$, $\eta_p^2 = 0.11$) was found. Post-hoc analyses showed that, in the VSD group, higher maternal proactive parenting behavior at t1 was significantly associated with lower anxiety ratings at t2 ($r = -0.460$, $p = 0.041$). There was no significant correlation between maternal proactive parenting behavior and anxiety symptoms in the control group.

ADHD. Self-ratings on ADHD showed no significant main group or interaction effects.

Antisocial behavior. A slightly significant main group main occurred (Model A_{t2}: $F(1,41) = 3.26$, $p = 0.078$, $\eta_p^2 = 0.07$): children with VSDs reported higher antisocial behavior than non-affected controls. Additionally, a marginally significant interaction effect between group and maternal anxiety at t2 could be demonstrated (Model A_{t2}: $F(1,41) = 3.34$, $p = 0.075$, $\eta_p^2 = 0.08$). However, post-hoc analyses revealed no significant associations.

5.3.2. Children's Hair Cortisol

Results are shown in Table 5. A slightly significant main group effect was observed (Model B_{t2}: $F(1,28) = 3.09$, $p = 0.090$, $\eta_p^2 = 0.10$), demonstrating that children with VSDs had lower hair cortisol values compared to non-affected controls. Marginally significant interaction effects could be shown (Model B_{t1}: $F(1,28) = 3.73$, $p = 0.064$, $\eta_p^2 = 0.12$; Model B_{t2}: $F(1,28) = 3.94$, $p = 0.057$, $\eta_p^2 = 0.12$). In the control group, higher maternal proactive parenting behavior at t1 was significantly correlated with higher hair cortisol levels at t2 ($r = 0.451$, $p = 0.053$). In the VSD group, higher maternal proactive parenting behavior at t2 was significantly associated with children's lower hair cortisol values at t2 ($r = -0.804$, $p = 0.002$).

Table 5. ANCOVA-Tested Differences between the VSD group and Controls. Covariate Maternal Anxiety (Model $A_{t1/t2}$) or Maternal Parenting (Model $B_{t1/t2}$).

	VSD		Controls		Statistics F (η^2_p)			
	M	SD	M	SD				
Adolescent's psychopathology rating					group		group × anxiety t1	
Depression$_{t2}$	0.31	0.33	0.34	0.36	1.36	(0.03)	1.31	(0.03)
Anxiety$_{t2}$	0.34	0.42	0.38	0.35	0.33	(0.01)	0.27	(0.01)
ADHD$_{t2}$	0.40	0.36	0.16	0.22	0.00	(0.00)	0.32	(0.01)
Antisocial$_{t2}$	0.19	0.20	0.18	0.10	0.92	(0.02)	1.03	(0.03)
							group × anxiety t2	
Depression$_{t2}$	0.32	0.32	0.34	0.36	0.09	(0.00)	0.10	(0.00)
Anxiety$_{t2}$	0.34	0.41	0.38	0.35	0.03	(0.00)	0.02	(0.00)
ADHD$_{t2}$	0.40	0.36	0.16	0.22	0.93	(0.02)	0.39	(0.01)
Antisocial$_{t2}$	0.19	0.20	0.18	0.10	3.26 $^+$	(0.07)	3.34 $^+$	(0.08)
							group × parenting t1	
Depression$_{t2}$	0.31	0.32	0.33	0.37	6.56 *	(0.15)	6.87 *	(0.15)
Anxiety$_{t2}$	0.34	0.42	0.38	0.36	3.98 $^+$	(0.10)	4.42 *	(0.11)
ADHD$_{t2}$	0.40	0.36	0.16	0.23	1.61	(0.04)	0.76	(0.02)
Antisocial$_{t2}$	0.19	0.20	0.17	0.10	1.64	(0.04)	10.57	(0.04)
							group × parenting t2	
Depression$_{t2}$	0.34	0.32	0.34	0.36	1.23	(0.03)	1.33	(0.03)
Anxiety$_{t2}$	0.36	0.42	0.38	0.35	0.09	(0.00)	0.12	(0.00)
ADHD$_{t2}$	0.44	0.38	0.16	0.22	0.11	(0.00)	0.04	(0.00)
Antisocial$_{t2}$	0.19	0.20	0.18	0.10	0.30	(0.01)	0.28	(0.01)
Cortisol Adolescent					group		group × anxiety t1	
	0.18	0.67	0.67	0.60	0.03	0.00	0.03	(0.00)
							group × anxiety t2	
	0.17	0.64	0.67	0.60	0.07	0.00	0.00	(0.00)
							group × parenting t1	

Table 5. Cont.

	VSD		Controls				Statistics F (η^2_p)	
	M	SD	M	SD				
	0.18	0.67	0.65	0.61	2.58	0.08	3.73 +	(0.12)
							group × parenting t2	
	0.27	0.62	0.67	0.60	3.09 +	0.10	3.94 +	(0.12)

Note. + $p < 0.10$, * $p < 0.05$. Adolescent's psychopathology rating at t2: Diagnostic System for Psychiatric Disorders according to ICD-10/DSM-IV, DYSIPS [18]—0, 'not at all'; 1, 'a little bit'; 2, 'to a great extent'; 3, 'particularly'. Sample size (n): VSD: psychopathology self-ratings, Depression $n = 18$–20, Anxiety $n = 19$–21, ADHD $n = 18$–22 Antisocial $n = 19$–21, Cortisol $n = 12$–14; Controls: psychopathology self-ratings, Depression $n = 23$–24, Anxiety $n = 21$–22, ADHD $n = 23$–24, Antisocial $n = 23$–24, Cortisol $n = 12$–14. Degrees of freedom in ANCOVAs (df_F) Depression $df_F = 38$–40, Anxiety $df_F = 37$–39, ADHD $df_F = 38$–40, Antisocial $df_F = 39$–41, Cortisol $df = 28$–30 $df_H = 1$. Adolescent cortisol at t2: ln-transformed hair cortisol concentration. VSD = ventricular septal defect ADHD = attention deficit/hyperactivity disorder, Antisocial = antisocial behavior. η^2_p, partial eta-squared, effect size measure: ≥0.01 small effect, ≥0.06 medium effect, ≥0.14 large effect.

6. Discussion

The aim of this follow-up study was to explore the long-term consequences of early surgical VSD correction on children's neurodevelopment, internalizing and externalizing problems, HRQOL, and hair cortisol levels from primary school age to adolescence, as well as to additionally reveal the role of maternal characteristics (proactive parenting behavior and maternal anxiety) in child development. Children with early surgically repaired isolated VSDs were examined in comparison to a matched, non-affected control group.

6.1. Long-Term Psychological Adjustment

Neurodevelopment. This study hypothesized no differences in cognitive development between children with VSDs and non-affected controls except for poorer language outcomes in the VSD group. In line with the results when children were primary school-aged, as already published by Eichler et al. [50], this study found no differences in cognitive development between children with VSDs and typically developing children in adolescence Other studies reported an association between the severity of CHD and the degree of cognitive impairment and predicted cognitive outcomes in adolescence [15,76,77]. As VSDs are considered to be a mild form of CHD, our result is in line with previous findings showing that cognitive development in mild CHDs seems to be comparable to the non-affected population, also in adolescence [57]. In this study, children with VSDs showed tendentially lower language scores compared to non-affected controls at primary school age (as already shown by Eichler et al. [50]), though not in adolescence. Fourdain, et al. [78] also found no global neurodevelopmental impairment in children with CHD, but a discrepancy between language and cognitive development was observed. The authors discussed delayed development in the frontal and temporal cortical areas (areas associated with speech production and comprehension) and prenatal and postnatal white matter alterations as causative factors of specific language impairment. This effect is not very stable, as it could only be shown when maternal proactive parenting behavior was considered as a potential moderator. Therefore, the results must be replicated. However, contrary to our initial assumption, the finding of this study suggests that the difference in language abilities between children with VSDs and typically developing children evens out during adolescence. Since this effect occurred when both moderators were taken into account, it could be considered as stable. Additionally, a moderate effect showed that higher maternal anxiety at t1 seemed to only be a risk factor for language impairment in children with VSDs when they were primary school-aged, and not during adolescence. Nevertheless, the result should be replicated as it could only be shown in one model (when considering maternal anxiety as a potential moderator).

Emotional and behavioral problems. The present study aimed to investigate whether VSD-affected children show more internalizing and externalizing symptoms than non-affected controls in adolescence while not showing differences during childhood (see

Eichler et al. [50]). Mothers of children with VSDs reported at least marginally more internalizing problems (depression and anxiety) in their children during childhood and adolescence compared to mothers of non-affected controls, which is in line with most studies on this matter [23,56]. In this context, in the VSD but not in the control group, maternal anxiety at primary school age t1 acted as a significant moderator of child development. When mothers had higher anxiety scores, they also described their children to have more depressive and anxiety symptoms, both at primary school age and in adolescence. This finding is interesting as only in the VSD group (and not in controls) did maternal anxiety levels decrease from primary school age to adolescence. In addition, regardless of group, all maternal anxiety levels were in a normal range and not clinically apparent. However, even at this low level of maternal anxiety, it seems to be relevant for children's and adolescents' mental health after early surgical VSD correction. There might be at least two explanations for these findings. First, elevated maternal anxiety might lead to higher internalizing symptoms in the vulnerable group of children with surgically corrected VSDs. In line with this thought, Eichler and colleagues [50] found higher maternal anxiety to be a risk factor for developing more anxious symptoms in children with surgically corrected VSD when they were primary school-aged, and maternal anxiety thus served as a risk factor. Second, mothers who have had the experience of having a child with a VSD and associated cardiac surgery and medical treatments and who have experienced higher anxiety symptoms might be subject to different perceptions of children's internalizing symptomatology than mothers of typically developing children. Such an altered perception due to their own anxiety symptomatology could lead to a stronger rating of child internalizing behavior problems. To sum up, our findings support the assumptions of several current studies that emphasize the important role of maternal characteristics (e.g., parenting stress, maternal mental health) in the psychological adjustment of children with VSDs [47,79,80]. With regard to our results, this effect seems to outlast childhood and remain until adolescence. The group difference in anxiety symptoms occurred under both moderators and can therefore be interpreted as stable. The other results on internalizing problems should be replicated, as they could only be demonstrated when maternal anxiety was taken into account.

Mothers' reports on their children's externalizing problems (ADHD and antisocial behavior) revealed no differences between the VSD and control group. This result is contrary to various studies showing an increased risk of ADHD for children with CHD [12,22]. A current review of behavioral problems in children with CHD found these children to be at greater risk of internalizing but not externalizing problems and discussed method differences in this context (e.g., type of questionnaire) as a potential cause [81]. Methodological differences in assessing internalizing and externalizing problems might not be relevant in our study as we used symptom-specific subtests of one questionnaire. Dahlawi et al. [23] found younger children with CHD to be at greater risk of behavior problems compared to older children, which is in line with the results of this study showing that ADHD symptoms decreased over time and that the difference in ADHD symptoms between primary school age and adolescence was larger in the VSD group. An explanation for this matter could be a temporal association between the occurrence of risk factors (e.g., children's physical health) and externalizing behavior problems, as found by Kjeldsen, et al. [82]. If the surgical correction for the VSD is performed in early childhood, it may no longer account for the externalizing behavior problems in adolescence. Additionally, a highly engaged parenting style at t1 was associated with lower ADHD symptoms in primary school-aged children. This correlation was not significant but showed a moderate effect size, indicating the potential protective role of proactive parenting behavior on ADHD symptoms in children with VSDs. The results regarding externalizing problems should be replicated, as they could only be demonstrated when maternal proactive parenting behavior was considered as a potential moderator. The model is therefore only slightly stable.

HRQOL. In line with our assumptions and the already published results for primary school-aged children [50], mothers of children with VSDs reported higher HRQOL in their children compared to mothers of typically developing children. Several studies have reported on decreased HRQOL as a function of the severity of the CHD; in less severe CHDs, higher HRQOL compared to non-affected control groups might be expected [19,29,32]. Conversely, in our sample of children who underwent surgical VSD correction, even higher HRQOL than in typically developing children was found. Eichler et al. [50] explained that a mother's experience of having a newborn with a serious disease might influence their reference level in terms of their child's quality of life. As children with VSDs also showed higher self-ratings for HRQOL than controls, this modified reference level may also account for these self-report differences.

Maternal proactive parenting behavior (assessed when children were primary school-aged) was found to influence the development of children's HRQOL. In the group with typically developing children, both mothers and children reported an association between maternal proactive parenting behavior and HRQOL; higher proactive parenting behavior was associated with lower HRQOL. In contrast, this relation did not show up in the VSD group. Maternal proactive parenting behavior is described as greater engagement in mother–child interactions, including more sensitive, stimulating, and supporting behavior [70]. We suppose that children with VSDs, who have experienced a life-threatening disease in their early childhood, require higher maternal proactive parenting behavior to develop similarly to their non-affected peers [50]. Thus, highly proactive parenting behavior might be a protective factor in at-risk contexts, such as in the case of early surgical VSD corrections, and may be prone to an overdose effect in unaffected controls, especially in adolescence. Whether maternal proactive parenting behavior actually has a different function for children with an early surgically corrected VSD and non-affected children should be the subject of future studies. The effects on children's HRQOL only occurred when maternal proactive parenting behavior was taken into account and should therefore be replicated in future studies.

In summary, the results of this study showed that the long-term effects of an early surgically corrected VSD on psychological adjustment in children and adolescents must be considered in a differentiated manner. The sole presence of a VSD does not automatically lead to behavior problems and lower HRQOL in children and adolescents. We could observe that internalizing behavior problems seemed to be present and stable over time, especially when maternal anxiety during primary school was high. By contrast, there was no evidence of the presence of externalizing behavior problems in adolescence. However, there was an indication that high maternal engagement in mother–child interaction could act as a protective factor regarding ADHD symptoms in children with VSDs.

6.2. Children's Self-Reported Psychological Adjustment and Stress System in Adolescence

This study aimed to investigate if VSD-affected children differ in terms of their self-reported psychological adjustment and hair cortisol values from typically developing children. In adolescence, children with VSDs reported lower depression and anxiety symptoms during adolescence compared to typically developing children. Several studies found similar findings by demonstrating no difference in self-reported psychological adjustment between adolescents with VSDs and non-affected controls [83,84]. As already mentioned, the intensity of psychopathological symptoms is related to the severity of the CHD, as children with more severe CHD are at higher risk of developing psychosocial impairments [8].

Interestingly, the control group showed a comparable interaction with maternal proactive parenting behavior at t1 in terms of depressive symptoms, as was already shown for HRQOL. Non-affected children reported higher depressive symptoms in adolescence when mothers showed a pronounced engagement in mother–child interaction. In childhood, high maternal proactive parenting behavior is important for child development and leads to stronger mother–child attachment and a more sensitive perception of one's own emotions, as described above [70,85]. In adolescence, as a natural effect of puberty, children detach themselves from their parents and become more independent [86], which is why conflicts between children and parents increase [87]. Therefore, adolescents who experienced pronounced maternal involvement in childhood have to actively detach themselves from their close maternal bond, which is a developmentally appropriate step towards reaching individualization. Thus, high maternal engagement might be perceived as a stress factor in typically developing adolescents in this study. Further, for adolescents with VSDs, an opposite association was demonstrated. When mothers were more engaged in mother–child interaction, children with VSDs reported lower anxiety symptoms in adolescence. When mothers of children with VSDs managed to control the fears surrounding their children and establish a proactive parenting style, this had a positive effect on their children's development, (such as with language outcome results in a study by Eichler et al. [50]). In adolescence, the following questions arise: Why do children with VSDs not show the same developmental steps as their non-affected peers? Why do children with VSDs not experience the same difficulties and why is pronounced maternal engagement not perceived as a stress factor in adolescence? Developmental gaps could be an explanation. It is possible that this developmental stage is delayed in children with VSDs or is omitted altogether. Another explanation might lay in the age difference between the VSD and control group, as the non-affected children were older than those in the VSD group. Children with VSDs may also have a closer bond with their mothers because of their condition. In any case, future studies should be dedicated to these questions.

Regarding self-ratings for externalizing problems, adolescents with VSDs showed slightly higher symptoms of antisocial behavior compared to controls, while there were no differences in ADHD. Since antisocial behavior is mainly associated with the onset of puberty, it is not surprising that the differences between children with VSDs and controls only emerge in adolescence [88]. It is also known that early adverse life events are associated with antisocial behavior in adolescence [89,90], and several studies were able to show more pronounced externalizing problems in adolescents with VSDs compared to non-affected controls [46,91]. In this context, we also identified maternal anxiety shaping self-ratings of antisocial behavior in adolescents with surgically corrected VSDs. High maternal anxiety (assessed when children were in primary school) was related to lower symptoms of antisocial behavior. Conversely, this association was not found in the control group. This might be explained by the authors of [92], who suggested that mothers with more anxiety symptoms use a more overprotective parenting style. In turn, overprotective behavior could serve a positive developmental function in children with a chronic disease [93]. Therefore, future research should focus on how maternal characteristics might shape child development differently in children with and without CHD.

In this study, both the VSD and the control group had hair cortisol levels in the normal range. Interestingly, children with VSDs showed marginally lower hair cortisol values compared to the control group. Cortisol levels in the normal range for children with VSDs have also been observed in other studies [51,94] and indicate development comparable to non-affected peers. Golub, et al. [95] demonstrated that children with a chronic disease display hypocortisolism. Even though children with a surgically corrected VSDs have to be regarded as somatically healthy and not as chronically ill, our sample might also react with comparable hypocortisolism. In the VSD group, children's self-reports on their better psychological adjustments fit very well with the findings regarding their lower cortisol levels in comparison to typically developing children. Additionally, in children with VSDs, lower cortisol levels were slightly associated with more pronounced maternal proactive parenting behavior, while the association was reversed in the control group. In line with the results regarding internalizing behavior problems, a highly engaged parenting style seems to be a stress factor for non-affected adolescents, which is a developmentally appropriate step towards reaching individualization. Again, further studies are needed to clarify the following question: Why do adolescents with VSDs not show the same development steps as their peers?

In general, the ratings provided by adolescents with VSDs regarding their internalizing and externalizing problems did not match their mothers' ratings in this study. The discrepancy in self-reports and proxy ratings found in our study corresponds to the study of Spijkerboer, et al. [96], who showed that parents of children with CHD reported higher internalizing behavior problems than their children, with children rating themselves comparably to (or even better than) their non-affected peers. The discrepancy between self-reports and proxy ratings of behavior problems has been demonstrated in several studies, with the difference explained by increased autonomy and therefore less behavioral observation from parents [97,98]. These findings emphasize the need for both self-reports and proxy ratings when trying to realize a better understanding of psychological adjustment in children with VSDs.

All effects on children's psychological adjustments and hair cortisol values occurred under only one of the two moderators, not in both models. Therefore, the effects should be interpreted as slightly stable and should be replicated.

7. Strengths and Limitations

A clear strength of the present study is the multi-level approach towards data collection. In addition to maternal ratings, we also collected self-ratings in order to obtain several perspectives on the children's psychological adjustments and relied on standardized tests for assessing children's neurocognitive development, which were performed by trained researchers. Further, children's hair cortisol levels were evaluated in order to gain information on children's physiological stress system. This provided comprehensive insight into the children's psychological development.

An additional strength of this study is the longitudinal approach to assessing children's psychological adjustment over time in a homogeneous group of children with an isolated surgically corrected VSD and a matched non-affected control group. Longitudinal studies always carry the risk of participants dropping out and may result in smaller sample sizes. For example, in this case, it could be that mothers who were concerned about the development of their children chose to continue participating in the study more than mothers who were less concerned, which may exaggerate the results. Therefore, results should be interpreted carefully. The consistently medium to high effect sizes indicate the practical relevance of our results and should be replicated in future studies with larger sample sizes.

One limitation of the present study might lay in the age difference between the VSD and control group, as the non-affected children were older than the VSD group. However, the control group was still well matched regarding other sample characteristics.

Furthermore, an important issue to discuss is the approach taken to testing our hypotheses. To analyze one hypothesis, we conducted four (rm) ANCOVAs separately for each outcome variable and moderator. We chose this data analyzing approach by including as few variables as possible in each model to increase test power due to the small sample size. In the case of multiple testing, α-levels have to be corrected. However, we decided against an alpha correction because of the explorative character of our study. The results have to be interpreted cautiously while taking effect size measures into account. For this reason, the presented findings should be replicated with a larger sample.

Another limitation is not including data from fathers, which leads to a one-sided parental perspective and hides potential protective or risk factors. Future studies should include fathers' perceptions of their children's health and explore the role of paternal characteristics in child development for children with surgically corrected VSDs.

8. Conclusions

The results of this study indicate that children with an early surgically repaired VSDs have the potential for age-typical development in terms of intellectual abilities, psychological adjustment, and stress response. This seems to remain stable over time, as the results of this follow-up study replicated findings from primary school-aged children with surgically corrected VSDs (cf. [50]). In general, the sample of this study was clinically not suspicious. All outcomes for VSD-affected and unaffected children were within a normal non-pathological range. There are some relevant factors supporting the age-typical development of children after an early surgical VSD repair, such as lower maternal anxiety symptoms and proactive parenting behavior. The relevance of these factors was already shown during childhood in a previous cohort [50], and the effect lasts into adolescence. Maternal proactive parenting behavior proved to be an important factor associated with positive psychological adjustment in children with VSDs and is thus a promising approach for future interventions. Conversely, mothers of children with surgically repaired VSDs still reported heightened internalizing problems in adolescence. Even though the amount of maternal anxiety experienced by mothers of children with surgical VSD correction decreased from primary school age to adolescence, relatively high levels of maternal anxiety still acted as an amplifying factor in this context. Based on the differences between self-reports and proxy ratings of children's psychopathological symptoms and the association found between emotional and behavioral problems and maternal anxiety, one can deduce that the psychological long-term consequences of an early corrected VSD are more likely to manifest in the mothers, instead of in the children. Mothers were exposed to enormous trauma through diagnosis of and early operation on their child. Therefore, they might find it difficult to let go and have confidence in the positive psychological and somatic development of their children. This highlights the importance of further studies on the psychological well-being of mothers of children with CHD and how they can be adequately supported from the beginning.

Author Contributions: Conceptualization, R.A.C., A.P., O.K., G.H.M. and A.E.; methodology, R.A.C., A.P., O.K. and A.E.; software, L.L. and J.G.; validation, R.A.C., O.K. and A.E.; formal analysis, L.L., J.G., A.-C.P. and A.E.; investigation, L.L., J.G. and A.-C.P.; resources, O.K. and G.H.M.; data curation, J.G. and A.E.; writing—original draft preparation, L.L.; writing—review and editing, R.A.C., A.P., O.K., G.H.M., A.-C.P., L.L., J.G. and A.E.; visualization, L.L.; supervision, R.A.C., O.K., J.G. and A.E.; project administration, A.E.; funding acquisition, A.E. The present work was performed in (partial) fulfilment of the requirements for obtaining the degree "Dr. med." (L.L.). All authors have read and agreed to the published version of the manuscript.

Funding: This research was funded by the Robert-Enke Foundation, Barsinghausen, Germany, with EUR 41000 provided, and by the German Foundation of Heart Research, Frankfurt am Main, Germany, with EUR 58000 (F/28/19) provided to A.E.

Institutional Review Board Statement: The study was conducted in accordance with the Declaration of Helsinki and approved by the Ethics Committee of the Erlangen University Hospital, Friedrich-Alexander-Universität Erlangen-Nürnberg (353_18B, 12 April 2019).

Informed Consent Statement: Informed consent was obtained from all mothers involved in the study and assent of the children was obtained.

Data Availability Statement: Data are available upon reasonable request.

Acknowledgments: We would like to thank all participating children and their families for being part of this study. Additionally, we want to thank Jörg Distler for his valuable assistance in hair cortisol analyses.

Conflicts of Interest: The authors declare no conflict of interest.

References

1. Dakkak, W.; Oliver, T.I. Ventricular Septal Defect. In *StatPearls*; StatPearls Publishing LLC: Treasure Island, FL, USA, 2021.
2. Leirgul, E.; Fomina, T.; Brodwall, K.; Greve, G.; Holmstrøm, H.; Vollset, S.E.; Tell, G.S.; Øyen, N. Birth prevalence of congenital heart defects in Norway 1994–2009—A nationwide study. *Am. Heart J.* **2014**, *168*, 956–964. [CrossRef] [PubMed]
3. Liu, Y.; Chen, S.; Zühlke, L.; Babu-Narayan, S.V.; Black, G.C.; Choy, M.K.; Li, N.; Keavney, B.D. Global prevalence of congenital heart disease in school-age children: A meta-analysis and systematic review. *BMC Cardiovasc. Disord.* **2020**, *20*, 488. [CrossRef] [PubMed]
4. Centers for Disease Control and Prevention. Congenital Heart Defects (CHDs). Available online: https://www.cdc.gov/ncbddd/heartdefects/data.html (accessed on 14 August 2022).
5. Amedro, P.; Gavotto, A.; Guillaumont, S.; Bertet, H.; Vincenti, M.; De La Villeon, G.; Bredy, C.; Acar, P.; Ovaert, C.; Picot, M.C.; et al. Cardiopulmonary fitness in children with congenital heart diseases versus healthy children. *Heart* **2018**, *104*, 1026–1036. [CrossRef] [PubMed]

6. Moodie, D. Adult congenital heart disease: Past, present, and future. *Tex. Heart Inst. J.* **2011**, *38*, 705–706. [PubMed]
7. Zhao, Q.M.; Niu, C.; Liu, F.; Wu, L.; Ma, X.J.; Huang, G.Y. Spontaneous Closure Rates of Ventricular Septal Defects (6,750 Consecutive Neonates). *Am. J. Cardiol.* **2019**, *124*, 613–617. [CrossRef] [PubMed]
8. Clancy, T.; Jordan, B.; de Weerth, C.; Muscara, F. Early emotional, behavioural and social development of infants and young children with congenital heart disease: A systematic review. *J. Clin. Psychol. Med. Settings* **2019**, *27*, 686–703. [CrossRef] [PubMed]
9. Huisenga, D.; La Bastide-Van Gemert, S.; Van Bergen, A.; Sweeney, J.; Hadders-Algra, M. Developmental outcomes after early surgery for complex congenital heart disease: A systematic review and meta-analysis. *Dev. Med. Child Neurol.* **2021**, *63*, 29–46. [CrossRef]
10. Bucholz, E.M.; Sleeper, L.A.; Sananes, R.; Brosig, C.L.; Goldberg, C.S.; Pasquali, S.K.; Newburger, J.W. Trajectories in Neurodevelopmental, Health-Related Quality of Life, and Functional Status Outcomes by Socioeconomic Status and Maternal Education in Children with Single Ventricle Heart Disease. *J. Pediatr.* **2021**, *229*, 289–293.e3. [CrossRef]
11. Hoskote, A.; Ridout, D.; Banks, V.; Kakat, S.; Lakhanpaul, M.; Pagel, C.; Franklin, R.C.; Witter, T.; Lakhani, R.; Tibby, S.M. Neurodevelopmental status and follow-up in preschool children with heart disease in London, UK. *Arch. Dis. Child.* **2021**, *106*, 263–271. [CrossRef]
12. Siciliano, R.E.; Murphy, L.K.; Prussien, K.V.; Henry, L.M.; Watson, K.H.; Patel, N.J.; Lee, C.A.; McNally, C.M.; Markham, L.W.; Compas, B.E.; et al. Cognitive and Attentional Function in Children with Hypoplastic Left Heart Syndrome: A Pilot Study. *J. Clin. Psychol. Med. Settings* **2021**, *28*, 619–626. [CrossRef]
13. Venchiarutti, M.; Vergine, M.; Zilli, T.; Sommariva, G.; Gortan, A.J.; Crescentini, C.; Urgesi, C.; Fabbro, F.; Cogo, P. Neuropsychological Impairment in Children With Class 1 Congenital Heart Disease. *Percept. Mot. Ski.* **2019**, *126*, 797–814. [CrossRef]
14. Jacobsen, R.M. Outcomes in Adult Congenital Heart Disease: Neurocognitive Issues and Transition of Care. *Pediatr. Clin. North Am.* **2020**, *67*, 963–971. [CrossRef] [PubMed]
15. Matos, S.M.; Sarmento, S.; Moreira, S.; Pereira, M.M.; Quintas, J.; Peixoto, B.; Areias, J.C.; Areias, M.E. Impact of fetal development on neurocognitive performance of adolescents with cyanotic and acyanotic congenital heart disease. *Congenit. Heart Dis.* **2014**, *9*, 373–381. [CrossRef] [PubMed]
16. Abda, A.; Bolduc, M.E.; Tsimicalis, A.; Rennick, J.; Vatcher, D.; Brossard-Racine, M. Psychosocial Outcomes of Children and Adolescents With Severe Congenital Heart Defect: A Systematic Review and Meta-Analysis. *J. Pediatr. Psychol.* **2019**, *44*, 463–477. [CrossRef]
17. Brosig, C.L.; Bear, L.; Allen, S.; Hoffmann, R.G.; Pan, A.; Frommelt, M.; Mussatto, K.A. Preschool Neurodevelopmental Outcomes in Children with Congenital Heart Disease. *J. Pediatr.* **2017**, *183*, 80–86.e81. [CrossRef]
18. Döpfner, M.; Görtz-Dorten, A. *Diagnostik-System für psychische Störungen nach ICD-10 und DSM-IV für Kinder und Jugendliche*; Hogrefe: Göttingen, Germany, 2017.
19. Coelho, R.; Teixeira, F.; Silva, A.M.; Vaz, C.; Vieira, D.; Proença, C.; Moura, C.; Viana, V.; Areias, J.C.; Areias, M.E.G. Psychosocial adjustment, psychiatric morbidity and quality of life in adolescents and young adults with congenital heart disease. *Rev. Port. Cardiol.* **2013**, *32*, 657–664. [CrossRef]
20. Freitas, I.R.; Castro, M.; Sarmento, S.L.; Moura, C.; Viana, V.; Areias, J.C.; Areias, M.E.G. A cohort study on psychosocial adjustment and psychopathology in adolescents and young adults with congenital heart disease. *BMJ Open* **2013**, *3*, e001138. [CrossRef]
21. Holland, J.E.; Cassidy, A.R.; Stopp, C.; White, M.T.; Bellinger, D.C.; Rivkin, M.J.; Newburger, J.W.; DeMaso, D.R. Psychiatric Disorders and Function in Adolescents with Tetralogy of Fallot. *J. Pediatr.* **2017**, *187*, 165–173. [CrossRef]
22. Holst, L.M.; Kronborg, J.B.; Jepsen, J.R.; Christensen, J.Ø.; Vejlstrup, N.G.; Juul, K.; Bjerre, J.V.; Bilenberg, N.; Ravn, H.B. Attention-deficit/hyperactivity disorder symptoms in children with surgically corrected Ventricular Septal Defect, Transposition of the Great Arteries, and Tetralogy of Fallot. *Cardiol. Young* **2020**, *30*, 180–187. [CrossRef] [PubMed]
23. Dahlawi, N.; Milnes, L.J.; Swallow, V. Behaviour and emotions of children and young people with congenital heart disease: A literature review. *J. Child Health Care* **2020**, *24*, 317–332. [CrossRef]
24. Opić, P.; Roos-Hesselink, J.W.; Cuypers, J.A.; Witsenburg, M.; van den Bosch, A.; van Domburg, R.T.; Bogers, A.J.; Utens, E.M. Longitudinal development of psychopathology and subjective health status in CHD adults: A 30- to 43-year follow-up in a unique cohort. *Cardiol. Young* **2016**, *26*, 547–555. [CrossRef] [PubMed]
25. Ernst, M.M.; Marino, B.S.; Cassedy, A.; Piazza-Waggoner, C.; Franklin, R.C.; Brown, K.; Wray, J. Biopsychosocial Predictors of Quality of Life Outcomes in Pediatric Congenital Heart Disease. *Pediatr. Cardiol.* **2018**, *39*, 79–88. [CrossRef] [PubMed]
26. Marino, B.S.; Cassedy, A.; Drotar, D.; Wray, J. The Impact of Neurodevelopmental and Psychosocial Outcomes on Health-Related Quality of Life in Survivors of Congenital Heart Disease. *J. Pediatr.* **2016**, *174*, 11–22.e12. [CrossRef]
27. Abassi, H.; Huguet, H.; Picot, M.-C.; Vincenti, M.; Guillaumont, S.; Auer, A.; Werner, O.; De La Villeon, G.; Lavastre, K.; Gavotto, A. Health-related quality of life in children with congenital heart disease aged 5 to 7 years: A multicentre controlled cross-sectional study. *Health Qual. Life Outcomes* **2020**, *18*, 366. [CrossRef]
28. Mishra, T.A.; Sharma, P. Health Related Quality of Life of Children with Congenital Heart Disease Attending at Tertiary Level Hospital. *J. Nepal Health Res. Counc.* **2019**, *17*, 288–292. [CrossRef]
29. Silva, A.M.; Vaz, C.; Areias, M.E.; Vieira, D.; Proença, C.; Viana, V.; Moura, C.; Areias, J.C. Quality of life of patients with congenital heart diseases. *Cardiol Young* **2011**, *21*, 670–676. [CrossRef]

20. Holst, L.M.; Kronborg, J.B.; Idorn, L.; Bjerre, J.V.; Vejlstrup, N.; Juul, K.; Ravn, H.B. Impact of congenital heart surgery on quality of life in children and adolescents with surgically corrected Ventricular Septal Defect, Tetralogy of Fallot, and Transposition of the Great Arteries. *Cardiol. Young* **2019**, *29*, 1082–1087. [CrossRef]
21. Hövels-Gürich, H. Psychomotor and Cognitive Development and Quality of Life in Children and Adolescents with Congenital Heart Defect. *Klin. Padiatr.* **2019**, *231*, 183–190. [CrossRef]
22. Mellion, K.; Uzark, K.; Cassedy, A.; Drotar, D.; Wernovsky, G.; Newburger, J.W.; Mahony, L.; Mussatto, K.; Cohen, M.; Limbers, C.; et al. Health-related quality of life outcomes in children and adolescents with congenital heart disease. *J. Pediatr.* **2014**, *164*, 781–788.e1. [CrossRef] [PubMed]
23. Ferguson, M.K.; Kovacs, A.H. Quality of life in children and young adults with cardiac conditions. *Curr. Opin. Cardiol.* **2013**, *28*, 115–121. [CrossRef] [PubMed]
24. Huang, J.-S.; Huang, S.-T.; Sun, K.-P.; Hong, Z.-N.; Chen, L.-W.; Kuo, Y.-R.; Chen, Q. Health-related quality of life in children and adolescents undergoing intraoperative device closure of isolated perimembranous ventricular septal defects in southeastern China. *J. Cardiothorac. Surg.* **2019**, *14*, 218. [CrossRef]
25. Juruena, M.F.; Eror, F.; Cleare, A.J.; Young, A.H. The Role of Early Life Stress in HPA Axis and Anxiety. *Adv. Exp. Med. Biol.* **2020**, *1191*, 141–153. [CrossRef] [PubMed]
26. McGauran, M.; Jordan, B.; Beijers, R.; Janssen, I.; Franich-Ray, C.; de Weerth, C.; Cheung, M. Long-term alteration of the hypothalamic-pituitary-adrenal axis in children undergoing cardiac surgery in the first 6 months of life. *Stress* **2017**, *20*, 505–512. [CrossRef]
27. Raymond, C.; Marin, M.F.; Majeur, D.; Lupien, S. Early child adversity and psychopathology in adulthood: HPA axis and cognitive dysregulations as potential mechanisms. *Prog. Neuropsychopharmacol. Biol. Psychiatry* **2018**, *85*, 152–160. [CrossRef] [PubMed]
28. Jackson, A.C.; Frydenberg, E.; Koey, X.M.; Fernandez, A.; Higgins, R.O.; Stanley, T.; Liang, R.P.-T.; Le Grande, M.R.; Murphy, B.M. Enhancing parental coping with a child's heart condition: A co-production pilot study. *Compr. Child Adolesc. Nurs.* **2020**, *43*, 314–333. [CrossRef] [PubMed]
29. Parker, R.; Houghton, S.; Bichard, E.; McKeever, S. Impact of congenital heart disease on siblings: A review. *J. Child Health Care* **2020**, *24*, 297–316. [CrossRef] [PubMed]
30. Nayeri, N.D.; Roddehghan, Z.; Mahmoodi, F.; Mahmoodi, P. Being parent of a child with congenital heart disease, what does it mean? A qualitative research. *BMC Psychol.* **2021**, *9*, 33. [CrossRef] [PubMed]
31. Lee, S.; Ahn, J.-A. Experiences of Mothers Facing the Prognosis of Their Children with Complex Congenital Heart Disease. *Int. J. Environ. Res. Public Health* **2020**, *17*, 7134. [CrossRef] [PubMed]
32. Lemacks, J.; Fowles, K.; Mateus, A.; Thomas, K. Insights from parents about caring for a child with birth defects. *Int. J. Environ. Res. Public Health* **2013**, *10*, 3465–3482. [CrossRef]
33. Gardner, F.; Freeman, N.; Black, A.; Angelini, G. Disturbed mother-infant interaction in association with congenital heart disease. *Heart* **1996**, *76*, 56–59. [CrossRef]
34. Biber, S.; Andonian, C.; Beckmann, J.; Ewert, P.; Freilinger, S.; Nagdyman, N.; Kaemmerer, H.; Oberhoffer, R.; Pieper, L.; Neidenbach, R.C. Current research status on the psychological situation of parents of children with congenital heart disease. *Cardiovasc. Diagn. Ther.* **2019**, *9*, 369–376. [CrossRef]
35. Jilek, E.; Shields, A.; Zhang, L.; Simpson, P.; Bear, L.; Martins, S.A.; Mussatto, K.A.; Brosig, C.L. Predictors of behavioural and emotional outcomes in toddlers with congenital heart disease. *Cardiol. Young* **2021**, *32*, 1216–1221. [CrossRef] [PubMed]
36. Chang, L.-Y.; Wang, C.-C.; Weng, W.-C.; Chiu, S.-N.; Chang, H.-Y. Age differences in the mediating effects of parenting stress on the relationship between cyanotic congenital heart disease and externalizing problems in children and adolescents. *J. Cardiovasc. Nurs.* **2021**, *36*, 293–303. [CrossRef] [PubMed]
37. Guan, G.; Liu, H.; Wang, Y.; Han, B.; Jin, Y. Behavioural and emotional outcomes in school-aged children after surgery or transcatheter closure treatment for ventricular septal defect. *Cardiol. Young* **2014**, *24*, 910–917. [CrossRef]
38. McCusker, C.G.; Doherty, N.N.; Molloy, B.; Casey, F.; Rooney, N.; Mulholland, C.; Sands, A.; Craig, B.; Stewart, M. Determinants of neuropsychological and behavioural outcomes in early childhood survivors of congenital heart disease. *Arch. Dis. Child.* **2007**, *92*, 137–141. [CrossRef]
39. Burek, B.; Ford, M.K.; Hooper, M.; Green, R.; Kohut, S.A.; Andrade, B.F.; Ravi, M.; Sananes, R.; Desrocher, M.; Miller, S.P. Transdiagnostic feasibility trial of internet-based parenting intervention to reduce child behavioural difficulties associated with congenital and neonatal neurodevelopmental risk: Introducing I-InTERACT-North. *Clin. Neuropsychol.* **2021**, *35*, 1030–1052. [CrossRef]
40. Eichler, A.; Köhler-Jonas, N.; Stonawski, V.; Purbojo, A.; Moll, G.H.; Heinrich, H.; Cesnjevar, R.A.; Kratz, O. Child neurodevelopment and mental health after surgical ventricular septal defect repair: Risk and protective factors. *Dev. Med. Child Neurol.* **2019**, *61*, 152–160. [CrossRef]
41. Stonawski, V.; Vollmer, L.; Köhler-Jonas, N.; Rohleder, N.; Golub, Y.; Purbojo, A.; Moll, G.H.; Heinrich, H.; Cesnjevar, R.A.; Kratz, O.; et al. Long-term Associations of an Early Corrected Ventricular Septal Defect and Stress Systems of Child and Mother at Primary School Age. *Front. Pediatr.* **2018**, *5*, 293. [CrossRef]
42. Canivez, G.L.; Watkins, M.W. Long-term stability of the Wechsler Intelligence Scale for Children—Third Edition. *Psychol. Assess.* **1998**, *10*, 285. [CrossRef]

53. Rushton, J.L.; Forcier, M.; Schectman, R.M. Epidemiology of depressive symptoms in the National Longitudinal Study of Adolescent Health. *J. Am. Acad. Child Adolesc. Psychiatry* **2002**, *41*, 199–205. [CrossRef]
54. Kessler, R.C.; Berglund, P.; Demler, O.; Jin, R.; Merikangas, K.R.; Walters, E.E. Lifetime prevalence and age-of-onset distributions of DSM-IV disorders in the National Comorbidity Survey Replication. *Arch. Gen. Psychiatry* **2005**, *62*, 593–602. [CrossRef] [PubMed]
55. Schwarz, S.W. *Adolescent Mental Health in the United States: Facts for Policymakers*; National Center for Child in Poverty: New York NY, USA, 2009.
56. DeMaso, D.R.; Calderon, J.; Taylor, G.A.; Holland, J.E.; Stopp, C.; White, M.T.; Bellinger, D.C.; Rivkin, M.J.; Wypij, D.; Newburger J.W. Psychiatric Disorders in Adolescents With Single Ventricle Congenital Heart Disease. *Pediatrics* **2017**, *139*, e20162241 [CrossRef] [PubMed]
57. Karsdorp, P.A.; Everaerd, W.; Kindt, M.; Mulder, B.J. Psychological and cognitive functioning in children and adolescents with congenital heart disease: A meta-analysis. *J. Pediatr. Psychol.* **2007**, *32*, 527–541. [CrossRef]
58. Taşar, S.; Dikmen, N.; Bulut, İ.; Haskılıç, Y.E.; Saç, R.Ü.; Şenes, M.; Taşar, M.A.; Taşar, M. Potential role of salivary cortisol levels to reflect stress response in children undergoing congenital heart surgery. *Cardiol. Young* **2022**, *32*, 1–7. [CrossRef] [PubMed]
59. Zänkert, S.; Bellingrath, S.; Wüst, S.; Kudielka, B.M. HPA axis responses to psychological challenge linking stress and disease What do we know on sources of intra- and interindividual variability? *Psychoneuroendocrinology* **2019**, *105*, 86–97. [CrossRef] [PubMed]
60. Wennig, R. Potential problems with the interpretation of hair analysis results. *Forensic Sci. Int.* **2000**, *107*, 5–12. [CrossRef] [PubMed]
61. Eichler, A.; Grunitz, J.; Grimm, J.; Walz, L.; Raabe, E.; Goecke, T.W.; Beckmann, M.W.; Kratz, O.; Heinrich, H.; Moll, G.H.; et al. Did you drink alcohol during pregnancy? Inaccuracy and discontinuity of women's self-reports: On the way to establish meconium ethyl glucuronide (EtG) as a biomarker for alcohol consumption during pregnancy. *Alcohol* **2016**, *54*, 39–44. [CrossRef]
62. Grob, A.; Meyer, C.; Hagmann-von Arx, P. *Intelligence and Development Scales (Ids)*; Huber: Bern, Switzerland, 2009.
63. Peterman, F.H. *Wechsler Intelligence Scale for Children (WISC—V)—Fifth Edition*; Übersetzung und Adaptation der WISC-V von David Wechsler; Pearson Assessment: Frankfurt, Germany, 2017.
64. Franiek, S.; Reichle, B. Elterliches Erziehungsverhalten und Sozialverhalten im Grundschulalter. *Kindh. Und Entwickl.* **2007**, *16*, 240–249. [CrossRef]
65. Shelton, K.K.; Frick, P.J.; Wootton, J. Assessment of parenting practices in families of elementary school-age children. *J. Clin. Child Psychol.* **1996**, *25*, 317–329. [CrossRef]
66. Derogatis, L.R. *Brief Symptom Inventory (BSI). Administration, Scoring, and Procedures Manual*; National Computer Systems: Minneapolis, MN, USA, 1993.
67. Grob, A.; Hagmann-von Arx, P.; Meyer, C.S. *Intelligence and Development Scales: (IDS); Intelligenz-und Entwicklungsskalen für Kinder von 5–10 Jahren*; Huber: Bern, Switzerland, 2009.
68. Ravens-Sieberer, U.; Ellert, U.; Erhart, M. [Health-related quality of life of children and adolescents in Germany. Norm data from the German Health Interview and Examination Survey (KiGGS)]. *Bundesgesundheitsblatt Gesundh. Gesundh.* **2007**, *50*, 810–818. [CrossRef]
69. Ravens-Sieberer, U.; The KIDSCREEN Group Europe. *The KIDSCREEN Questionnaires—Quality of Life Questionnaires for Children and Adolescents—Handbook*; Pabst Science Publishers: Lengerich, Germany, 2006.
70. Reichle, B.; Franiek, S. Erziehungsstil aus Elternsicht: Deutsche erweiterte Version des Alabama Parenting Questionnaire für Grundschulkinder (DEAPQ-EL-GS). *Z. Für Entwickl. Und Pädagogischen Psychol.* **2009**, *41*, 12–25. [CrossRef]
71. Frisch, N.; Eichler, A.; Plank, A.C.; Golub, Y.; Moll, G.H.; Kratz, O. Exploring Reference Values for Hair Cortisol: Hair Weight versus Hair Protein. *Drug Monit.* **2020**, *42*, 902–908. [CrossRef]
72. Davenport, M.D.; Tiefenbacher, S.; Lutz, C.K.; Novak, M.A.; Meyer, J.S. Analysis of endogenous cortisol concentrations in the hair of rhesus macaques. *Gen. Comp. Endocrinol.* **2006**, *147*, 255–261. [CrossRef] [PubMed]
73. Slominski, R.; Rovnaghi, C.R.; Anand, K.J. Methodological Considerations for Hair Cortisol Measurements in Children. *Ther. Drug Monit.* **2015**, *37*, 812–820. [CrossRef]
74. Grimm, J.; Stemmler, M.; Golub, Y.; Schwenke, E.; Goecke, T.W.; Fasching, P.A.; Beckmann, M.W.; Kratz, O.; Moll, G.H.; Kornhuber, J.; et al. The association between prenatal alcohol consumption and preschool child stress system disturbance. *Dev. Psychobiol.* **2021**, *63*, 687–697. [CrossRef]
75. Cohen, J. *Statistical Power Analysis for the Behavioral Sciences*; Lawrence Erlbaum Associates: Hillsday, NY, USA, 1988; pp. 20–26.
76. Feldmann, M.; Bataillard, C.; Ehrler, M.; Ullrich, C.; Knirsch, W.; Gosteli-Peter, M.A.; Held, U.; Latal, B. Cognitive and Executive Function in Congenital Heart Disease: A Meta-analysis. *Pediatrics* **2021**, *148*, e2021050875. [CrossRef]
77. Verrall, C.E.; Blue, G.M.; Loughran-Fowlds, A.; Kasparian, N.; Gecz, J.; Walker, K.; Dunwoodie, S.L.; Cordina, R.; Sholler, G.; Badawi, N.; et al. 'Big issues' in neurodevelopment for children and adults with congenital heart disease. *Open Heart* **2019**, *6*, e000998. [CrossRef]
78. Fourdain, S.; St-Denis, A.; Harvey, J.; Birca, A.; Carmant, L.; Gallagher, A.; Trudeau, N. Language development in children with congenital heart disease aged 12-24 months. *Eur. J. Paediatr. Neurol.* **2019**, *23*, 491–499. [CrossRef]
79. Perricone, G.; Polizzi, C.; De Luca, F. Self-representation of children suffering from congenital heart disease and maternal competence. *Pediatr. Rep.* **2013**, *5*, e1. [CrossRef]

80. Hsiao, L.C.; Chiu, S.N.; Chang, L.Y.; Wang, C.C.; Weng, W.C.; Chang, H.Y. Patterns and Correlates of Changes in Emotional and Behavioral Problems Among Children with Congenital Heart Disease. *J. Dev. Behav. Pediatr.* **2022**, *43*, e399–e406. [CrossRef]
81. Finkel, G.G.; Sun, L.S.; Jackson, W.M. Children with Congenital Heart Disease Show Increased Behavioral Problems Compared to Healthy Peers: A Systematic Review and Meta-Analysis. *Pediatr. Cardiol.* **2022**, *43*, 1–8. [CrossRef]
82. Kjeldsen, A.; Nes, R.B.; Sanson, A.; Ystrom, E.; Karevold, E.B. Understanding trajectories of externalizing problems: Stability and emergence of risk factors from infancy to middle adolescence. *Dev. Psychopathol.* **2021**, *33*, 264–283. [CrossRef] [PubMed]
83. Schaefer, C.; von Rhein, M.; Knirsch, W.; Huber, R.; Natalucci, G.; Caflisch, J.; Landolt, M.A.; Latal, B. Neurodevelopmental outcome, psychological adjustment, and quality of life in adolescents with congenital heart disease. *Dev. Med. Child Neurol.* **2013**, *55*, 1143–1149. [CrossRef]
84. Latal, B.; Helfricht, S.; Fischer, J.E.; Bauersfeld, U.; Landolt, M.A. Psychological adjustment and quality of life in children and adolescents following open-heart surgery for congenital heart disease: A systematic review. *BMC Pediatr.* **2009**, *9*, 6. [CrossRef] [PubMed]
85. Dexter, C.A.; Wong, K.; Stacks, A.M.; Beeghly, M.; Barnett, D. Parenting and attachment among low-income African American and Caucasian preschoolers. *J. Fam. Psychol.* **2013**, *27*, 629. [CrossRef] [PubMed]
86. Frank, R.A.; Cohen, D.J. Preadolescent development: Case studies in twins. *Yale J. Biol. Med.* **1980**, *53*, 471–483. [PubMed]
87. Marceau, K.; Ram, N.; Susman, E. Development and Lability in the Parent-Child Relationship During Adolescence: Associations With Pubertal Timing and Tempo. *J. Res. Adolesc.* **2015**, *25*, 474–489. [CrossRef]
88. Patton, G.C.; Viner, R. Pubertal transitions in health. *Lancet* **2007**, *369*, 1130–1139. [CrossRef]
89. Yazgan, I.; Hanson, J.L.; Bates, J.E.; Lansford, J.E.; Pettit, G.S.; Dodge, K.A. Cumulative early childhood adversity and later antisocial behavior: The mediating role of passive avoidance. *Dev. Psychopathol.* **2021**, *33*, 340–350. [CrossRef]
90. Mackey, S.; Chaarani, B.; Kan, K.J.; Spechler, P.A.; Orr, C.; Banaschewski, T.; Barker, G.; Bokde, A.L.W.; Bromberg, U.; Büchel, C.; et al. Brain Regions Related to Impulsivity Mediate the Effects of Early Adversity on Antisocial Behavior. *Biol. Psychiatry* **2017**, *82*, 275–282. [CrossRef]
91. Areias, M.E.G.; Pinto, C.I.; Vieira, P.F.; Teixeira, F.; Coelho, R.; Freitas, I.; Matos, S.; Castro, M.; Sarmento, S.; Viana, V. Long term psychosocial outcomes of congenital heart disease (CHD) in adolescents and young adults. *Transl. Pediatr.* **2013**, *2*, 90. [CrossRef] [PubMed]
92. Jones, L.B.; Hall, B.A.; Kiel, E.J. Systematic review of the link between maternal anxiety and overprotection. *J. Affect. Disord.* **2021**, *295*, 541–551. [CrossRef] [PubMed]
93. Colletti, C.J.; Wolfe-Christensen, C.; Carpentier, M.Y.; Page, M.C.; McNall-Knapp, R.Y.; Meyer, W.H.; Chaney, J.M.; Mullins, L.L. The relationship of parental overprotection, perceived vulnerability, and parenting stress to behavioral, emotional, and social adjustment in children with cancer. *Pediatric. Blood Cancer* **2008**, *51*, 269–274. [CrossRef] [PubMed]
94. Caprirolo, G.; Ghanayem, N.S.; Murkowski, K.; Nugent, M.L.; Simpson, P.M.; Raff, H. Circadian rhythm of salivary cortisol in infants with congenital heart disease. *Endocrine* **2013**, *43*, 214–218. [CrossRef]
95. Golub, Y.; Kuitunen-Paul, S.; Panaseth, K.; Stonawski, V.; Frey, S.; Steigleder, R.; Grimm, J.; Goecke, T.W.; Fasching, P.A.; Beckmann, M.W.; et al. Salivary and hair cortisol as biomarkers of emotional and behavioral symptoms in 6-9 year old children. *Physiol. Behav.* **2019**, *209*, 112584. [CrossRef] [PubMed]
96. Spijkerboer, A.W.; Utens, E.M.; Bogers, A.J.; Verhulst, F.C.; Helbing, W.A. Long-term behavioural and emotional problems in four cardiac diagnostic groups of children and adolescents after invasive treatment for congenital heart disease. *Int. J. Cardiol.* **2008**, *125*, 66–73. [CrossRef]
97. Lansford, J.E.; Godwin, J.; Bornstein, M.H.; Chang, L.; Deater-Deckard, K.; Di Giunta, L.; Dodge, K.A.; Malone, P.S.; Oburu, P.; Pastorelli, C.; et al. Parenting, culture, and the development of externalizing behaviors from age 7 to 14 in nine countries. *Dev. Psychopathol.* **2018**, *30*, 1937–1958. [CrossRef]
98. Yang, P.; Schlomer, G.L.; Lippold, M.A.; Feinberg, M.E. Longitudinal Discrepancy in Adolescent Aggressive Behavior Problems: Differences by Reporter and Contextual Factors. *J. Youth Adolesc.* **2021**, *50*, 1564–1581. [CrossRef]

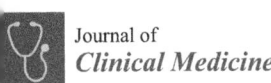

Review

Artificial Intelligence in Pediatric Cardiology: A Scoping Review

Yashendra Sethi [1,2], Neil Patel [1,3], Nirja Kaka [1,3], Ami Desai [4], Oroshay Kaiwan [1,5,*], Mili Sheth [6], Rupal Sharma [7], Helen Huang [8], Hitesh Chopra [9], Mayeen Uddin Khandaker [10], Maha M. A. Lashin [11], Zuhal Y. Hamd [12,*] and Talha Bin Emran [13,14,*]

1. PearResearch, Dehradun 248001, India
2. Department of Medicine, Government Doon Medical College, Dehradun 248001, India
3. Department of Medicine, GMERS Medical College, Himmatnagar 383001, India
4. Department of Medicine, SMIMER Medical College, Surat 395010, India
5. Department of Medicine, Northeast Ohio Medical University, Rootstown, OH 44272, USA
6. Department of Medicine, GMERS Gandhinagar, Gandhinagar 382012, India
7. Department of Medicine, Government Medical College, Nagpur 440003, India
8. Faculty of Medicine and Health Science, Royal College of Surgeons in Ireland, D02 YN77 Dublin, Ireland
9. Chitkara College of Pharmacy, Chitkara University, Rajpura 140401, India
10. Centre for Applied Physics and Radiation Technologies, School of Engineering and Technology, Sunway University, Bandar Sunway 47500, Malaysia
11. Department of Biomedical Engineering, College of Engineering, Princess Nourah bint Abdulrahman University, P.O. 84428, Riyadh 11671, Saudi Arabia
12. Department of Radiological Sciences, College of Health and Rehabilitation Sciences, Princess Nourah bint Abdulrahman University, P.O. 84428, Riyadh 11671, Saudi Arabia
13. Department of Pharmacy, BGC Trust University Bangladesh, Chittagong 4381, Bangladesh
14. Department of Pharmacy, Faculty of Allied Health Sciences, Daffodil International University, Dhaka 1207, Bangladesh
* Correspondence: okaiwan@neomed.edu (O.K.); zyhamd@pnu.edu.sa (Z.Y.H.); talhabmb@bgctub.ac.bd (T.B.E.)

Abstract: The evolution of AI and data science has aided in mechanizing several aspects of medical care requiring critical thinking: diagnosis, risk stratification, and management, thus mitigating the burden of physicians and reducing the likelihood of human error. AI modalities have expanded feet to the specialty of pediatric cardiology as well. We conducted a scoping review searching the Scopus, Embase, and PubMed databases covering the recent literature between 2002–2022. We found that the use of neural networks and machine learning has significantly improved the diagnostic value of cardiac magnetic resonance imaging, echocardiograms, computer tomography scans, and electrocardiographs, thus augmenting the clinicians' diagnostic accuracy of pediatric heart diseases. The use of AI-based prediction algorithms in pediatric cardiac surgeries improves postoperative outcomes and prognosis to a great extent. Risk stratification and the prediction of treatment outcomes are feasible using the key clinical findings of each CHD with appropriate computational algorithms. Notably, AI can revolutionize prenatal prediction as well as the diagnosis of CHD using the EMR (electronic medical records) data on maternal risk factors. The use of AI in the diagnostics, risk stratification, and management of CHD in the near future is a promising possibility with current advancements in machine learning and neural networks. However, the challenges posed by the dearth of appropriate algorithms and their nascent nature, limited physician training, fear of over-mechanization, and apprehension of missing the 'human touch' limit the acceptability. Still, AI proposes to aid the clinician tomorrow with precision cardiology, paving a way for extremely efficient human-error-free health care.

Keywords: artificial intelligence; pediatric cardiology; pediatric cardiac surgery; machine learning; congenital heart diseases

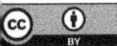

1. Introduction

The discipline of pediatric cardiology has evolved as a specialty over the past 60 years deriving its roots from attempts to treat congenital heart diseases [1]. Congenital heart diseases (CHD), in the wake of the burden of mortality and morbidity they bring in have always been an issue of concern. A total of 3.12 million babies in the United States were born with congenital heart disease, and around 13.3 million individuals are living with congenital heart anomalies [2]. CHD has a multifactorial etiology that consists of environmental stressors and genetic factors and accounts for 80% of all forms of CHD [3]. Pediatric heart diseases remain a global burden on health services and are associated with lifelong comorbidities that carry into adulthood, ultimately decreasing the quality of life for children [4]. The last decade has seen the increasing prevalence of hypertension and other 'adult' heart diseases among the pediatric population, especially adolescents, which has counterpoised the falling burden of rheumatic heart disease in the same age group.

Advancements in pediatric cardiology care and surgical technology have helped with significant reductions in mortality [5,6]. However, while high-income countries saw the mortality rates of CHD reduce by half, the needs for surgical care and advanced imaging for pediatric patients are unmet in middle- and lower-income countries [7]. The absence of a timely diagnosis for suspected pediatric heart diseases significantly delays timely treatment and often presents a diagnostic dilemma. The clinically suspected diagnosis of CHD is confirmed by echocardiography, which can even be conducted during pre- and postnatal screening [8,9]. The diagnosis thus requires adequate clinical suspicion, health infrastructure, and a skilled workforce [10].

The growth of artificial intelligence (AI) in the context of medicine has contributed immensely to the streamlining of clinical processes and decision making in health care since 1960 [11,12]. The concept of machine learning (ML) is integral to the evolution of AI. ML is defined as the ability of machines to learn tasks from a large amount of previous data and be able to predict the same for future instances [12]. As a result, AI has multiple key applications in the diagnosis, surveillance, prevention, and intervention of congenital heart diseases and has created major advancements in pediatric cardiology as a specialty [13]. Due to its widespread ability to improve the diagnostic value of cardiac magnetic resonance imaging (MRI), echocardiograms (ECHO), computer tomography (CT) scans, and electrocardiographs (ECG), AI can augment the diagnostic accuracy of pediatric heart diseases [14,15].

While AI has already found its applications in a multitude of specialties, the notion of its use in almost any medical specialty is conceivable. CHD is an interesting area where AI can be applied owing to the burden of CHDs in pediatric and adult populations. AI-based algorithms have expanded their application in various domains of pediatric cardiology including but not limited to screening, clinical examination, diagnosis, image processing, prognosis, risk stratification, and precision medicine [12]. Surprisingly, the full extent of AI applications in all stages of care for patients with congenital heart diseases has not yet been discussed. Evolving literature has pinpointed the efficiency of machine-learning algorithms in the interpretation of heart murmurs, a common sign of congenital heart diseases [16–18]. The recent utilization of deep-learning computer networks has demonstrated the ability to perform MRI segmentation, allowing clinicians to detect valvular defects simultaneously in all four of the heart's chambers [19,20].

Based on our knowledge, there is only one systematic analysis of a case series of atrial septal defect repair with robotic assistance and AI; the full extent of AI applications in all stages of care for patients with CHD has not yet been discussed. The objective of this systematic review is to compile all existing literature on AI applications in the specialty of pediatric cardiology with a focus on CHD. The review will attempt to appraise the evolving literature and compile clinically relevant data that can serve as a source of health information for clinicians.

2. Materials and Methods

We conducted a scoping review in line with the PRISMA (Preferred Reporting Items for Systematic Reviews and Meta-Analyses) guidelines.

2.1. Data Sources and Searches

A literature search was conducted on PubMed, Scopus, and Embase by two authors (YS, NK) based on the following search terms: ("Artificial intelligence" OR "machine learning" OR "Deep learning") AND ("Pediatric cardiology" OR "congenital heart disease"). The search was also refined using the MeSH Major Topic term "artificial intelligence".

2.2. Article Selection

Duplicate studies were eliminated after the initial search, and two reviewers (NK, YS) independently evaluated the title and abstract to see if the articles qualified for a full-text review. An adjudicator (NP) overcame any disagreements. Both reviewers further evaluated the entire article in accordance with the inclusion and exclusion criteria for each potentially eligible study. A comprehensive review was ensured by screening the references to include additional studies (Figure 1).

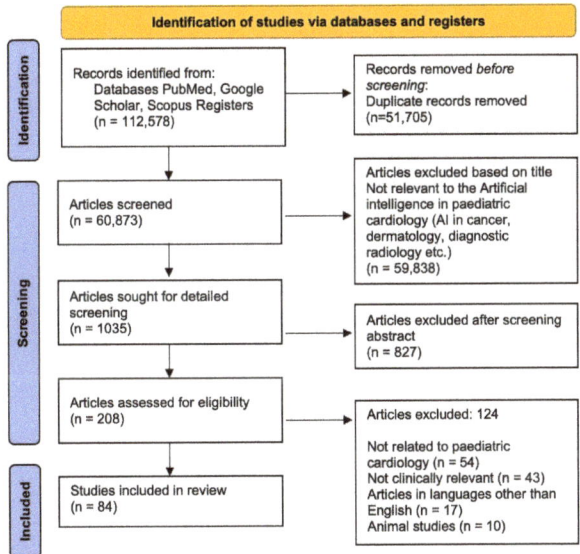

Figure 1. Flow diagram showing selection process of studies included.

2.3. Inclusion and Exclusion Criteria

The initial search was narrowed down by limiting the search to the English language and excluding animal studies. We limited our search to studies published between January 2002 and March 2022 because of the rise in interest in AI in the field of pediatric cardiology over the last 20 years. The inclusion criteria included observational studies (case–control, case series, and cross-sectional studies), experimental studies (randomized control trials), reviews, and expert opinions on the application of AI in pediatric cardiology. Studies were excluded if they lacked direct relevance to AI or were aimed at a population other than the pediatric (18 years) age group. Studies with no full text available, conference abstracts, papers, and book chapters were also excluded.

3. Results

The studies describing the role of AI in pediatric cardiology are compiled in Table 1, while Table 2 describes AI algorithms in pediatric cardiology.

Table 1. Pediatric Heart diseases and the role of AI.

Serial No.	Authors	Study Design	References	Pediatric Heart Diseases Covered	Applications of AI			
					AI in Diagnosis/Fetal Imaging	AI in Prognosis/Risk Stratification	AI in Cardiac Intervention
1	Jef Van den Eynde et al.	Review	[12]	General description	Clinical examination and diagnosis; image processing	Cardiovascular intervention planning and management; prognosis and risk classification.	Omics and precision medicine; fetal cardiology
2	Jingjing Lv et al.	Observational study	[21]	CHD	AI-AA platform revealed similar results to the experts' face-to-face auscultation and reported high auscultation accuracy in detecting aberrant heart sounds.	-	-
3	Rhodri Davies et al.	Editorial	[22]	General description	Minor discernible fluctuations when ejection fraction was evaluated by a cardiac MRI expert were 8.7%, owing primarily to poor repeatability. Deep learning enables more accurate and precise analysis with quantifiable levels of confidence in the outcomes.	-	-
4	Sharib Gaffar et al.	Review	[15]	General description	-	With the aid of precise predictive risk calculators, ongoing health monitoring from wearables, and precision medicine, AI can assist in providing the best possible patient care.	-

Table 1. Cont.

Serial No.	Authors	Study Design	References	Pediatric Heart Diseases Covered	Applications of AI		
					AI in Diagnosis/Fetal Imaging	AI in Prognosis/Risk Stratification	AI in Cardiac Intervention
5	Yeo et al.	Observational study	[23]	General description	FINE is an intelligent navigation technique that automatically acquires several anatomical views of the fetal heart during echocardiography to identify anomalies therein. In four cases, the instrument was able to show fetal heart structural malformations.	-	-
6	Arnaout et al.	Observational study	[24]	General description	Using 685 echocardiograms of fetuses between 18 and 24 weeks of gestation, supervised fully convolutional DL was used to (1) identify the 5 most crucial views of the fetal heart; (2) segment and measure the cardiac structures; and (3) differentiate between normal hearts, tetralogy of Fallot, and hypoplastic left heart syndrome.	-	-
7	Dimitris Bertsimas et al.	Observational study	[25]	CHD	-	For patients who underwent congenital heart surgery, machine learning (ML) models can predict mortality, postoperative mechanical ventilatory support time (MVST), and hospital length of stay (congenital heart surgery).	-

Table 1. *Cont.*

Serial No.	Authors	Study Design	References	Pediatric Heart Diseases Covered	AI in Diagnosis/Fetal Imaging	AI in Prognosis/Risk Stratification	AI in Cardiac Intervention
						Applications of AI	
8	Ulrich Bodenhofer et al.	Editorial	[25]	CHD	-	In comparison with existing risk scores based on logistic regression on pre-selected factors, advanced machine learning is more accurate at predicting the results of valve surgery treatments. This strategy enables training models for the cohorts of certain institutions and is generalizable to other elective high-risk procedures.	-
9	Shaine A. Morris et al.	Expert opinion	[26]	CHD	Congenital illness, the most prevalent and fatal birth defect, could be more accurately diagnosed during pregnancy thanks to recent developments in machine learning.	-	-
10	Siti Nurmaini et al.	Observational study	[20]	CHD	Studies based on 1149 fetal heart images to predict 24 objects, including 3 congenital heart defect instances, 17 heart-chamber objects in each view, and 4 conventional fetal heart view shapes showed that the suggested model worked satisfactorily for segmenting standard views, with an intersection over union of 79.97% and a Dice coefficient similarity of 89.70%. Automatic segmentation and detection methods could significantly increase the number of CHD diagnoses.	-	-

Table 1. *Cont.*

Serial No.	Authors	Study Design	References	Pediatric Heart Diseases Covered	Applications of AI		
					AI in Diagnosis/Fetal Imaging	AI in Prognosis/Risk Stratification	AI in Cardiac Intervention
11	Ai Dozen et al.	Observational study	[27]	VSD	To calibrate the output of U-net, cropping-segmentation-calibration (CSC) uses the time-series information of videos and specific section information. The mean intersections over union (mIoU) of 0.0224, 0.1519, and 0.5543, respectively, were used to assess the segmentation outcomes of DeepLab v3+, U-net, and CSC.	-	-
12	Makoto Nishimori et al.	Scientific report	[28]	Accessory pathway and WPW syndrome	A multimodal deep learning model based on 1D-CNN using ECG waveforms supported with CXR showed great accuracy in identifying AP location.	-	-
13	Tao Wang et al.	Observational study	[29]	General description	The adversarial learning mechanism focusing on the overall spatial structure and context consistency of myocardium showed more accuracy than the conventional method.	-	-
14	Yichen Ding et al.	Observational study	[30]	General description	The complete 3-D imaging of cardiac architecture and mechanics is made possible using light-sheet fluorescence microscopy. This innovative approach offers a solid foundation for post-light-sheet image processing and supports data-driven machine learning for the automated measurement of cardiac ultra-structure.	-	-

Table 1. *Cont.*

Serial No.	Authors	Study Design	References	Pediatric Heart Diseases Covered	Applications of AI			
					AI in Diagnosis/Fetal Imaging	AI in Prognosis/Risk Stratification	AI in Cardiac Intervention
15	C Decourt et al.	Observational study	[31]	General description	The identification of the left ventricle in pediatric MRI using a generative adversarial network (GAN) segmentation approach was useful for the automatic analysis of cardiac MRI and for carrying out large-scale investigations based on MRI reading with a limited amount of training data.	-	-
16	Aapo L. Aro et al.	Editorial	[32]	ECG	Based on a single 12-lead electrocardiogram, AI may identify structural heart problems (AI-ECG).	-	-
17	W. Reid Thompson et al.	Observational study	[33]	CHD	An objective evaluation of an AI-based murmur detection algorithm showed promising results with a Sensitivity of 93% (CI 90–95%), specificity of 81% (CI 75–85%), with accuracy 88% (CI 85–91%) for the detection of pathologic cases. They also suggested that it could be used to compare the efficacy of other algorithms on the same particular dataset.	-	-
18	Saeed Karimi-Bidhendi et al.	Observational study	[34]	CHD	A GAN was devised that could accurately to synthetically augment the training dataset via generating synthetic CMR images and their corresponding chamber segmentations successfully.	-	-

Table 1. *Cont.*

Serial No.	Authors	Study Design	References	Pediatric Heart Diseases Covered	Applications of AI			
					AI in Diagnosis/Fetal Imaging	AI in Prognosis/Risk Stratification	AI in Cardiac Intervention
19	Hiroki Mori et al.	Observational study	[35]		Using a deep learning model comprising a CNN and LTSMs, the researchers identified that the AI algorithm could identify the disease accurately with more sensitivity and specificity than pediatric cardiologists using electrocardiograms.	-	-
20	Benovoy M et al.	Observational study	[36]	Kawasaki disease		The degree of optical coherence tomography (OCT) observations of KD-related CA damage correlates with the degree of distensibility changes in the coronary artery (CA) of Kawasaki disease (KD) patients. When observed longitudinally, this reduced distensibility peaks at 1 year in KD patients and is more severe in those with persisting CA aneurysms.	-
21	Sweatt et al.	Observational study	[37]	Pulmonary arterial hypertension	Patients are categorized using machine learning (consensus clustering) into proteomic immune groups (cytokines, chemokines, and factors using multiplex immunoassay).	-	Different PAH immunological phenotypes with varying clinical risks are identified by blood cytokine patterns. These characteristics may help with mechanistic research on the pathobiology of disease and offer a framework for analysing patient responses to newly developed immunotherapy treatments.

Table 1. Cont.

Serial No.	Authors	Study Design	References	Pediatric Heart Diseases Covered	Applications of AI		
					AI in Diagnosis/Fetal Imaging	AI in Prognosis/Risk Stratification	AI in Cardiac Intervention
22	Diller et al.	Observational study	[38]	CHD (transposition of great arteries—after atrial switch procedure or congenitally corrected TGA).	Use of deep machine learning algorithms trained on routine echocardiographic to detect the diagnosis.	-	Using machine learning algorithms that have been trained on common echocardiographic datasets, it is possible to determine the underlying cause of complex CHD and to perform a continuous, automated evaluation of ventricular function.
23	Li et al.	Observational study	[39]	CHD	-	To find the predictors that were substantially linked with CHD, ANN models such as univariate logistic regression studies and the traditional feed-forward back-propagation neural network (BPNN) model were used. Additionally, BPNN can be utilized to forecast a person's risk of CHD.	-
24	Liu et al.	Observational study	[7]	CHD	-	An RCRnet model can preliminarily identify specific types of left-to-right shunt CHD and improve screening detection rate.	-
25	Tandon et al.	Observational study	[40]	CHD (rTOF)	-	-	The new mostly structurally normal (MSN) algorithm + rTOF algorithm showed improvements in LV epicardial and RV endocardial contours

Table 1. Cont.

Serial No.	Authors	Study Design	References	Pediatric Heart Diseases Covered	AI in Diagnosis/Fetal Imaging	AI in Prognosis/Risk Stratification	AI in Cardiac Intervention
						Applications of AI	
26	Samad et al.	Observational study	[41]	CHD (rTOF)	-	Regression analysis previously failed to recognize the value of baseline variables, but machine learning pipeline did. Predictive models could help organise early interventions in high-risk individuals.	-
27	Diller et al.	Observational study	[42]	CHD	Deep learning (DL) algorithms enhance the de-noising of transthoracic echocardiographic images and removing acoustic shadowing artefacts.		-
28	Montalt-Tordera et al.	Observational study	[43]	CHD	Deep learning can improve contrast in LD cardiovascular magnetic resonance angiography (MRA) without sacrificing clinical utility.		-
29	Junior et al.	Observational study	[44]	CHD	-	Random forest (0.902) (a statistical model to ascertain mortality risk) gave top performing area under the curve and gave predictive variables that represented 67.8% of importance for the risk of mortality in the random forest algorithm.	-
30	Siontis et al.	Observational study	[45]	Hypertrophic cardiomyopathy	A deep-learning AI model can accurately identify juvenile HCM using a typical 12 lead ECG.	-	-

Table 1. Cont.

Serial No.	Authors	Study Design	References	Pediatric Heart Diseases Covered	Applications of AI			
					AI in Diagnosis/Fetal Imaging	AI in Prognosis/Risk Stratification	AI in Cardiac Intervention
31	Tan et al.	Observational study	[46]	CHD	It is anticipated that a novel convolution neural network-based classification algorithm for CHD will be used in machine-assisted auscultation because it has increased heart sound classification accuracy, specificity, and robustness.	-	-
32	Baris Bozkurt et al.	Observational study	[47]	CHD	For automatic structural heart abnormality risk detection from digital phonocardiogram (PCG) signals, sub-band envelopes are preferred to the most often utilized features, and period synchronous windowing is preferred over asynchronous windowing.	-	-
33	Shaan Khurshid et al.	Observational study	[48]	General description	Estimates of the left ventricle's mass-produced by deep learning from 12-lead ECGs and associated with incident cardiovascular disease.	-	-
34	Sabine Ernst et al.	Observational study	[49]	Intra-atrial baffle anatomy	-	-	SVTs might be safely and effectively eliminated using remote-controlled catheter ablation by magnetic navigation employing a retrograde strategy and precise 3D image integration.
35	Thomas Ernest Perry et al.	Observational study	[49]	General description	To effectively and efficiently utilize the potential of textual predictors, the Laplacian eigenmap technique embeds textual predictors into a low-dimensional Euclidean space.	-	-

Table 1. Cont.

Serial No.	Authors	Study Design	References	Pediatric Heart Diseases Covered	AI in Diagnosis/Fetal Imaging	Applications of AI		
						AI in Prognosis/Risk Stratification	AI in Cardiac Intervention	
36	Nikolaos Papoutsidakis et al.	Observational study	[50]	Inherited Cardiomyopathies	In order to effectively keep providers informed about pathogenicity assessments for any previously found genetic variant, the Machine-Assisted Genotype Update System (MAGUS) method of accessing ClinVar without specification to any specific gene or variant is proposed.	-	-	
37	Shu-Hui Yao et al.	Observational study	[51]	PDA	-	-	When therapeutic drug monitoring is unavailable, the nine-parameter ANN model is the best alternative to predict serum digoxin concentrations in PDA.	
38	Zhoupeng Ren et al.	Observational study	[52]	CHD	-	-	This study's use of two machine models reveals a link between CHDs in Beijing and maternal exposure to ambient particulate matter with an aerodynamic diameter of less than 10 m (PM10).	
39	Hui Shi et al.	Observational study	[53]	CHD	-	The ML model assists in deciding on specific therapy and nutritional follow-up strategies while making early forecasts of malnutrition in children with CHD at 1 year postoperative.	-	

Table 1. Cont.

Serial No.	Authors	Study Design	References	Pediatric Heart Diseases Covered	Applications of AI		
					AI in Diagnosis/Fetal Imaging	AI in Prognosis/Risk Stratification	AI in Cardiac Intervention
40	Lei Huang et al.	Observational study	[54]	CHD	-	-	In post-Glenn shunt patients with suspected mean pulmonary arterial pressure >15 mmHg, the preoperative cardiac computed tomography (CT)-based RF model exhibits good performance in the prediction of mean pulmonary arterial pressure, potentially reducing the requirement for right heart catheterization.
41	Andreas Hauptmann et al.	Observational study	[55]	CHD	Real-time radial data artefact suppression using a residual U-Net could aid in the widespread use of real-time CMR in clinical settings. Children and sick people who are unable to hold their breath would benefit most from this.	-	-
42	Gerhard-Paul Diller et al.	Observational study	[56]	ACHD	-	-	Machine learning algorithms that have been trained on big datasets can be useful for estimating prognosis and possibly directing therapy in ACHD.

Table 1. Cont.

Serial No.	Authors	Study Design	References	Pediatric Heart Diseases Covered	Applications of AI		
					AI in Diagnosis/Fetal Imaging	AI in Prognosis/Risk Stratification	AI in Cardiac Intervention
43	Weize Xu et al.	Observational study	[57]	CHD	The precise classification of CHD is completed using a heart sound segmentation method based on PCG segment to achieve the segmentation of cardiac cycles. The accuracy, sensitivity, specificity, and f1-score of classification for CHD are, respectively, 0.953, 0.946, 0.961, and 0.953, which demonstrate that the suggested technique performs competitively.	-	-
44	Daniel Ruiz-Fernández et al.	Observational study	[58]	Pediatric cardiac surgery	-	Future difficulties, or even death, could be prevented with the use of AI-based decision support algorithms when classifying the risk of congenital heart surgery.	-
45	Sukrit Narula et al.	Observational study	[59]	HOCM	Using echocardiographic data, machine learning algorithms can help distinguish between physiological and pathological remodelling patterns in hypertrophic cardiomyopathy (HCM) and physiological hypertrophy seen in athletes (ATH).	-	-
46	Sumeet Gandhi et al.	Review	[60]	Cardiology	Automation has been introduced into many vendor software systems to increase the precision and effectiveness of human echocardiogram tracings.	-	-

Table 1. Cont.

Serial No.	Authors	Study Design	References	Pediatric Heart Diseases Covered	Applications of AI			
					AI in Diagnosis/Fetal Imaging	AI in Prognosis/Risk Stratification	AI in Cardiac Intervention	
47	Kipp W Johnson et al.	Review	[61]	Cardiology	Because doctors will be able to analyze a greater volume of data in greater depth than ever before, AI will result in better patient care. Physicians will benefit from the streamlined clinical treatment provided by reinforcement learning algorithms. Unsupervised learning developments will allow for a far more thorough definition of patients' problems, which will ultimately result in a better choice of treatments and better results.	-	-	
48	Peter Kokol et al.	Review	[62]	Pediatric developmental disorders, oncology, emergencies	The use of AI in pediatrics led to better clinical outcomes, more precise and swifter diagnoses, better decision making, and more sensitive and specific identification of high-risk patients.	-	-	
49	Chen Chen et al.	Review	[63]	General	Different cardiac anatomical features, such as the heart ventricle, atria, and vessels, can be segmented using deep learning algorithms that are applied in three main imaging modalities: MRI, CT, and ultrasound.	-	-	
50	Chang AC et al.	Editorial	[64]	Pediatric heart diseases	The subspecialty that will gain the most from future technologies and AI approaches is pediatric cardiology, hands down.	-	-	

Table 1. Cont.

Serial No.	Authors	Study Design	References	Pediatric Heart Diseases Covered	Applications of AI		
					AI in Diagnosis/Fetal Imaging	AI in Prognosis/Risk Stratification	AI in Cardiac Intervention
51	Diller GP et al.	Observational study	[65]	TOF	-	Automated evaluation of cardiac magnetic resonance (CMR) imaging parameters using machine learning techniques based in two dimensions to predict prognosis in TOF.	In patients with corrected tetralogy of Fallot, automated analysis using machine learning algorithms may replace labor-intensively obtained imaging parameters from cardiac magnetic resonance (CMR) (ToF).
52	Eynde J et al.	Perspective article	[12]	CHD	-	When AI is combined with mechanistic models to describe complicated interactions among variables, medically based data can be utilized to identify trends and predict late problems such arrhythmias and congestive heart failure as well as survival.	
53	Zhang et al.	Observational study	[66]	TOF	-	-	The patch size, shape, and position optimization technique used in pulmonary artery-enlarging repair surgery using generative adversarial networks (GANs) is more accurate and produces superior clinical results.

Table 1. Cont.

Serial No.	Authors	Study Design	References	Pediatric Heart Diseases Covered	Applications of AI		
					AI in Diagnosis/Fetal Imaging	AI in Prognosis/Risk Stratification	AI in Cardiac Intervention
54	Asmare MH et al.	Observational study	[67]	RHD	The automatic auscultation and categorization of the heart sound as being normal or rheumatic is performed using a deep learning method based on convolutional neural networks. It is not necessary to extract the first, second, or systolic and diastolic heart sounds when classifying un-segmented data.	-	-
55	Lakhe A et al.	Observational study	[68]	CHD	An adaptive line enhancement approach is used by a digital stethoscope to digitally amplify, record, examine, play back, and process heart sounds.	-	-
56	A. Arafati	Review	[69]	CHD	AI-based methods for analyzing cardiac MRI data have the potential to be very effective and error-free.	-	-
57	Pyles Lee at al	Observational study	[70]	CHD	The viability of using the cloud-based HeartLink system to distinguish between pathologic murmurs caused by CHD and typical functional cardiac murmurs was demonstrated in the proof-of-concept study.	-	-
58	Andrisevic N et al.	RCT	[71]	CHD	With a specificity of 70.5% and a sensitivity of 64.7%, an AI-based diagnostic system can distinguish between healthy, normal heart sounds and abnormal heart sounds.	-	-

Table 1. Cont.

Serial No.	Authors	Study Design	References	Pediatric Heart Diseases Covered	Applications of AI			
					AI in Diagnosis/Fetal Imaging	AI in Prognosis/Risk Stratification	AI in Cardiac Intervention	
59	M El-Segaier et al.	RCT	[72]	CHD	First and second heart sounds are detected by an AI algorithm. As benchmarks for detection, R- and T-waves were used.	-	-	
60	Sukryool Kang et al.	Observational study	[73]	CHD	With 84–93% sensitivity and 91–99% specificity, the discussed AI algorithm correctly diagnosed Still's murmur using the jackknife approach based on 87 Still's murmurs and 170 non-murmurs.	-	-	
61	Patricia Garcia-Canadilla et al.	Observational study	[74]	CHD	By enhancing picture capture, quantification, and segmentation, ML methods can enhance the evaluation of fetal cardiac function and help with the early detection of fetal cardiac anomalies and remodelling.	-	-	
62	Hong S et al.	Review	[75]	General	ECG tasks including disease diagnosis, localization, sleep staging, biometric human identification, and denoising have all been tackled using deep learning systems.	-	-	
63	Bodenhofer U et al.	Observational study	[76]	CHD	Machine learning technologies can more accurately predict the results of valve surgery treatments.	-	Machine learning technologies can more accurately predict the results of valve surgery treatments.	
64	Sravani Gampala et al.	Review	[77]	CHD	AI may be useful to radiologists, but it will not replace them.	-	-	
65	J. van den Eynde et al.	Perspective	[78]	CHD	Medicine-based evidence has the potential to transform medical decision making.	-	-	

Table 1. Cont.

Serial No.	Authors	Study Design	References	Pediatric Heart Diseases Covered	Applications of AI			
					AI in Diagnosis/Fetal Imaging	AI in Prognosis/Risk Stratification	AI in Cardiac Intervention
66	Mingming Ma et al.	Observational study	[79]	Dilated Obstructed Right Ventricle	Using intelligent navigation technology to STIC volume datasets, FINE can produce and show three unique aberrant fetal echocardiogram images with display rates of 84.0%, 76.0%, and 84.0%, respectively, and therefore may be utilised for screening and remote consultation of fetal DORV.	-	-
67	Zeng X et al.	Review	[80]	CHD	-	-	For effectively predicting problems during pediatric congenital heart surgery, the machine-learning-based model incorporates patient demographics, surgical factors, and intraoperative blood pressure data.
68	Lo Muzio FP et al.	Observational study	[81]	CHD	-	-	AI algorithms can assist surgeons in making decisions during open-chest surgery.
69	Simona Aufiero et al.		[82]	Congenital long QT syndrome	DL models have the potential to help cardiologists diagnose LQTS.	-	-
70	Dias RD et al.	Review	[83]	Cardiology	Machine learning will be used in high-tech operating rooms to improve intra-operative and post-operative outcomes.	-	-

Table 1. Cont.

Serial No.	Authors	Study Design	References	Pediatric Heart Diseases Covered	Applications of AI			
					AI in Diagnosis/Fetal Imaging	AI in Prognosis/Risk Stratification	AI in Cardiac Intervention
71	Wang T et al.	Observational study	[84]	Kawasaki Disease	A machine learning-based model based on patient data predicts intravenous immunoglobulin resistance in Kawasaki disease.	-	-
72	João Francisco B S Martins et al.	Observational study	[85]	RHD	When the advantage of a 3D convolutional neural network was compared with the benefit of 2D convolutional neural network, the accuracy was 72.77%.	-	-
73	Ghosh P et al.	Review	[86]	MIS-C and Kawasaki disease	Targetable cytokine pathways revealed by the ViP signatures in MIS-C and Kawasaki pinpoint crucial clinical (reduced cardiac function) and laboratory (thrombocytopenia and eosinophenia) indicators to assist monitor severity.	-	-

Table 2. AI algorithms in Pediatric Cardiology.

Serial No.	Authors	Reference	AI Algorithms	Algorithm Functions	Pediatric Pathology Assessed
1	Rima Arnaout et. al	[68]	DL Classifier	A deep learning classifier model predicting probable diagnostic outcomes based on real-time imaging or retrospective data	Congenital heart diseases
2	Mori H, Inai K, et. al.	[35]	Convolutional Neural Networks (CNN) & Long Short-term Memory Models (LSTM)	ECG data utilized by CNN to extract waveform shapes that are further classified by LSTM to find ECG features predicting pathology	Atrial septal defect
3	Zuercher M, Ufkes S, et.al.	[69]	Echo-Net Dynamic Model	Using an echocardiogram databank with other cardiac parameter data, the model predicts left ventricular ejection fractions.	LVEF defects in dilated cardiomyopathies
4	Sepehri AA, Hancq J, et. al.	[70]	Arash-Band Method	Specific frequency bands, Arash bands, are used to analyze heart sound energy from pathological murmurs to predict CHDs.	Congenital heart diseases
5	Wang SH, Wu K, Chu T, et al.	[29]	Structurally optimized Stochastic pooling convolutional neural network	Cardiac magnetic imaging data are classified based on a trained convolutional neural network that allows TOF diagnosis.	Tetralogy of Fallot
6	Ko WY, Siontis KC, Attia ZI, et al.	[71]	Convolutional Neural Network enabled ECG	Utilizing 12-lead ECG data to train a convolutional neural network resulting in a model that ascertains HCM diagnosis	Hypertrophic cardiomyopathy
7	DeGroff CG, Bhatikar S, et al.	[72]	Artificial Neural Network (ANN)	Auscultatory data fed into a trained artificial neural network allows classification of normal vs. pathological heart sounds	Pediatric heart murmurs
8	Na JY, Kim D, Kwon AM, et al.	[73]	Light Gradient-Boosting machine (L-GBM)	A decision tree-based algorithm that utilizes prior weaker models to classify data and predict a diagnosis	Patent ductus arteriosus
9	Sepehri AA, Gharehbaghi A, et. al.	[74]	Multi-layer Perceptron (MLP) Neural Network Classifier	An artificial neural network that processes input data through hidden layers to extract and sort data leading to precise segmentation of heart sounds	Pediatric heart sounds
10	Chou, FS., Ghimire, L.V.	[75]	Random Forest Algorithm	A supervised ML algorithm that uses decision trees that are trained using a combination of learning models to aid in precision diagnostic indicators	Pediatric myocarditis
11	Ali F, Hasan B, Ahmad H, et al.	[76]	Long short-term memory (LSTM) recurrent neural network	A recurrent neural network which is trained to retain and utilize past input with concurrent data to recognize patterns for diagnostic predictions	Pediatric rheumatic heart disease

3.1. AI and Heart Murmurs

AI has the potential to improve the validity of auscultatory findings for diagnosing CHD [87–89]. The limitations of objective performance data have restricted wide acceptability so far [90–92]. The auscultatory findings of CHD are integral to the clinical diagnosis and have the benefit of being a low-cost tool, but are subject to clinical expertise, which becomes a limitation in resource-limited countries and creates a need for support to the clinician [93–96] that is objective and reportable by even peripheral health workers. The lack of trained cardiologists at the peripheral level leads to an unavoidable miss of a timely clinical diagnosis of CHD, contributing to delayed intervention and thus a poor prognosis [97]. The emergence of AI-based digital stethoscopes and cloud reporting for telemedicine has helped with the timely diagnosis and early intervention of CHD in reported samples [68,70]. The AI-based technologies also seem affordable, helping the current interest. The use of an intelligent diagnostic system based on AI algorithms such as wavelet analysis and artificial neural networks (Figure 2) has shown a specificity of 70.5% and a sensitivity of 64.7% [71,72]. The developments in AI for detecting cardiac murmurs have shown promise in terms of sensitivity but still require clinical validation before wide clinical recommendation [73,98].

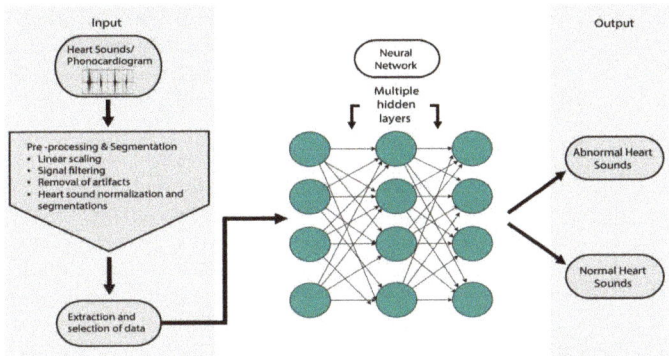

Figure 2. A model of application of neural networks in pediatric cardiology.

3.2. Image Processing with AI

3.2.1. Chest X-ray

CHDs present with some classical chest x-ray signs that can help with suspicion of the disease, including boot-shaped heart (Tetralogy of Fallot), egg-on-string (Transposition of Great Arteries), snowman sign (Total Anomalous Pulmonary Venous Return), scimitar sign (Partial Anomalous Pulmonary Venous Return), gooseneck sign (Endocardial cushion defects), a figure of three (Coarctation of Aorta) and box-shaped hear (Ebstein anomaly) [99]. Chest radiography being easy, cost-effective, and readily available allows a direct or collaborative diagnostic approach to CHD. The evolution of deep learning models and machine learning models and the establishment of defined pediatric datasets have allowed the entry of AI for use in the pediatric population [74]. AI can be immensely beneficial in various steps of imaging such as ordering tests, reporting communication, enhancing the quality of images, and aiding radiologists in interpreting images [77].

3.2.2. MRI

Cardiac MRI has evolved as a precise method for structural and functional evaluations of the heart [100]. The technology has evolved over the years from traditional techniques such as cardiac gating and the suspension of breathing to newer advanced techniques of high-field-strength magnets, high-performance gradient hardware and ultrafast pulse sequences. In the discipline of magnetic resonance imaging, the advancement of AI has allowed for shorter scan times, resulting in higher patient satisfaction; it also reduces errors by minimizing motion artefacts caused by patient movement. The segmentation of cardiac chambers helps visualize them better and aids in diagnosis. Currently, we do this manually, and a shift to AI will help with a faster diagnosis and reduce variation between different analysts [69].

3.2.3. Echocardiography

New AI-based technologies have revolutionized modern medicine in obtaining fetal echocardiograms with improved precision and accuracy. Combining it with machine learning has been quintessential in making predictions of future variables associated with disease progression using retrospective patient data. It has helped in eliminating limitations associated with a lack of expertise in fetal echocardiology, fetal movements, and fetal heart size [19,74]. Machine learning-based systems have been useful in differentiating pathological versus physiological hypertrophic remodeling of the heart [59]. Deep learning models have demonstrated superiority in terms of sensitivity and specificity up to 76% and 88%, respectively, in diagnosing atrial septal defect (ASD) compared with pediatric cardiologists who demonstrated sensitivity and specificity of 53% $\pm$ 0.04 and 67% $\pm$ 0.10 respectively [35]. Automation, AI, and machine learning are game-changing as complementary tools to physicians and in areas with limited expert medical personnel or cardiologists [60]. Fetal intelligent navigation echocardiography (FINE) has presented as a novel method for fetal echocardiography using "intelligent navigation" technology to obtain nine standard views—four-chamber, aortic arch, three vessels, and trachea—and display abnormalities with great sensitivity helping to detect CHD [23,79].

3.2.4. ECG

The use of deep learning (DL), an application of AI, in the field of adult cardiology has been well studied [64]. Its application in pediatric cardiology has become especially relevant due to its potential for allowing early diagnosis, and thus better prognosis, in congenital heart diseases (CHDs). DL models such as convolutional neural network (CNN) and recurrent neural network (RNN) are used in conjunction with electrocardiograms, which remain the staple diagnostic tool for CHDs, to provide enhanced diagnostic information that is otherwise only deduced with input from specialists [35]. Convolutional neural networks can perform image processing and classification, providing an advantage of extracting additional ECG information that would otherwise either be undetected [82]. While the efficiency and utility of using AI models with ECGs for CHDs is evident, the enhancement of the interpretability and training of deep learning models is still needed for widespread implementation [75].

3.3. Prognosis and Risk Stratification

AI-based algorithms have proven to be of great help for pediatric cardiology in the clinical examination, diagnosis, procedural planning, and management of cardiac interventions [12]. AI models have also aided with the extraction of patient data for risk stratification and ambulatory health monitoring from wearables [15]. Machine learning (ML)-based models such as optimal classification trees (OCTs) have accurately predicted mortality, postoperative mechanical ventilatory support time (MVST), and hospital length of stay (LOS) even with nonlinear data in patients with a history of congenital heart surgery [25]. Similarly, ML algorithm-based models, extreme gradient boosting (XGBoost), and RCRnet have accurately predicted preoperative mortality odds in patients with CHDs and statistically significant prognostic indicators along with risk stratification markers in patients with Tetralogy of Fallot and left-to-right shunt CHDs, respectively [41,53]. Importantly, the far-reaching utility of AI-based models in risk stratification and prognostic predictions is the trainability of models to work with various data cohorts [76].

3.4. Planning and Management of Cardiac Interventions

The current approach to planning and the execution of interventions in CHD relies primarily on generic treatment protocols derived from biological data and set guidelines.

As such, there is a lack of tailor-made interventions based on each patient, which would drastically improve outcomes and post-intervention prognosis [78]. Artificial intelligence (AI), with its applications in the form of machine learning (ML) and deep learning (DL) among many, has emerged as a tool aiding the creation of personalized intervention plans as well as an accurate data extractor to ascertain potential post-operative sequelae [80]. The supervised machine learning models such as k-nearest neighbor classifier (KNN) and support vector machine classifier (SVM) have also aided in the intra-operative assessment of cardiac fluid kinematics, which are significant determinants of successful congenital heart surgeries [81]. The subsequent post-operative management of CHDs is imperative for maintaining the structural fluid dynamics and thus the prognosis. This could be done seamlessly with the help of recurrent neural networks based on ML models and deep learning models, allowing for an integrated system that can enhance survival outcomes in pediatric patients [101].

3.5. AI in Cardiac Surgeries

AI can revolutionize pediatric surgery in all stages of surgery: preoperative, intraoperative and post-operative. Preoperative risk assessment and decision-making can be made easier by the tremendous processing and analyzing capacity of AI-enabled algorithms. Surgical decision support systems using ANN can predict post-op outcomes and can prevent morbidity and mortality arising from poor risk assessment pre-operatively.

Tech-enhanced (Hitech) operation theaters can enable intraoperative interventions and decision support [83,102] and bring about a paradigm shift in telesurgery; it is especially useful in cardiac surgeries, where manual segmentation of retrieved images (CT/MRI) can take an unreasonable amount of time. Humans embarked on this path successfully when Xiaowei Xu et al. utilized AI to perform a cardiac surgery remotely in a patient having complications of long-standing ASD through the backbone of 5G technology. This was possible since AI replaced manual segmentation and provided accurate results in just two minutes compared to the traditional manual segmentation which takes 2–3 h even by experts [69]. In this situation, the authors helped a patient who could not be transported to another hospital due to her frail condition; we can extend the same advantage to a remote inaccessible location especially in rural areas and developing countries [103].

Postoperative AI can help in various aspects such as ambulatory patient monitoring post-discharge with AI wearables and automated risk stratification of patients to enable stricter follow-ups. Mahayni AA et al. described an ECG based AI algorithm that predicts ventricular dysfunction post-surgery, predicts long-term mortality in cardiac surgeries. Such algorithms can be developed and implemented for pediatric surgical procedures and drastically improve surgical outcomes [104].

3.6. AI in other Pediatric Heart Diseases

Kawasaki disease (KD) is an acquired pediatric vasculitis that can lead to coronary artery aneurysms and acute coronary syndrome [105]. Very little is known about the pathogenesis of Kawasaki disease but a recent study using AI-guided signatures reveals a shared pathology with Multisystem inflammatory syndrome in children (MIS-C), COVID-19 associated vasculitis in children. Both these syndromes share systemic inflammatory storm with similar cytokines such as IL15/IL15RA. Such AI-based investigative approaches will further elucidate its complex pathogenesis and help decipher novel diagnostic and therapeutic targets [86].

The appropriate and timely management of Kawasaki disease can significantly reduce the coronary complications associated with Kawasaki disease which contribute greatly to mortality in adulthood [106]. AI-based approaches can prove to be extremely crucial in predicting the risk of developing a coronary aneurysm. It is widely known that Kawasaki patients with intravenous immunoglobulin resistance are at a higher risk of developing coronary artery aneurysms, but most scoring models present for predicting the resistance are impractical. Wang T et al. describe a machine learning-based model on patient data that can predict intravenous immunoglobulin resistance in Kawasaki disease patients successfully. The scope for several such prediction models is possible with the advent of AI and can support clinical decisions to improve patient outcomes [84].

Distensibility changes in a coronary artery can be used to predict acute coronary disease in these patients. Benovoy M et al. calculated these changes in KD using an automated deep learning approach and correlated it with the severity of OCT (Optical coherence tomography) findings of KD-related CA damage [36]. Despite, the limited studies using AI-based approaches, AI has the potential to revolutionize risk stratification and prognosis estimation of Kawasaki disease as well as paving way for newer drug targets by elucidating the pathogenesis.

RHD—The screening of RHD requires the clinician's expertise, and hence the grass-root level is limited by a lack of skilled human resources. Automatic diagnosis of echo-detected RHD is feasible and can form the core of the screening programs of the future covering the workload of experts [85]. Recent data has also shown promise for a convolutional neural network-based deep learning algorithm to identify heart sounds as 'rheumatic with an overall accuracy of 96.1% having 94.0% sensitivity and 98.1% specificity [67]. Therefore, AI can form the backbone of future global screening programs for RHD.

3.7. AI Algorithms in Pediatric Cardiology

In many areas of pediatric cardiology, AI-based algorithms can be beneficial, including: (1) clinical examination and diagnosis, (2) image processing, (3) fetal cardiology, (4) prognosis and risk stratification, (5) precision cardiology, and (6) planning and management of cardiac interventions. Machine learning algorithms are a very promising tool for diagnosing and assessing critical and non-critical CHD; however, extensive research is still required to develop interpretable, robust, and generalizable models for clinical application, especially in light of the extreme heterogeneity of complex CHD. Various such AI algorithm models have gained interest over the past decade, and the present time has seen many motivating developments. The most relevant ones for our discussion are summarized in Table 2 and Figure 3.

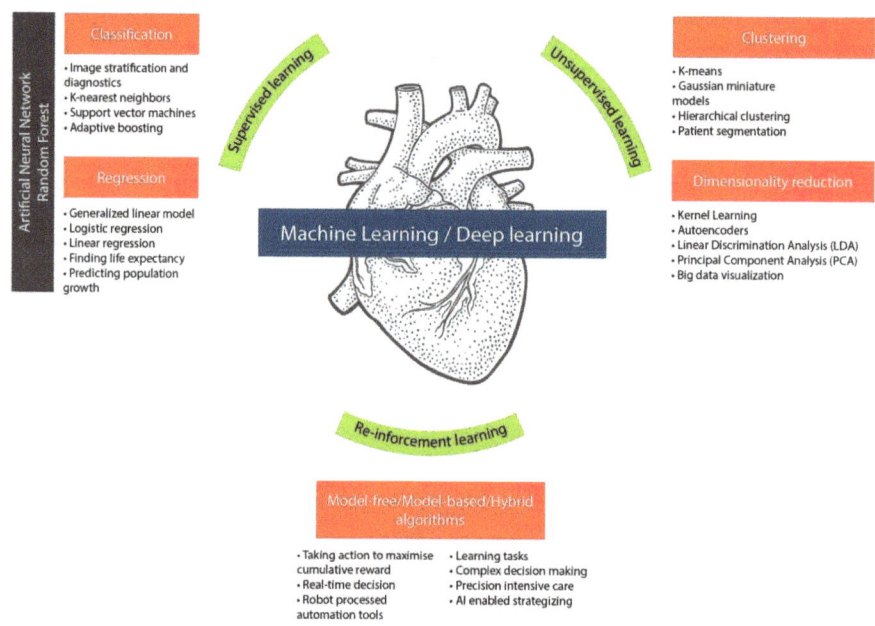

Figure 3. AI-based algorithms and pediatric cardiology.

4. Discussion

AI is rapidly growing, and its significance in clinical practice cannot be negated. It plays a crucial part in augmenting and standardizing care by adding to a physician's skills and expertise. The role of AI in pediatric cardiology has greatly evolved over the past two decades (Figure 4). It picks up subtle or unrecognizable features, preventing missed diagnoses and leading to a better prognosis. Physicians can combine their clinical expertise with AI to enhance their outputs in the domains of prevention, predictive intervention, and health maintenance. AI can make use of continuous data received from wearable devices to offer insight into patients' behaviors and health trends. These features of AI empower the professional to provide the best care to the patient earlier in the course of the disease, helping to improve prognosis and leading to better outcomes.

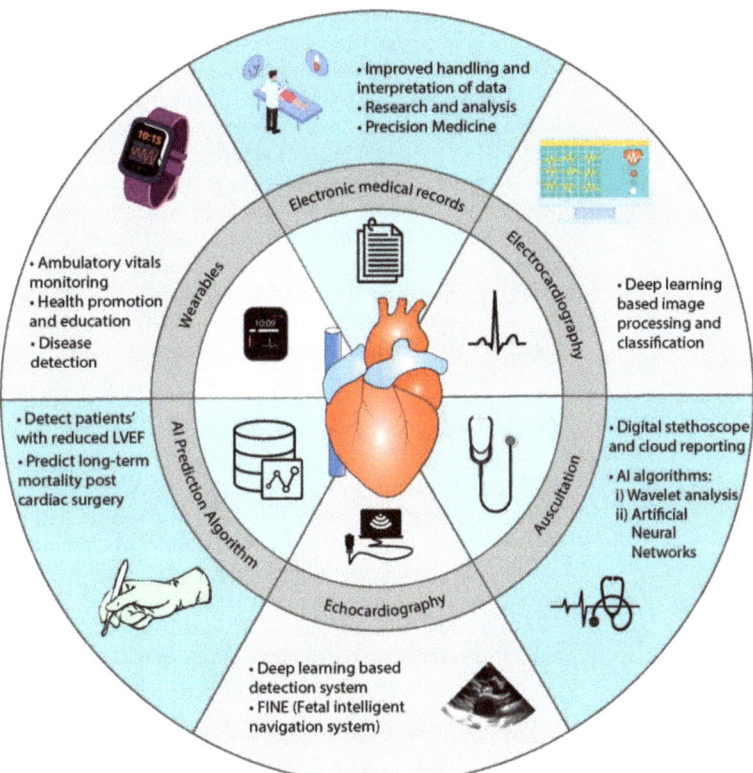

Figure 4. Diagnostic and prognostic applications of AI in Pediatric Cardiology.

The current AI-based applications have greatly enhanced the diagnostics and prognostic areas of pediatric cardiology. The applications with the most promising potential are:

(1) AI prediction algorithms: AI prediction algorithms can help assess patients' risk based on left ventricular ejection fraction and predict post-surgery mortality outcomes based on predefined criteria.
(2) Wearables: Wearables and mobile monitoring devices can help with ambulatory monitoring and early diagnosis. They can also help in educating patients about lifestyle modifications and health promotion.
(3) EMR: Real-time analysis and the clustering of patients through EMR can help formulate research questions and aid the applicability of precision medicine.

(4) Electrocardiography: ECG processing and classification based on deep learning-based algorithms can aid diagnosis.
(5) Echocardiography: Deep learning-based programs such as FINE can also help process echo images to enhance the precision of detection of abnormalities.
(6) Auscultation: AI algorithms such as wavelet analysis and ANN with digital stethoscopes promise to improve the accuracy of detecting abnormal heart sounds (murmurs).

AI seems to be the tool of rich and economically advanced countries, but it can be the magic wand for risk stratification troubles in lower- and middle-income countries (LMICs). AI has the potential to reduce global health inequalities [107]. It can help serve LMICs by bridging gaps in equity, availability, affordability, and accessibility [108]. For instance, the major addition of AI is a reduction in the costs of dimensions requiring expensive equipment and specialized expertise, including tools of screening and planning that are unavailable in most hospitals, especially in LMICs. AI-based innovations can help overcome resource-constrained environments.

The advent of AI has allowed smart tools to assist peripheral health workers in helping with a rough screening at the doorstep and in peripheral areas having poor doctor–patient ratios [60]. The availability of skilled cardiologists to diagnose CHD in remote locations will require a giant leap in these countries. AI-based medical equipment can aid peripheral health care providers in helping with screening and referral. It can also help in terms of teleconsultation and remote radiology [109]. Furthermore, with the availability of AI-based chatbots or virtual avatars and characters, we can offer greater help to populations suffering from stigmatizing pathologies (such as HIV/AIDS and psychiatric pathologies). This therefore can aid in improving access to health care and follow-up services. One of the biggest challenges to health care is language, with improving translation tools, AI can help cover this area well too [110].

4.1. AI: An Efficient Physician Assistant

The full-blown implementation of AI still is resisted by physicians and health care staff fearing inaccuracies, the exclusion of social variables, and possible unemployment. The mechanization of health care, loss of empathy, and human touch to this extent often invite skepticism from the traditional medical community. Despite the fear-mongering and skepticism of loss of human touch and jobs, we opine AI can be an efficient aid to physicians rather than a replacement [111]. It can streamline insurance reviews, provide real-time data analysis, and assist in research. It can reduce the burden on physicians and burnout rates in the medical community. Thus, application in appropriate areas can contribute to the overall enhancement of health care delivery and experience [13].

4.2. Challenges to AI in Pediatric Cardiology

The incorporation of AI into pediatric cardiology has several challenges. The data available for pediatric cardiology is still very limited which is necessary to train AI algorithms to identify, assess and reduce inherent biases and overfitting. Furthermore, the heterogeneity in cardiac anatomy and the rarity of individual disease entities make data accessibility and AI incorporation into pediatric cardiology difficult. We can cater to this limitation by pooling data from all the different hospitals to get a large data set [19]. Imaging in the pediatric population has another challenge owing to their smaller size and frequent movements during imaging, which lead to higher motion artifacts. This poses a technical challenge, for instance, requiring higher spatial resolution in the MRI [69].

The doctor and patient may hesitate to use AI to replace the current protocols. The incorporation of AI will require health care providers to learn interpret data and accurately understand the many model parameters or model architectures. This challenge is being tackled in different ways. For example, some works have incorporated more intuitive interfaces in the models aiding easier interpretation [75].

Additionally, AI is evolving and several ethical concerns are arising. These concerns include informed consent to data access, data security and privacy, algorithm fairness and biases, and transparency [112]. Currently, there are no well-defined laws or regulations in place to address the legal and ethical issues that may arise with AI use in health care settings. However, as AI continues to grow and be used, laws and regulations can certainly be explored to ensure algorithmic transparency and protect data privacy.

5. Conclusions

AI can be touted as the next revolution in medicine. From making physicians' lives easier to enabling research with ease, it has variegated applications in the working environment as well as in the management of patients. Pediatric cardiology is a specialty requiring a great skill set in cognition and interpretation which makes it an ideal candidate for AI incorporation. AI has been successfully integrated into clinical examination, image interpretation, diagnoses, prognosis, risk stratification, precision medicine, and treatment in pediatric cardiology. The advent of AI has facilitated medicine to be more accurate and precise, but it is still a work in progress with challenges and limitations. Despite the roadblocks, we optimistically opine that AI with its current pace will streamline approaches in pediatric cardiology.

Author Contributions: Conceptualization, methodology, visualization, formal analysis and writing—Y.S., N.P. and N.K.; original draft preparation—Y.S., N.P., N.K., A.D., O.K., M.S., R.S. and H.H.; validation and writing—review and editing—Y.S., N.P., N.K., O.K., A.D., H.C., M.U.K., M.M.A.L., Z.Y.H. and T.B.E.; software, investigation, resources and data curation, Y.S., N.P., N.K., A.D., O.K. and M.S.; supervision and project administration—Y.S., N.P., N.K., M.U.K., M.M.A.L., Z.Y.H. and T.B.E. All authors have read and agreed to the published version of the manuscript.

Funding: This research was funded by the Deanship of Scientific Research at Princess Nourah bint Abdulrahman University through the Fast-track Research Funding Program.

Institutional Review Board Statement: Not applicable.

Informed Consent Statement: Not applicable.

Data Availability Statement: All data available within this manuscript.

Acknowledgments: Our gratitude goes out to Deanship of Scientific Research at Princess Nourah bint Abdulrahman University through the Fast-track Research Funding Program.

Conflicts of Interest: The authors declare no conflict of interest.

References

1. Noonan, J.A. A History of Pediatric Specialties: The Development of Pediatric Cardiology. *Pediatr. Res.* **2004**, *56*, 298–306. [CrossRef] [PubMed]
2. van der Linde, D.; Konings, E.E.M.; Slager, M.A.; Witsenburg, M.; Helbing, W.A.; Takkenberg, J.J.M.; Roos-Hesselink, J.W. Birth Prevalence of Congenital Heart Disease Worldwide. *J. Am. Coll. Cardiol.* **2011**, *58*, 2241–2247. [CrossRef] [PubMed]
3. Roth, G.A.; Mensah, G.A.; Johnson, C.O.; Addolorato, G.; Ammirati, E.; Baddour, L.M.; Barengo, N.C.; Beaton, A.Z.; Benjamin, E.J.; Benziger, C.P.; et al. Global Burden of Cardiovascular Diseases and Risk Factors, 1990–2019. *J. Am. Coll. Cardiol.* **2020**, *76*, 2982–3021. [CrossRef] [PubMed]
4. Blue, G.M.; Kirk, E.P.; Sholler, G.F.; Harvey, R.P.; Winlaw, D.S. Congenital Heart Disease: Current Knowledge about Causes and Inheritance. *Med. J. Aust.* **2012**, *197*, 155–159. [CrossRef] [PubMed]
5. Gilboa, S.M.; Devine, O.J.; Kucik, J.E.; Oster, M.E.; Riehle-Colarusso, T.; Nembhard, W.N.; Xu, P.; Correa, A.; Jenkins, K.; Marelli, A.J. Congenital Heart Defects in the United States. *Circulation* **2016**, *134*, 101–109. [CrossRef] [PubMed]
6. van der Bom, T.; Zomer, A.C.; Zwinderman, A.H.; Meijboom, F.J.; Bouma, B.J.; Mulder, B.J.M. The Changing Epidemiology of Congenital Heart Disease. *Nat. Rev. Cardiol.* **2011**, *8*, 50–60. [CrossRef]
7. Liu, Y.; Chen, S.; Zühlke, L.; Black, G.C.; Choy, M.; Li, N.; Keavney, B.D. Global Birth Prevalence of Congenital Heart Defects 1970–2017: Updated Systematic Review and Meta-Analysis of 260 Studies. *Int. J. Epidemiol.* **2019**, *48*, 455–463. [CrossRef]
8. Higashi, H.; Barendregt, J.J.; Kassebaum, N.J.; Weiser, T.G.; Bickler, S.W.; Vos, T. The Burden of Selected Congenital Anomalies Amenable to Surgery in Low and Middle-Income Regions: Cleft Lip and Palate, Congenital Heart Anomalies and Neural Tube Defects. *Arch. Dis. Child.* **2015**, *100*, 233–238. [CrossRef]

9. Lytzen, R.; Vejlstrup, N.; Bjerre, J.; Petersen, O.B.; Leenskjold, S.; Dodd, J.K.; Jørgensen, F.S.; Søndergaard, L. Live-Born Major Congenital Heart Disease in Denmark. *JAMA Cardiol.* **2018**, *3*, 829. [CrossRef]
10. Mcleod, G.; Shum, K.; Gupta, T.; Chakravorty, S.; Kachur, S.; Bienvenu, L.; White, M.; Shah, S.B. Echocardiography in Congenital Heart Disease. *Prog. Cardiovasc. Dis.* **2018**, *61*, 468–475. [CrossRef]
11. Ramos Nascimento, B.; Zawacki Beaton, A. Improved Standardisation of Training Needed to Achieve the Potential of Handheld Echocardiography. *Heart* **2021**, *107*, 1772–1773. [CrossRef] [PubMed]
12. van den Eynde, J.; Kutty, S.; Danford, D.A.; Manlhiot, C. Artificial Intelligence in Pediatric Cardiology: Taking Baby Steps in the Big World of Data. *Curr. Opin. Cardiol.* **2022**, *37*, 130–136. [CrossRef] [PubMed]
13. Basu, K.; Sinha, R.; Ong, A.; Basu, T. Artificial Intelligence: How Is It Changing Medical Sciences and Its Future? *Indian J. Dermatol.* **2020**, *65*, 365. [CrossRef] [PubMed]
14. Mathur, P.; Srivastava, S.; Xu, X.; Mehta, J.L. Artificial Intelligence, Machine Learning, and Cardiovascular Disease. *Clin. Med. Insights Cardiol.* **2020**, *14*, 117954682092740. [CrossRef]
15. Gaffar, S.; Gearhart, A.S.; Chang, A.C. The Next Frontier in Pediatric Cardiology. *Pediatr. Clin. N. Am.* **2020**, *67*, 995–1009. [CrossRef]
16. Lemaire, J.B.; Schaefer, J.P.; Martin, L.A.; Faris, P.; Ainslie, M.D.; Hull, R.D. Effectiveness of the Quick Medical Reference as a Diagnostic Tool. *CMAJ* **1999**, *161*, 725–728.
17. Begic, E.; Gurbeta Pokvic, L.; Begic, Z.; Begic, N.; Dedic, M.; Mrsic, D.; Jamakovic, M.; Vila, N.; Badnjevic, A. From Heart Murmur to Echocardiography—Congenital Heart Defects Diagnostics Using Machine-Learning Algorithms. *Psychiatr. Danub.* **2021**, *33*, 236–246.
18. Liu, J.; Wang, H.; Yang, Z.; Quan, J.; Liu, L.; Tian, J. Deep Learning-Based Computer-Aided Heart Sound Analysis in Children with Left-to-Right Shunt Congenital Heart Disease. *Int. J. Cardiol.* **2022**, *348*, 58–64. [CrossRef]
19. Helman, S.M.; Herrup, E.A.; Christopher, A.B.; Al-Zaiti, S.S. The Role of Machine Learning Applications in Diagnosing and Assessing Critical and Non-Critical CHD: A Scoping Review. *Cardiol. Young* **2021**, *31*, 1770–1780. [CrossRef]
20. Nurmaini, S.; Rachmatullah, M.N.; Sapitri, A.I.; Darmawahyuni, A.; Tutuko, B.; Firdaus, F.; Partan, R.U.; Bernolian, N. Deep Learning-Based Computer-Aided Fetal Echocardiography: Application to Heart Standard View Segmentation for Congenital Heart Defects Detection. *Sensors* **2021**, *21*, 8007. [CrossRef]
21. Lv, J.; Dong, B.; Lei, H.; Shi, G.; Wang, H.; Zhu, F.; Wen, C.; Zhang, Q.; Fu, L.; Gu, X.; et al. Artificial Intelligence-Assisted Auscultation in Detecting Congenital Heart Disease. *Eur. Heart J. Digit. Health* **2021**, *2*, 119–124. [CrossRef]
22. Davies, R.; Babu-Narayan, S.V. Deep Learning in Congenital Heart Disease Imaging: Hope but Not Haste. *Heart* **2020**, *106*, 960–961. [CrossRef] [PubMed]
23. Yeo, L.; Romero, R. Fetal Intelligent Navigation Echocardiography (FINE): A Novel Method for Rapid, Simple, and Automatic Examination of the Fetal Heart. *Ultrasound Obstet. Gynecol.* **2013**, *42*, 268–284. [CrossRef] [PubMed]
24. Arnaout, R.; Curran, L.; Chinn, E.; Zhao, Y.; Moon-Grady, A. Deep-Learning Models Improve on Community-Level Diagnosis for Common Congenital Heart Disease Lesions. *arXiv* **2018**, arXiv:1809.06993. [CrossRef]
25. Bertsimas, D.; Zhuo, D.; Dunn, J.; Levine, J.; Zuccarelli, E.; Smyrnakis, N.; Tobota, Z.; Maruszewski, B.; Fragata, J.; Sarris, G.E. Adverse Outcomes Prediction for Congenital Heart Surgery: A Machine Learning Approach. *World J. Pediatr. Congenit. Heart Surg.* **2021**, *12*, 453–460. [CrossRef] [PubMed]
26. Morris, S.A.; Lopez, K.N. Deep Learning for Detecting Congenital Heart Disease in the Fetus. *Nat. Med.* **2021**, *27*, 764–765. [CrossRef] [PubMed]
27. Dozen, A.; Komatsu, M.; Sakai, A.; Komatsu, R.; Shozu, K.; Machino, H.; Yasutomi, S.; Arakaki, T.; Asada, K.; Kaneko, S.; et al. Image Segmentation of the Ventricular Septum in Fetal Cardiac Ultrasound Videos Based on Deep Learning Using Time-Series Information. *Biomolecules* **2020**, *10*, 1526. [CrossRef] [PubMed]
28. Nishimori, M.; Kiuchi, K.; Nishimura, K.; Kusano, K.; Yoshida, A.; Adachi, K.; Hirayama, Y.; Miyazaki, Y.; Fujiwara, R.; Sommer, P.; et al. Accessory Pathway Analysis Using a Multimodal Deep Learning Model. *Sci. Rep.* **2021**, *11*, 8045. [CrossRef]
29. Wang, T.; Wang, J.; Zhao, J.; Zhang, Y. A Myocardial Segmentation Method Based on Adversarial Learning. *Biomed. Res. Int.* **2021**, *2021*, 6618918. [CrossRef]
30. Ding, Y.; Gudapati, V.; Lin, R.; Fei, Y.; Packard, R.R.S.; Song, S.; Chang, C.-C.; Baek, K.I.; Wang, Z.; Roustaei, M.; et al. Saak Transform-Based Machine Learning for Light-Sheet Imaging of Cardiac Trabeculation. *IEEE Trans. Biomed. Eng.* **2021**, *68*, 225–235. [CrossRef] [PubMed]
31. Decourt, C.; Duong, L. Semi-Supervised Generative Adversarial Networks for the Segmentation of the Left Ventricle in Pediatric MRI. *Comput. Biol. Med.* **2020**, *123*, 103884. [CrossRef]
32. Aro, A.L.; Jaakkola, I. Artificial Intelligence in ECG Screening: Ready for Prime Time? *Int. J. Cardiol.* **2021**, *344*, 111–112. [CrossRef]
33. Thompson, W.R.; Reinisch, A.J.; Unterberger, M.J.; Schriefl, A.J. Artificial Intelligence-Assisted Auscultation of Heart Murmurs: Validation by Virtual Clinical Trial. *Pediatr. Cardiol.* **2019**, *40*, 623–629. [CrossRef]
34. Karimi-Bidhendi, S.; Arafati, A.; Cheng, A.L.; Wu, Y.; Kheradvar, A.; Jafarkhani, H. Fully-automated Deep-learning Segmentation of Pediatric Cardiovascular Magnetic Resonance of Patients with Complex Congenital Heart Diseases. *J. Cardiovasc. Magn. Reson.* **2020**, *22*, 80. [CrossRef]
35. Mori, H.; Inai, K.; Sugiyama, H.; Muragaki, Y. Diagnosing Atrial Septal Defect from Electrocardiogram with Deep Learning. *Pediatr. Cardiol.* **2021**, *42*, 1379–1387. [CrossRef]

36. Benovoy, M.; Dionne, A.; McCrindle, B.W.; Manlhiot, C.; Ibrahim, R.; Dahdah, N. Deep Learning-Based Approach to Automatically Assess Coronary Distensibility Following Kawasaki Disease. *Pediatr. Cardiol.* **2022**, *43*, 807–815. [CrossRef]
37. Sweatt, A.J.; Hedlin, H.K.; Balasubramanian, V.; Hsi, A.; Blum, L.K.; Robinson, W.H.; Haddad, F.; Hickey, P.M.; Condliffe, R.; Lawrie, A.; et al. Discovery of Distinct Immune Phenotypes Using Machine Learning in Pulmonary Arterial Hypertension. *Circ. Res.* **2019**, *124*, 904–919. [CrossRef]
38. Diller, G.-P.; Babu-Narayan, S.; Li, W.; Radojevic, J.; Kempny, A.; Uebing, A.; Dimopoulos, K.; Baumgartner, H.; Gatzoulis, M.A.; Orwat, S. Utility of Machine Learning Algorithms in Assessing Patients with a Systemic Right Ventricle. *Eur. Heart J. Cardiovasc. Imaging* **2019**, *20*, 925–931. [CrossRef]
39. Li, H.; Luo, M.; Zheng, J.; Luo, J.; Zeng, R.; Feng, N.; Du, Q.; Fang, J. An Artificial Neural Network Prediction Model of Congenital Heart Disease Based on Risk Factors. *Medicine* **2017**, *96*, e6090. [CrossRef]
40. Tandon, A.; Mohan, N.; Jensen, C.; Burkhardt, B.E.U.; Gooty, V.; Castellanos, D.A.; McKenzie, P.L.; Zahr, R.A.; Bhattaru, A.; Abdulkarim, M.; et al. Retraining Convolutional Neural Networks for Specialized Cardiovascular Imaging Tasks: Lessons from Tetralogy of Fallot. *Pediatr. Cardiol.* **2021**, *42*, 578–589. [CrossRef]
41. Samad, M.D.; Wehner, G.J.; Arbabshirani, M.R.; Jing, L.; Powell, A.J.; Geva, T.; Haggerty, C.M.; Fornwalt, B.K. Predicting Deterioration of Ventricular Function in Patients with Repaired Tetralogy of Fallot Using Machine Learning. *Eur. Heart J. Cardiovasc. Imaging* **2018**, *19*, 730–738. [CrossRef]
42. Diller, G.-P.; Lammers, A.E.; Babu-Narayan, S.; Li, W.; Radke, R.M.; Baumgartner, H.; Gatzoulis, M.A.; Orwat, S. Denoising and Artefact Removal for Transthoracic Echocardiographic Imaging in Congenital Heart Disease: Utility of Diagnosis Specific Deep Learning Algorithms. *Int. J. Cardiovasc. Imaging* **2019**, *35*, 2189–2196. [CrossRef]
43. Montalt-Tordera, J.; Quail, M.; Steeden, J.A.; Muthurangu, V. Reducing Contrast Agent Dose in Cardiovascular MR Angiography with Deep Learning. *J. Magn. Reson. Imaging* **2021**, *54*, 795–805. [CrossRef]
44. Chang, J.C.; Binuesa, F.; Caneo, L.F.; Turquetto, A.L.R.; Arita, E.C.T.C.; Barbosa, A.C.; Fernandes, A.M.D.S.; Trindade, E.M.; Jatene, F.B.; Dossou, P.-E.; et al. Improving Preoperative Risk-of-Death Prediction in Surgery Congenital Heart Defects Using Artificial Intelligence Model: A Pilot Study. *PLoS ONE* **2020**, *15*, e0238199. [CrossRef]
45. Siontis, K.C.; Liu, K.; Bos, J.M.; Attia, Z.I.; Cohen-Shelly, M.; Arruda-Olson, A.M.; Zanjirani Farahani, N.; Friedman, P.A.; Noseworthy, P.A.; Ackerman, M.J. Detection of Hypertrophic Cardiomyopathy by an Artificial Intelligence Electrocardiogram in Children and Adolescents. *Int. J. Cardiol.* **2021**, *340*, 42–47. [CrossRef]
46. Tan, Z.; Wang, W.; Zong, R.; Pan, J.; Yang, H. Classification of Heart Sound Signals in Congenital Heart Disease Based on Convolutional Neural Network. *Sheng Wu Yi Xue Gong Cheng Xue Za Zhi* **2019**, *36*, 728–736. [CrossRef]
47. Bozkurt, B.; Germanakis, I.; Stylianou, Y. A Study of Time-Frequency Features for CNN-Based Automatic Heart Sound Classification for Pathology Detection. *Comput. Biol. Med.* **2018**, *100*, 132–143. [CrossRef]
48. Khurshid, S.; Friedman, S.; Pirruccello, J.P.; di Achille, P.; Diamant, N.; Anderson, C.D.; Ellinor, P.T.; Batra, P.; Ho, J.E.; Philippakis, A.A.; et al. Deep Learning to Predict Cardiac Magnetic Resonance–Derived Left Ventricular Mass and Hypertrophy from 12-Lead ECGs. *Circ. Cardiovasc. Imaging* **2021**, *14*, e012281. [CrossRef]
49. Ernst, S.; Babu-Narayan, S.V.; Keegan, J.; Horduna, I.; Lyne, J.; Till, J.; Kilner, P.J.; Pennell, D.; Rigby, M.L.; Gatzoulis, M.A. Remote-Controlled Magnetic Navigation and Ablation with 3D Image Integration as an Alternative Approach in Patients with Intra-Atrial Baffle Anatomy. *Circ. Arrhythm. Electrophysiol.* **2012**, *5*, 131–139. [CrossRef]
50. Papoutsidakis, N.; Heitner, S.B.; Mannello, M.C.; Rodonski, A.; Campbell, W.; McElheran, K.; Jacoby, D.L. Machine-Assisted Genotype Update System (MAGUS) for Inherited Cardiomyopathies. *Circ. Cardiovasc. Qual. Outcomes* **2018**, *11*, e004835. [CrossRef]
51. Yao, S.-H.; Tsai, H.-T.; Lin, W.-L.; Chen, Y.-C.; Chou, C.; Lin, H.-W. Predicting the Serum Digoxin Concentrations of Infants in the Neonatal Intensive Care Unit through an Artificial Neural Network. *BMC Pediatr.* **2019**, *19*, 517. [CrossRef]
52. Ren, Z.; Zhu, J.; Gao, Y.; Yin, Q.; Hu, M.; Dai, L.; Deng, C.; Yi, L.; Deng, K.; Wang, Y.; et al. Maternal Exposure to Ambient PM10 during Pregnancy Increases the Risk of Congenital Heart Defects: Evidence from Machine Learning Models. *Sci. Total Environ.* **2018**, *630*, 1–10. [CrossRef]
53. Shi, H.; Yang, D.; Tang, K.; Hu, C.; Li, L.; Zhang, L.; Gong, T.; Cui, Y. Explainable Machine Learning Model for Predicting the Occurrence of Postoperative Malnutrition in Children with Congenital Heart Disease. *Clin. Nutr.* **2022**, *41*, 202–210. [CrossRef] [PubMed]
54. Huang, L.; Li, J.; Huang, M.; Zhuang, J.; Yuan, H.; Jia, Q.; Zeng, D.; Que, L.; Xi, Y.; Lin, J.; et al. Prediction of Pulmonary Pressure after Glenn Shunts by Computed Tomography–Based Machine Learning Models. *Eur. Radiol.* **2020**, *30*, 1369–1377. [CrossRef]
55. Hauptmann, A.; Arridge, S.; Lucka, F.; Muthurangu, V.; Steeden, J.A. Real-time Cardiovascular MR with Spatio-temporal Artifact Suppression Using Deep Learning–Proof of Concept in Congenital Heart Disease. *Magn. Reason. Med.* **2019**, *81*, 1143–1156. [CrossRef] [PubMed]
56. Diller, G.-P.; Kempny, A.; Babu-Narayan, S.V.; Henrichs, M.; Brida, M.; Uebing, A.; Lammers, A.E.; Baumgartner, H.; Li, W.; Wort, S.J.; et al. Machine Learning Algorithms Estimating Prognosis and Guiding Therapy in Adult Congenital Heart Disease: Data from a Single Tertiary Centre Including 10,019 Patients. *Eur. Heart J.* **2019**, *40*, 1069–1077. [CrossRef]
57. Xu, W.; Yu, K.; Ye, J.; Li, H.; Chen, J.; Yin, F.; Xu, J.; Zhu, J.; Li, D.; Shu, Q. Automatic Pediatric Congenital Heart Disease Classification Based on Heart Sound Signal. *Artif. Intell. Med.* **2022**, *126*, 102257. [CrossRef]

58. Ruiz-Fernández, D.; Monsalve Torra, A.; Soriano-Payá, A.; Marín-Alonso, O.; Triana Palencia, E. Aid Decision Algorithms to Estimate the Risk in Congenital Heart Surgery. *Comput. Methods Programs Biomed.* **2016**, *126*, 118–127. [CrossRef]
59. Narula, S.; Shameer, K.; Salem Omar, A.M.; Dudley, J.T.; Sengupta, P.P. Machine-Learning Algorithms to Automate Morphological and Functional Assessments in 2D Echocardiography. *J. Am. Coll. Cardiol.* **2016**, *68*, 2287–2295. [CrossRef]
60. Gandhi, S.; Mosleh, W.; Shen, J.; Chow, C.-M. Automation, Machine Learning, and Artificial Intelligence in Echocardiography: A Brave New World. *Echocardiography* **2018**, *35*, 1402–1418. [CrossRef]
61. Johnson, K.W.; Torres Soto, J.; Glicksberg, B.S.; Shameer, K.; Miotto, R.; Ali, M.; Ashley, E.; Dudley, J.T. Artificial Intelligence in Cardiology. *J. Am. Coll. Cardiol.* **2018**, *71*, 2668–2679. [CrossRef] [PubMed]
62. Kokol, P.; Završnik, J.; Blažun Vošner, H. Artificial Intelligence and Pediatrics: A Synthetic Mini Review. *Pediatr. Dimens.* **2017**, *2*. [CrossRef]
63. Chen, C.; Qin, C.; Qiu, H.; Tarroni, G.; Duan, J.; Bai, W.; Rueckert, D. Deep Learning for Cardiac Image Segmentation: A Review. *Front. Cardiovasc. Med.* **2020**, *7*, 25. [CrossRef] [PubMed]
64. Chang, A. Artificial Intelligence in Pediatric Cardiology and Cardiac Surgery: Irrational Hype or Paradigm Shift? *Ann. Pediatr. Cardiol.* **2019**, *12*, 191. [CrossRef] [PubMed]
65. Diller, G.P.; Orwat, S.; Vahle, J.; Bauer, U.M.M.; Urban, A.; Sarikouch, S.; Berger, F.; Beerbaum, P.; Baumgartner, H. Prediction of Prognosis in Patients with Tetralogy of Fallot Based on Deep Learning Imaging Analysis. *Heart* **2020**, *106*, 1007–1014. [CrossRef]
66. Zhang, G.; Mao, Y.; Li, M.; Peng, L.; Ling, Y.; Zhou, X. The Optimal Tetralogy of Fallot Repair Using Generative Adversarial Networks. *Front. Physiol.* **2021**, *12*, 613330. [CrossRef] [PubMed]
67. Asmare, M.H.; Woldehanna, F.; Janssens, L.; Vanrumste, B. Rheumatic Heart Disease Detection Using Deep Learning from Spectro-Temporal Representation of Un-Segmented Heart Sounds. In Proceedings of the 2020 42nd Annual International Conference of the IEEE Engineering in Medicine & Biology Society (EMBC), Montreal, QC, Canada, 20–24 July 2020; pp. 168–171.
68. Lakhe, A.; Sodhi, I.; Warrier, J.; Sinha, V. Development of Digital Stethoscope for Telemedicine. *J. Med. Eng. Technol.* **2016**, *40*, 20–24. [CrossRef]
69. Arafati, A.; Hu, P.; Finn, J.P.; Rickers, C.; Cheng, A.L.; Jafarkhani, H.; Kheradvar, A. Artificial Intelligence in Pediatric and Adult Congenital Cardiac MRI: An Unmet Clinical Need. *Cardiovasc. Diagn. Ther.* **2019**, *9*, S310–S325. [CrossRef] [PubMed]
70. Pyles, L.; Hemmati, P.; Pan, J.; Yu, X.; Liu, K.; Wang, J.; Tsakistos, A.; Zheleva, B.; Shao, W.; Ni, Q. Initial Field Test of a Cloud-Based Cardiac Auscultation System to Determine Murmur Etiology in Rural China. *Pediatr. Cardiol.* **2017**, *38*, 656–662. [CrossRef] [PubMed]
71. Andrisevic, N.; Ejaz, K.; Rios-Gutierrez, F.; Alba-Flores, R.; Nordehn, G.; Burns, S. Detection of Heart Murmurs Using Wavelet Analysis and Artificial Neural Networks. *J. Biomech. Eng.* **2005**, *127*, 899–904. [CrossRef]
72. El-Segaier, M.; Lilja, O.; Lukkarinen, S.; Sörnmo, L.; Sepponen, R.; Pesonen, E. Computer-Based Detection and Analysis of Heart Sound and Murmur. *Ann. Biomed. Eng.* **2005**, *33*, 937–942. [CrossRef] [PubMed]
73. Kang, S.; Doroshow, R.; McConnaughey, J.; Shekhar, R. Automated Identification of Innocent Still's Murmur in Children. *IEEE Trans. Biomed. Eng.* **2017**, *64*, 1326–1334. [CrossRef]
74. Garcia-Canadilla, P.; Sanchez-Martinez, S.; Crispi, F.; Bijnens, B. Machine Learning in Fetal Cardiology: What to Expect. *Fetal Diagn. Ther.* **2020**, *47*, 363–372. [CrossRef]
75. Hong, S.; Zhou, Y.; Shang, J.; Xiao, C.; Sun, J. Opportunities and Challenges of Deep Learning Methods for Electrocardiogram Data: A Systematic Review. *Comput. Biol. Med.* **2020**, *122*, 103801. [CrossRef] [PubMed]
76. Bodenhofer, U.; Haslinger-Eisterer, B.; Minichmayer, A.; Hermanutz, G.; Meier, J. Machine Learning-Based Risk Profile Classification of Patients Undergoing Elective Heart Valve Surgery. *Eur. J. Cardiothorac. Surg.* **2021**, *60*, 1378–1385. [CrossRef]
77. Gampala, S.; Vankeshwaram, V.; Gadula, S.S.P. Is Artificial Intelligence the New Friend for Radiologists? A Review Article. *Cureus* **2020**, *12*, e11137. [CrossRef]
78. van den Eynde, J.; Manlhiot, C.; van de Bruaene, A.; Diller, G.-P.; Frangi, A.F.; Budts, W.; Kutty, S. Medicine-Based Evidence in Congenital Heart Disease: How Artificial Intelligence Can Guide Treatment Decisions for Individual Patients. *Front. Cardiovasc. Med.* **2021**, *8*, 1792. [CrossRef]
79. Ma, M.; Li, Y.; Chen, R.; Huang, C.; Mao, Y.; Zhao, B. Diagnostic Performance of Fetal Intelligent Navigation Echocardiography (FINE) in Fetuses with Double-Outlet Right Ventricle (DORV). *Int. J. Cardiovasc. Imaging* **2020**, *36*, 2165–2172. [CrossRef] [PubMed]
80. Zeng, X.; Hu, Y.; Shu, L.; Li, J.; Duan, H.; Shu, Q.; Li, H. Explainable Machine-Learning Predictions for Complications after Pediatric Congenital Heart Surgery. *Sci. Rep.* **2021**, *11*, 17244. [CrossRef] [PubMed]
81. lo Muzio, F.P.; Rozzi, G.; Rossi, S.; Luciani, G.B.; Foresti, R.; Cabassi, A.; Fassina, L.; Miragoli, M. Artificial Intelligence Supports Decision Making during Open-Chest Surgery of Rare Congenital Heart Defects. *J. Clin. Med.* **2021**, *10*, 5330. [CrossRef]
82. Aufiero, S.; Bleijendaal, H.; Robyns, T.; Vandenberk, B.; Krijger, C.; Bezzina, C.; Zwinderman, A.H.; Wilde, A.A.M.; Pinto, Y.M. A Deep Learning Approach Identifies New ECG Features in Congenital Long QT Syndrome. *BMC Med.* **2022**, *20*, 162. [CrossRef] [PubMed]
83. Dias, R.D.; Shah, J.A.; Zenati, M.A. Artificial Intelligence in Cardiothoracic Surgery. *Minerva Cardioangiol.* **2020**, *68*, 532–538. [CrossRef] [PubMed]
84. Wang, T.; Liu, G.; Lin, H. A Machine Learning Approach to Predict Intravenous Immunoglobulin Resistance in Kawasaki Disease Patients: A Study Based on a Southeast China Population. *PLoS ONE* **2020**, *15*, e0237321. [CrossRef] [PubMed]

85. Martins, J.F.B.S.; Nascimento, E.R.; Nascimento, B.R.; Sable, C.A.; Beaton, A.Z.; Ribeiro, A.L.; Meira, W.; Pappa, G.L. Towards Automatic Diagnosis of Rheumatic Heart Disease on Echocardiographic Exams through Video-Based Deep Learning. *J. Am. Med. Inform. Assoc.* **2021**, *28*, 1834–1842. [CrossRef]
86. Ghosh, P.; Katkar, G.D.; Shimizu, C.; Kim, J.; Khandelwal, S.; Tremoulet, A.H.; Kanegaye, J.T.; Abe, N.; Austin-Page, L.; Bryl, A.; et al. An Artificial Intelligence-Guided Signature Reveals the Shared Host Immune Response in MIS-C and Kawasaki Disease. *Nat. Commun.* **2022**, *13*, 2687. [CrossRef] [PubMed]
87. Arnaout, R.; Curran, L.; Zhao, Y.; Levine, J.C.; Chinn, E.; Moon-Grady, A.J. An Ensemble of Neural Networks Provides Expert-Level Prenatal Detection of Complex Congenital Heart Disease. *Nat. Med.* **2021**, *27*, 882–891. [CrossRef] [PubMed]
88. Zuercher, M.; Ufkes, S.; Erdman, L.; Slorach, C.; Mertens, L.; Taylor, K. Retraining an Artificial Intelligence Algorithm to Calculate Left Ventricular Ejection Fraction in Pediatrics. *J. Cardiothorac. Vasc. Anesth.* **2022**, *36*, 3610–3616. [CrossRef]
89. Sepehri, A.A.; Hancq, J.; Dutoit, T.; Gharehbaghi, A.; Kocharian, A.; Kiani, A. Computerized Screening of Children Congenital Heart Diseases. *Comput. Methods Programs Biomed.* **2008**, *92*, 186–192. [CrossRef]
90. Ko, W.-Y.; Siontis, K.C.; Attia, Z.I.; Carter, R.E.; Kapa, S.; Ommen, S.R.; Demuth, S.J.; Ackerman, M.J.; Gersh, B.J.; Arruda-Olson, A.M.; et al. Detection of Hypertrophic Cardiomyopathy Using a Convolutional Neural Network-Enabled Electrocardiogram. *J. Am. Coll. Cardiol.* **2020**, *75*, 722–733. [CrossRef]
91. DeGroff, C.G.; Bhatikar, S.; Hertzberg, J.; Shandas, R.; Valdes-Cruz, L.; Mahajan, R.L. Artificial Neural Network–Based Method of Screening Heart Murmurs in Children. *Circulation* **2001**, *103*, 2711–2716. [CrossRef] [PubMed]
92. Na, J.Y.; Kim, D.; Kwon, A.M.; Jeon, J.Y.; Kim, H.; Kim, C.-R.; Lee, H.J.; Lee, J.; Park, H.-K. Artificial Intelligence Model Comparison for Risk Factor Analysis of Patent Ductus Arteriosus in Nationwide Very Low Birth Weight Infants Cohort. *Sci. Rep.* **2021**, *11*, 22353. [CrossRef]
93. Sepehri, A.A.; Gharehbaghi, A.; Dutoit, T.; Kocharian, A.; Kiani, A. A Novel Method for Pediatric Heart Sound Segmentation without Using the ECG. *Comput. Methods Programs Biomed.* **2010**, *99*, 43–48. [CrossRef]
94. Chou, F.-S.; Ghimire, L.V. Identification of Prognostic Factors for Pediatric Myocarditis with a Random Forests Algorithm-Assisted Approach. *Pediatr. Res.* **2021**, *90*, 427–430. [CrossRef] [PubMed]
95. Ali, F.; Hasan, B.; Ahmad, H.; Hoodbhoy, Z.; Bhuriwala, Z.; Hanif, M.; Ansari, S.U.; Chowdhury, D. Detection of Subclinical Rheumatic Heart Disease in Children Using a Deep Learning Algorithm on Digital Stethoscope: A Study Protocol. *BMJ Open* **2021**, *11*, e044070. [CrossRef]
96. Leng, S.; Tan, R.S.; Chai, K.T.C.; Wang, C.; Ghista, D.; Zhong, L. The Electronic Stethoscope. *Biomed. Eng. Online* **2015**, *14*, 66. [CrossRef]
97. Ma, X.-J.; Huang, G.-Y. Current Status of Screening, Diagnosis, and Treatment of Neonatal Congenital Heart Disease in China. *World J. Pediatr.* **2018**, *14*, 313–314. [CrossRef] [PubMed]
98. Ahmad, M.S.; Mir, J.; Ullah, M.O.; Shahid, M.L.U.R.; Syed, M.A. An Efficient Heart Murmur Recognition and Cardiovascular Disorders Classification System. *Australas. Phys. Eng. Sci. Med.* **2019**, *42*, 733–743. [CrossRef]
99. Ferguson, E.C.; Krishnamurthy, R.; Oldham, S.A.A. Classic Imaging Signs of Congenital Cardiovascular Abnormalities. *Radiographics* **2007**, *27*, 1323–1334. [CrossRef]
100. Sreedhar, C.; Ram, M.S.; Alam, A.; Indrajit, I. Cardiac MRI in Congenital Heart Disease—Our Experience. *Med. J. Armed Forces India* **2005**, *61*, 57–62. [CrossRef] [PubMed]
101. Garcia-Canadilla, P.; Isabel-Roquero, A.; Aurensanz-Clemente, E.; Valls-Esteve, A.; Miguel, F.A.; Ormazabal, D.; Llanos, F.; Sanchez-de-Toledo, J. Machine Learning-Based Systems for the Anticipation of Adverse Events after Pediatric Cardiac Surgery. *Front. Pediatr.* **2022**, *10*, 930913. [CrossRef]
102. Wilhelm, D.; Ostler, D.; Müller-Stich, B.; Lamadé, W.; Stier, A.; Feußner, H. Künstliche Intelligenz in Der Allgemein- Und Viszeralchirurgie. *Der Chir.* **2020**, *91*, 181–189. [CrossRef]
103. Xu, X.; Qiu, H.; Jia, Q.; Dong, Y.; Yao, Z.; Xie, W.; Guo, H.; Yuan, H.; Zhuang, J.; Huang, M.; et al. AI-CHD. *Commun. ACM* **2021**, *64*, 66–74. [CrossRef]
104. Mahayni, A.A.; Attia, Z.I.; Medina-Inojosa, J.R.; Elsisy, M.F.A.; Noseworthy, P.A.; Lopez-Jimenez, F.; Kapa, S.; Asirvatham, S.J.; Friedman, P.A.; Crestenallo, J.A.; et al. Electrocardiography-Based Artificial Intelligence Algorithm Aids in Prediction of Long-Term Mortality after Cardiac Surgery. *Mayo Clin. Proc.* **2021**, *96*, 3062–3070. [CrossRef] [PubMed]
105. Newburger, J.W.; Takahashi, M.; Burns, J.C. Kawasaki Disease. *J. Am. Coll. Cardiol.* **2016**, *67*, 1738–1749. [CrossRef] [PubMed]
106. Bayers, S.; Shulman, S.T.; Paller, A.S. Kawasaki Disease. *J. Am. Acad. Dermatol.* **2013**, *69*, 513.e1–513.e8. [CrossRef]
107. Santosh, K.C. AI-Driven Tools for Coronavirus Outbreak: Need of Active Learning and Cross-Population Train/Test Models on Multitudinal/Multimodal Data. *J. Med. Syst.* **2020**, *44*, 93. [CrossRef] [PubMed]
108. Benke, K.; Benke, G. Artificial Intelligence and Big Data in Public Health. *Int. J. Environ. Res. Public Health* **2018**, *15*, 2796. [CrossRef] [PubMed]
109. Mollura, D.J.; Culp, M.P.; Pollack, E.; Battino, G.; Scheel, J.R.; Mango, V.L.; Elahi, A.; Schweitzer, A.; Dako, F. Artificial Intelligence in Low- and Middle-Income Countries: Innovating Global Health Radiology. *Radiology* **2020**, *297*, 513–520. [CrossRef]
110. McCall, B. COVID-19 and Artificial Intelligence: Protecting Health-Care Workers and Curbing the Spread. *Lancet Digit. Health* **2020**, *2*, e166–e167. [CrossRef]

111. Malik, P.; Pathania, M.; Rathaur, V.K. Overview of Artificial Intelligence in Medicine. *J. Fam. Med. Prim. Care* **2019**, *8*, 2328–2331. [CrossRef]
112. Gerke, S.; Minssen, T.; Cohen, G. Ethical and Legal Challenges of Artificial Intelligence-Driven Healthcare. In *Artificial Intelligence in Healthcare*; Elsevier: Amsterdam, The Netherlands, 2020; pp. 295–336.

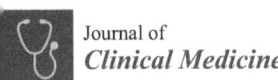

Article

Neuroimaging and Cerebrovascular Changes in Fetuses with Complex Congenital Heart Disease

Flaminia Vena [1,2,*], Lucia Manganaro [3], Valentina D'Ambrosio [1], Luisa Masciullo [1], Flavia Ventriglia [4], Giada Ercolani [3], Camilla Bertolini [5], Carlo Catalano [3], Daniele Di Mascio [1], Elena D'Alberti [1], Fabrizio Signore [6], Antonio Pizzuti [2] and Antonella Giancotti [1]

1. Department of Maternal and Child Health and Urological Sciences, Umberto I Hospital, Sapienza University of Rome, Viale del Policlinico 155, 00161 Rome, Italy
2. Department of Experimental Medicine, Umberto I Hospital, Sapienza University of Rome, Viale del Policlinico 155, 00161 Rome, Italy
3. Department of Radiological, Oncological and Pathological Sciences, Policlinico Umberto I, Sapienza University of Rome, Viale del Policlinico 155, 00161 Rome, Italy
4. Pediatric and Neonatology Unit, Maternal and Child Department, Sapienza University of Rome (Polo Pontino), 4100 Latina, Italy
5. Department of Radiology and Imaging Sciences, Santo Spirito Hospital, Lungotevere in Sassia 1, 00193 Rome, Italy
6. Obsetrics and Gynecology Department, USL Roma2, Sant'Eugenio Hospital, 00144 Rome, Italy
* Correspondence: flaminiavena89@gmail.com

Abstract: **Background:** Congenital heart diseases (CHDs) are often associated with significant neurocognitive impairment and neurological delay. This study aims to elucidate the correlation between type of CHD and Doppler velocimetry and to investigate the possible presence of fetal brain abnormalities identified by magnetic resonance imaging (MRI). **Methods:** From July 2010 to July 2020, we carried out a cross-sectional study of 63 singleton pregnancies with a diagnosis of different types of complex CHD: LSOL (left-sided obstructive lesions; RSOL (right-sided obstructive lesions) and MTC (mixed type of CHD). All patients underwent fetal echocardiography, ultrasound evaluation, a magnetic resonance of the fetal brain, and genetic counseling. **Results:** The analysis of 63 fetuses shows statistically significant results in Doppler velocimetry among the different CHD groups. The RSOL group leads to higher umbilical artery (UA-PI) pressure indexes values, whereas the LSOL group correlates with significantly lower values of the middle cerebral artery (MCA-PI) compared to the other subgroups ($p = 0.036$), whereas the RSOL group shows a tendency to higher pulsatility indexes in the umbilical artery (UA-PI). A significant correlation has been found between a reduced head circumference (HC) and the presence of brain injury at MRI ($p = 0.003$). **Conclusions:** Congenital left- and right-sided cardiac obstructive lesions are responsible for fetal hemodynamic changes and brain growth impairment. The correct evaluation of the central nervous system (CNS) in fetuses affected by CHD could be essential as prenatal screening and the prediction of postnatal abnormalities.

Keywords: congenital heart disease; brain abnormalities; Doppler velocimetry

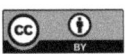

1. Introduction

Congenital heart diseases (CHDs) represent some of the most frequent fetal and neonatal abnormalities, which seem to affect 9 per 1000 live births [1]. These numbers may underestimate the real prevalence, which includes 20% of the spontaneous miscarriages and 10% of intrauterine demises [2]. CHD involves a huge variety of cardiovascular defects which could have a detrimental effect on neonatal and infant outcomes as well as a great impact on personal and family's quality of life [3]. An extensive body of evidence has already assessed an association between CHD and neurocognitive impairment, as a direct consequence of the postnatal cardiac surgery on brain development [4–6]. Interestingly, the use of neuroimaging techniques, such as magnetic resonance imaging (MRI) and functional-MRI (f-MRI), suggest the hypothesis of brain abnormalities even before birth [7–14].

Therefore, several authors have studied the hemodynamic changes in fetuses affected by various subtypes of CHD [15–20]: in particular, they evaluated the presence of hypoplastic left heart syndrome (HLHS) on the onset of cerebral abnormalities and cardiovascular changes. This CHD consists of an inadequate left cardiac output and a negligible flow into the ascending aorta [21]. This leads to a necessary redistribution of energetic substances, as a consequence of this impaired circulation [15–20]. This inadequate hemodynamic flow can severely compromise myelinization and growth of brain cells as well as its microstructure, leading to the risk of a white matter impairment [12,22].

Consequently, exploring the hemodynamic adaptation of CHD and the possible relationship between heart disease and neurological impairment becomes of paramount importance.

Therefore, the primary aim of this study is to detect potential correlations between the type of CHD and changes in Doppler velocimetry. The secondary aim is to investigate the presence of central nervous system (CNS) abnormalities in fetuses affected by complex CHD.

2. Materials and Methods

From July 2010 to July 2020, a cross-sectional study was carried out, recruiting pregnant women referred for fetal echocardiography. The inclusion criteria required a diagnosis of one of the following complex CHD:

1. LSOL (left-sided obstructive lesions): HLHS, aortic stenosis, aortic arch hypoplasia or coarctation.
2. RSOL (right-sided obstructive lesions): pulmonary atresia, tetralogy of Fallot, Ebstein's anomaly, Tricuspid atresia, pulmonary stenosis.
3. MTC (mixed type of CHD): double outlet right ventricle without pulmonary stenosis, single ventricle, truncus arteriosus, transposition of great arteries.
4. Others (e.g., cardiomyopathy, tumors).

Exclusion criteria included (1) gestational age less than 20 weeks or greater than 40 weeks, (2) cardiac lesion other than the ones listed in the inclusion criteria, (3) age less than 18 years (4) persistent non-sinus rhythm, (5) fetal anemia (6) maternal condition that might affect fetal hemodynamics, such as fetal growth restriction, gestational diabetes, thyroid disease, or pre-eclampsia, (7) presence of any kind of extracardiac anomalies or neurologic malformations detectable with US, MRI and invasive procedures such as amniocentesis, (8) monochorionic twins and (9) chromosomal and sub-chromosomal anomalies, analyzing amniotic fluid samples.

All patients included in the study group as part of a research protocol underwent:

1. Fetal echocardiography;
2. Ultrasound evaluation;
3. MRI of fetal brain;
4. Genetic counseling;
5. Amniocentesis.

2.1. Fetal Echocardiography

Fetal echocardiography was conducted according to the International Society of Ultrasound in Obstetrics and Gynecology guideline [23] using a WS80A Elite scanner (Samsung Electronics, Seoul, South Korea) equipped with a 6 MHz curvilinear transducer.

Second-level echocardiography was performed in all fetuses following the sequential and systematic approach of heart evaluation. Multiple two-dimensional views were obtained to evaluate fetal heart anatomy. Doppler flow was employed to evaluate valve competence, stenosis, and shunting. M-mode was used to assess the cardiac rhythm. Doppler color flow mapping was used to identify the umbilical vessels; subsequently, a reduced color scale was used to identify the circle of Willis and the middle cerebral artery (MCA). All the CHD prenatally diagnosed were confirmed with an echocardiography performed postnatally.

2.2. Ultrasound Evaluation

All ultrasound evaluations were performed with a Voluson 730 Expert GE or Samsung Elite WS80A machine. Two full-time certified sonographers (F.V., A.G.) performed all the ultrasound scans. A first-trimester evaluation assessed the exact gestational age using the last menstrual period or fetal crown–rump length (CRL) [24].

The following fetal biometric parameters were analyzed: biparietal diameter (BPD), head circumference (HC), abdominal circumference (AC) and femoral length (FL). Estimated fetal weight (EFW) was calculated according to the method of Hadlock et al. [24,25]; both estimated fetal weight and birth weight centile were obtained using local reference curves [26].

IUGR was defined as birth weight (BW) below the 10th percentile for gestational age or estimated fetal weight or abdominal circumference below the 5th percentile at the mid-trimester anomaly scan, in presence of maternal and/or fetal Doppler anomalies [27]. Conversely, a fetus was detected as small for gestational age if the EFW or AC were below the 10th percentile, according to gestational age, or if the Z-score was below 2 [28].

Pulsed-wave Doppler was used to determine blood flow velocities in the umbilical artery (UA) and MCA. The peak systolic velocity, peak diastolic velocity and mean velocity were measured from stable signals during fetal apnea. The pulsatility index (PI) is a measure of vascular resistance in the circulatory bed downstream from the point of Doppler sampling. It is calculated according to the relationship: PI = (systolic velocity − diastolic velocity)/mean velocity. The MCA-PI to UA-PI ratio was labeled as the cerebroplacental (CPR) ratio [29,30].

2.3. Magnetic Resonance Imaging

MRI examinations were acquired using a 1.5 T Magnet (Siemens Magnetom Avanto, Erlangen Germany) without maternal–fetal sedation with one or two surface coil phased arrays.

The study protocol included the following sequences with the multiplanar acquisition (axial, coronal, sagittal) [31]:

- T2-weighted HASTE: repetition time (TR) 1500 ms, echo time (TE) 151 ms; slices of 3 mm; FOV 260 × 350 mm; 256 × 256 matrices; time of acquisition (TA) 20 s.
- T1-weighted FLASH 2D: TR 362 ms; TE 4.8 ms; slices 5.5 mm; flip angle 70°; FOV 350 × 300 mm; 256 × 192 matrices; TA 25 to 30 s with and [29] without fat saturation.
- Diffusion weighted imaging: TR 8000 ms; TE 90 ms; inversion time 185 ms; slices of 5 mm; FOV 420 × 300 mm; 192 × 192 matrix; TA 45 s; 3 b-factor per floor: 0.200 and 700 mm^2/s.

The following parameters were evaluated: biometry (Fronto-Occipital Diameter, cerebral biparietal diameter (BPD), Transverse Cerebellar Diameter, height of the vermis, Antero-Posterior Diameter of the vermis and length of Corpus callosum), ventriculomegaly (VM), gyration, and signal intensity.

2.4. Genetic Counseling

Genetic counseling was proposed to all the couples in presence of CHD. Amniocentesis for karyotype and CGH-array was proposed in all CHD cases; fetuses showing chromosomal and copy number variations (CNV) were excluded from the conducted analysis.

2.5. Statistical Analysis

The statistical analysis was performed using the Statistical Product and Service Solutions software (SPSS) version 20 for Windows (SPSS Inc., Chicago, IL, USA). Descriptive analyses were presented as frequency with percentage, mean and standard deviation for all variables considered.

We converted the PI measurements into Z-scores using published normative data from a cohort of 72,387 healthy fetuses from the Fetal Medicine Foundation database (https://fetalmedicine.org, accessed on 21 March 2022) [20,32]. In this way, the conducted analyses turn out to be independent of the gestational age. A Z-score equal to 0 refers to the mean of the normal data and a Z-score equal to ±1 and ±2 is at 1 and 2 SDs from the mean, respectively.

Doppler indices were compared between diagnostic groups using one-way ANOVA to determine differences between two groups. Chi-square test and t-test were used for intergroup correlations. p-values < 0.05 were considered statistically significant.

2.6. Ethical Approval

The study was approved by the Institutional Review Board of the Department of Maternal and Child Health and Uro-gynecological Sciences, Sapienza, University of Rome, Policlinico Umberto I, Italy (Report No.: 45/2010) as a quality improvement study with anonymized data. All the patients provided a written informed consent form, and all the followed procedures were in line with the Helsinki declaration's principles of 1975, as revised in 2000.

3. Results

During the study period, 170 individual fetuses suspected of CHD were evaluated by echocardiography. In 143 fetuses, CHD was confirmed. Eighty fetuses were excluded for: gestational age less than 20 weeks (n = 3), extracardiac anomalies (n = 29), chromosomal anomalies (n = 33), non-sinus rhythm (n = 5), maternal condition (n = 8), and monochorionic twins (n = 1; 2 pairs). In particular 120/143 (83%) underwent amniocentesis and a chromosomal anomaly was found in 27% of cases. Sixty-three fetuses were finally included for the analysis and evaluated between 19 and 38 weeks. The specific CHD diagnoses and the mean gestational ages at the time of the fetal echocardiogram are listed in Table 1.

Table 1. Descriptive analysis of main patients' characteristics using mean and standard deviation (SD) or n (%).

Main Sample's Characteristics	Mean ± SD
Age (years)	33.6 (5.3)
Gestational age at evaluation (weeks)	31.7 (5.4)
Type of CHD	n (%)
LSOL	11 (17.5)
RSOL	6 (9.5)
MTC	26 (41.3)
Others	20 (31.7)

LSOL: left-sided obstructive lesions; RSOL: right-sided obstructive lesions; MTC: mixed type of CHD.

3.1. Cerebroplacental Doppler Data

Doppler values were obtained in 46/63 cases. The mean PI Z-scores for the UA and MCA and the mean CPR ratio Z-scores are shown in Table 2.

We did not observe a significant difference in the UA-PI values (p = 0.07), even with regard to the RSOL group, which had a higher UA-PI than the other groups. We found a significant difference in the MCA-PI (p = 0.036) values among all groups considered, with the LSOL group having a lower MCA-PI than the other ones. We did not observe statistically significant differences in the CPR values among all groups considered (p = 0.4343505). We observed a significant reduction in HC measures, as LSOL was associated with lower values.

Table 2. One-way ANOVA Kruskal–Wallis Test using the z-scores of the variables analyzed, according to different types of CHD. CHD: congenital heart disease, HC: head circumference; UA-PI: pulsatility index of umbilical artery; MCA-PI: pulsatility index of middle cerebral artery; CPR: cerebroplacental ratio; LSOL: left-sided obstructive lesions; RSOL: right-sided obstructive lesions; MTC: mixed type of CHD.

US Variables	LSOL Median (IQRSD)	RSOL Median (IQR) m SD	MTC Median (IQR) m SD	OTHERS Median (IQR) m SD	p-Value
UA-PI	0.38 (2.29)	0.87 (1.88)	−0.28 (2.09)	0.15 (1.50)	0.4076
MCA-PI	−0.78 (1.88)	0.93 (1.68)	−0.33 (1.20)	0.34 (1.24)	**0.036**
CPR	−1.28 (1.66)	−0.26 (1.42)	−0.43 (1.73)	−0.08 (1.32)	0.4343
HC	−1.36 (0.89)	−0.4 (0.80)	−0.81 (0.45)	−0.96 (1.00)	**0.0182**

3.2. Brain Abnormalities

MRI was performed in all fetuses. It was found that 36/63 (57.1%) fetuses had signs of brain abnormalities at MRI and in 27/63 (42.9%) brain MRI was normal. Brain alterations are listed in Table 3. Corpus callosum (CC) abnormalities and ventriculomegaly (VM) were present, respectively, in 16/36 (25.4%) and 13/36 (20.6%) of fetuses. We stratified the analysis according to the single groups of CHD (Table 3): most of the cases of brain abnormalities were detected in the MTC and Others groups.

Table 3. Frequencies of brain abnormalities according to the different types of CHD, using number (n) and percentage (%). CHD: congenital heart disease; LSOL: left-sided obstructive lesions; RSOL: right-sided obstructive lesions; MTC: mixed type of CHD.

Fetal Brain Abnormalities	LSOL n (%)	RSOL n (%)	MTC n (%)	OTHERS n (%)	TOTAL n (%)
Supratentorial diameter	0	1 (11.1)	5 (55.6)	3 (33.3)	9 (14.3)
Subtentorial diameter	3 (37.5)	1 (12.5)	4 (50)	0	8 (12.7)
Corpus callosum	5 (31.3)	0	6 (37.5)	5 (31.2)	16 (25.4)
Subarachnoid spaces	0	1 (12.5)	4 (50)	3 (37.5)	8 (12.7)
Gyrification abnormalities	2 (22.2)	3 (33.4)	4 (44.4)	0	9 (14.3)
Ventriculomegaly	3 (23)	0	6 (46.2)	4 (30.8)	13 (20.6)

We found a significant correlation between the reduced HC and the presence of brain alterations at MRI ($p = 0.003$). Conversely, we did not achieve statistical significance evaluating the correlation between the detection of brain anomalies and UA-PI, MCA-PI, and CPR values (Table 4).

Table 4. Correlations among US descriptors and the presence of brain injury at MRI, using mean (m) and standard deviation (SD). US: ultrasound; MRI: magnetic resonance imaging; CNS: central nervous system; HC: head circumference; UA-PI: pulsatility index of umbilical artery; MCA-PI: pulsatility index of middle cerebral artery; CPR: cerebroplacental ratio.

US Descriptors	No CNS Abnormalities m (SD)	CNS Abnormalities m (SD)	p-Value
HC	307.8 (44)	264 (49.5)	0.003
UA-PI	0.9 (0.18)	1.07 (0.24)	0.15
MCA-PI	1.78 (0.32)	1.72 (0.33)	0.59
CPR	1.88 (0.44)	1.67 (0.47)	0.13

4. Discussion

This study investigates the relationship between the fetal cerebrovascular hemodynamic changes and the presence of CNS abnormalities in fetuses affected by CHD. We have observed that RSOL and LSOL CHD might cause a considerable change in Doppler velocimetry: in our LSOL group, 6/11 (54.5%) fetuses had an HLHS and the analysis of their Dopplers showed low MCA-PI values ($p = 0.036$). Different studies reported the same trend but without significant difference [20,33]. Kaltman et al. [20] also found that only fetuses with HLHS had a lower PIMCA ($p = 0.001$): this result might be attributed to the severity of obstructive lesions of fetuses with LSOL, which was inversely proportional to the amount of cerebral blood delivery. Interestingly, the use of Z-score index was able to completely remove the affect related to gender and gestational age, providing more comparable results.

We also observed registered a tendency to higher elevated UA-PI in fetuses with RSOL ($p = 0.027$), whereas in a previous study, Kaltman et al. reported a similar finding in their study, despite a significant elevation of UA-PI only in fetuses with severe RSOL. This could be related to the severe obstruction of the outflow tracts which could impair the diastolic blood flow in the UA, elevating UA-PI [20].

Evaluating the impaired hemodynamic flow that affected IUGR fetuses instead of SG, we decided to exclude IUGR fetuses from our analysis, because of the possible bias in Doppler velocimetry's assessment that might intrinsically affect and compromise its course [29]. Evaluating the CPR values, we did not find any statistically significant difference among the CHD subgroups, except for a tendency of lower CPR values in fetuses with LSOL, compared to the other CHD types. Therefore, this could be explained by the assumption that an obstruction of the left outflow tract might impact downstream pulsatility. In light of the above, the use of CPR as an indication of the brain-sparing effect may be inappropriate in the setting of CHD.

The type of CHD contributes to a blood flow distribution, resulting in devastating effects on neurological development [34,35]. In our study, we have found a significant correlation between reduced HC and the presence of brain alterations at MRI: this is in line with the scientific literature which showed a reduction in frontal brain area of fetuses with CHD with neurodevelopmental delay (NDD), in comparison with normal controls [15–17,36–39]. The exclusion of IUGR fetuses from our study allows us to demonstrate that, in fetuses with CHD, the reduced HC is mainly due to hemodynamic alterations. The etiology of the neurological delay is likely to be complex and multifactorial: some attributed it as a complication of surgery; conversely, it has been already well-established that pre- and peri-operative risk factors account for roughly 30% of poor neuro-developmental outcomes [40,41]. A systematic review examined the prevalence of prenatal brain abnormalities in fetuses with CHD [42]: three studies reported a 28% rate of structural brain abnormalities in fetuses with CHD, including abnormalities in brain's structure, volume and blood flow. In our study we did not find any statistically significant correlation between the CNS morphological alterations and the type of CHD. The lack of statistically significant data could be related to the limited sample size of LSOL and RSOL subgroups.

Our statistical data analysis showed that up to 57% of fetuses with CHD had brain abnormalities; particularly in the groups of LSOL (63%) and Others (70%). The most frequent alteration was observed in the corpus callosum size, usually related to fetal biometry. This finding was also reported by Ng et al. who carried out a study using tensor-based morphometry: they found a high rate of brain's volume alteration in infants with CHD compared to healthy control infants. They detected different development in gray, white matter and corpus callosum size, without establishing a direct correlation between the CHD subtype and the morphologic abnormalities. It seems that the regional brain involvement could be related to different oxygen demand and cerebral hemodynamic changes that affected CHD samples [43].

The international guidelines allow the MRI brain evaluation only in fetuses affected by HLHS, despite the consolidated literature evidence of brain abnormalities present in more than 1/3 of CHD fetuses [44,45].

This research represents one of the few studies in the literature which investigate the hemodynamical changes and brain abnormalities in fetuses with complex CHD using two different imaging techniques: US and MRI. Our results confirm the advantages of performing fetal brain MRI in fetuses with complex CHD to characterize and manage the structural and hemodynamic brain modifications even before birth.

Conversely, there are few limitations: first, the relatively small number of cases for the single complex CHD categories, which has prevented a detailed analysis by a single type of CHD. Second, we did not include a control group and specific gestation windows to compare the Doppler velocimetry indexes; this limitation is partially overcome with the use of Z-scores, which allows us to view our data in the context of previously published normal values. The mean MCA-PI Z-scores for the LSOL and RSOL groups were -0.75 and 0.89, respectively. While these values are within the range of normal (within a Z-score range of ± 2), they suggest a deviation from the mean of the normal population. In addition, outcome data, such as HC, birth weight, and the MRI scans of the brain at birth, were not obtained due to our inability to follow the antenatal and postnatal progress of these fetuses.

5. Conclusions

Our data seem to support that complex CHD impairs the growth of the central nervous system. Left and right-sided cardiac obstructive lesions modify the fetal cerebrovascular resistance. We demonstrated that MCA-PI is lower in fetuses with LSOL, and, according to previous study, we registered higher UA-PI in fetuses with RSOL even if not statistically significant, due to the smaller sample of RSOL group than the other groups. Furthermore, we did not find any statistically significant correlation between the CNS morphological alterations and the type of CHD, but we underline the importance of the study of the fetal brain when a cardiac abnormality is present. Alterations in cerebrovascular blood flow distribution may be associated with the postnatal, neurological abnormalities found in some newborns with complex CHD. Results of the multicenter international children NEUROHEART ongoing study will compare and describe preoperative markers on CHD-affected fetuses in prenatal as well as postnatal brain functional monitoring.

Author Contributions: Conceptualization, F.V. (Flaminia Vena); data curation, L.M. (Lucia Manganaro) and E.D.; investigation, V.D. and L.M. (Luisa Masciullo); methodology, G.E.; supervision, C.C.; validation, F.V. (Flavia Ventriglia) and A.P.; writing—original draft, C.B. and D.D.M.; writing—review & editing, F.S. and A.G. All authors have read and agreed to the published version of the manuscript.

Funding: This research received no external funding.

Institutional Review Board Statement: The study was approved by the Institutional Review Board of the Department of Maternal and Child Health and Uro-gynecological Sciences, Sapienza, University of Rome, Policlinico Umberto I, Italy (Report No.: 45/2010) as a quality improvement study with anonymized data. All the followed procedures were in line with the Helsinki declaration's principles of 1975, as revised in 2000.

Informed Consent Statement: Written informed consent was obtained from all subjects involved in the study.

Data Availability Statement: Not applicable.

Conflicts of Interest: The authors declare no conflict of interest.

References

1. Goldmuntz, E. The epidemiology and genetics of congenital heart disease. *Clin. Perinatol.* **2001**, *28*, 1–10. [CrossRef]
2. Botto, L.D.; Correa, A.; Erickson, J.D. Racial and temporal variations in the prevalence of heart defects. *Pediatrics*. **2001**, *107*, E32 [CrossRef] [PubMed]
3. Majnemer, A.; Shevell, M.; Law, M.; Poulin, C.; Rosenbaum, P. Reliability in the ratings of quality of life between parents and their children of school age with cerebral palsy. *Qual. Life Res.* **2008**, *17*, 1163–1171. [CrossRef] [PubMed]
4. Newburger, J.W.; Jonas, R.A.; Wernovsky, G.; Wypij, D.; Hickey, P.R.; Kuban, K.C.; Farrell, D.M.; Holmes, G.L.; Helmers, S.L.; Constantinou, J.; et al. A comparison of the perioperative neurologic effects of hypothermic circulatory arrest versus low-flow cardiopulmonary bypass in infant heart surgery. *N. Engl. J. Med.* **1993**, *329*, 1057–1064. [CrossRef]
5. O'Hare, B.; Bissonnette, B.; Bohn, D.; Cox, P.; Williams, W. Persistent low cerebral blood flow velocity following profound hypothermic circulatory arrest in infants. *Can. J. Anaesth.* **1995**, *42*, 964–971. [CrossRef]
6. Ferry, P.C. Neurologic sequelae of open-heart surgery in children. An 'irritating question'. *Am. J. Dis. Child.* **1990**, *144*, 369–373. [CrossRef]
7. Ortinau, C.; Beca, J.; Lambeth, J.; Ferdman, B.; Alexopoulos, D.; Shimony, J.S.; Wallendorf, M.; Neil, J.; Inder, T. Regional alterations in cerebral growth exist preoperatively in infants with congenital heart disease. *J. Thorac. Cardiovasc. Surg.* **2012**, *143*, 1264–1270. [CrossRef]
8. Limperopoulos, C.; Majnemer, A.; Shevell, M.I.; Rosenblatt, B.; Rohlicek, C.; Tchervenkov, C. Neurologic status of newborns with congenital heart defects before open heart surgery. *Pediatrics* **1999**, *103*, 402–408. [CrossRef]
9. Limperopoulos, C.; Majnemer, A.; Shevell, M.I.; Rosenblatt, B.; Rohlicek, C.; Tchervenkov, C. Neurodevelopmental status of newborns and infants with congenital heart defects before and after open heart surgery. *J. Pediatr.* **2000**, *137*, 638–645. [CrossRef]
10. Beca, J.; Gunn, J.; Coleman, L.; Hope, A.; Whelan, L.-C.; Gentles, T.; Inder, T.; Hunt, R.; Shekerdemian, L. Pre-operative brain injury in newborn infants with transposition of the great arteries occurs at rates similar to other complex congenital heart disease and is not related to balloon atrial septostomy. *J. Am. Coll. Cardiol.* **2009**, *53*, 1807–1811. [CrossRef]
11. Andropoulos, D.B.; Hunter, J.V.; Nelson, D.P.; Stayer, S.A.; Stark, A.R.; McKenzie, E.D.; Jeffrey, S.H.; Daniel, E.G.; Charles, D.F., Jr Brain immaturity is associated with brain injury before and after neonatal cardiac surgery with high-flow bypass and cerebral oxygenation monitoring. *J. Thorac. Cardiovasc. Surg.* **2010**, *139*, 543–556. [CrossRef]
12. Miller, S.P.; McQuillen, P.S.; Vigneron, D.B.; Glidden, D.V.; Barkovich, A.J.; Ferriero, D.M.; Harmic, E.G.S.; Azakie, A.; Karl, R.T. Preoperative brain injury in newborns with transposition of the great arteries. *Ann. Thorac. Surg.* **2004**, *77*, 1698–1706. [CrossRef]
13. Owen, M.; Shevell, M.; Majnemer, A.; Limperopoulos, C. Abnormal Brain Structure and Function in Newborns with Complex Congenital Heart Defects Before Open Heart Surgery: A Review of the Evidence. *J. Child. Neurol.* **2011**, *26*, 743–755. [CrossRef]
14. Khalil, A.; Suff, N.; Thilaganathan, B.; Hurrell, A.; Cooper, D.; Carvalho, J.S. Brain abnormalities and neurodevelopmental delay in congenital heart disease: Systematic review and meta-analysis. *Ultrasound Obstet. Gynecol.* **2014**, *43*, 14–24. [CrossRef]
15. Donofrio, M.T.; Bremer, Y.A.; Schieken, R.M.; Gennings, C.; Morton, L.D.; Eidem, B.W.; Cetta, F.; Falkensammer, C.B.; Hihta, J.C.; Kleinman, C.S. Autoregulation of cerebral blood flow in fetuses with congenital heart disease: The brain sparing effect. *Pediatr Cardiol.* **2003**, *24*, 436–443. [CrossRef]
16. Kinnear, C.; Haranal, M.; Shannon, P.; Jaeggi, E.; Chitayat, D.; Mital, S. Abnormal fetal cerebral and vascular development in hypoplastic left heart syndrome. *Prenat. Diagn.* **2019**, *39*, 38–44. [CrossRef]
17. Clouchoux, C.; du Plessis, A.J.; Bouyssi-Kobar, M.; Tworetzky, W.; McElhinney, D.B.; Brown, D.W.; Ghoulipour, A.; Kudelski, D.; Warfield, S.K.; McCarter, R.J.; et al. Delayed cortical development in fetuses with complex congenital heart disease. *Cereb. Cortex.* **2013**, *23*, 2932–2943. [CrossRef]
18. Meise, C.; Germer, U.; Gembruch, U. Arterial Doppler ultrasound in 115 second- and third-trimester fetuses with congenital heart disease. *Ultrasound Obstet. Gynecol.* **2001**, *17*, 398–402. [CrossRef]
19. Mahle, W.T.; Tavani, F.; Zimmerman, R.A.; Nicolson, S.C.; Galli, K.K.; Gaynor, J.W.; Clancy, R.R.; Montenegro, M.L.; Spray, T.L.; Chiavacci, R.M.; et al. An MRI study of neurological injury before and after congenital heart surgery. *Circulation* **2002**, *106* (Suppl. S1), 109–114. [CrossRef]
20. Kaltman, J.R.; Di, H.; Tian, Z.; Rychik, J. Impact of congenital heart disease on cerebrovascular blood flow dynamics in the fetus. *Ultrasound Obstet. Gynecol.* **2005**, *25*, 32–36. [CrossRef]
21. McQuillen, P.S.; Miller, S.P. Congenital heart disease and brain development. *Ann. N. Y. Acad. Sci.* **2010**, *1184*, 68–86. [CrossRef] [PubMed]
22. Peyvandi, S.; Lim, J.M.; Marini, D.; Xu, D.; Reddy, V.M.; Barkovich, A.J.; Miller, S.; McQuillen, P.; Seed, M. Fetal brain growth and risk of postnatal white matter injury in critical congenital heart disease. *J. Thorac. Cardiovasc. Surg.* **2021**, *162*, 1007–1014.e1. [CrossRef] [PubMed]
23. International Society of Ultrasound in Obstetrics and Gynecology; Carvalho, J.S.; Allan, D.; Chaoui, R.; Copel, J.; DeVore, G.R.; Hecher, K.; Lee, W.; Munoz, H.; Paladini, D.; et al. ISUOG Practice Guidelines (updated): Sonographic screening examination of the fetal heart. *Ultrasound Obstet. Gynecol.* **2013**, *41*, 348–359. [CrossRef] [PubMed]
24. Robinson, H.P.; Sweet, E.M.; Adam, A.H. The accuracy of radiological estimates of gestational age using early fetal crown-rump length measurements by ultrasound as a basis for comparison. *Br. J. Obstet. Gynaecol.* **1979**, *86*, 525–528. [CrossRef] [PubMed]
25. Hadlock, F.P.; Harrist, R.B.; Sharman, R.S.; Deter, R.L.; Park, S.K. Estimation of fetal weight with the use of head, body, and femur measurements–a prospective study. *Am. J. Obstet. Gynecol.* **1985**, *151*, 333–337. [CrossRef]

26. Hadlock, F.P.; Harrist, R.B.; Shah, Y.P.; King, D.E.; Park, S.K.; Sharman, R.S. Estimating fetal age using multiple parameters: A prospective evaluation in a racially mixed population. *Am. J. Obstet. Gynecol.* **1987**, *156*, 955–957. [CrossRef]
27. D'Ambrosio, V.; Vena, F.; Boccherini, C.; Di Mascio, D.; Squarcella, A.; Corno, S.; Pajno, C.; Pizzuti, A.; Piccioni, M.G.; Brunelli, R.; et al. Obstetrical and perinatal outcomes in fetuses with early versus late sonographic diagnosis of short femur length: A single-center, prospective, cohort study. *Eur. J. Obstet. Gynecol. Reprod. Biol.* **2020**, *254*, 170–174. [CrossRef]
28. Lees, C.C.; Stampalija, T.; Baschat, A.; da Silva Costa, F.; Ferrazzi, E.; Figueras, F.; Hecher, K.; Kingdom, J.; Poon, L.C.; Unterschider, J. SUOG Practice Guidelines: Diagnosis and management of small-for-gestational-age fetus and fetal growth restriction. *Ultrasound Obstet. Gynecol.* **2020**, *56*, 298–312. [CrossRef]
29. Wladimiroff, J.W.; Tonge, H.M.; Stewart, P.A. Doppler ultrasound assessment of cerebral blood flow in the human fetus. *Br. J. Obstet. Gynaecol.* **1986**, *93*, 471–475. [CrossRef]
30. Gramellini, D.; Folli, M.C.; Raboni, S.; Vadora, E.; Merialdi, A. Cerebral-umbilical Doppler ratio as a predictor of adverse perinatal outcome. *Obstet. Gynecol.* **1992**, *79*, 416–420. [CrossRef]
31. Manganaro, L.; Bernardo, S.; Antonelli, A.; Vinci, V.; Saldari, M.; Catalano, C. Fetal MRI of the central nervous system: State-of-the-art. *Eur. J. Radiol.* **2017**, *93*, 273–283. [CrossRef]
32. The Fetal Medicine Foundation. Available online: https://fetalmedicine.org (accessed on 22 November 2020).
33. Guorong, L.; Shaohui, L.; Peng, J.; Huitong, L.; Boyi, L.; Wanhong, X.; Liya, L. Cerebrovascular blood flow dynamic changes in fetuses with congenital heart disease. *Fetal Diagn. Ther.* **2009**, *25*, 167–172. [CrossRef]
34. Habek, D.; Hodek, B.; Herman, R.; Jugović, D.; Cerkez Habek, J.; Salihagić, A. Fetal biophysical profile and cerebro-umbilical ratio in assessment of perinatal outcome in growth-restricted fetuses. *Fetal Diagn. Ther.* **2003**, *18*, 12–16. [CrossRef]
35. Limperopoulos, C.; Tworetzky, W.; McElhinney, D.B.; Newburger, J.W.; Brown, D.W.; Robertson, R.L., Jr.; Guizard, N.; McGrath, E.; Geva, J.; Annese, D.; et al. Brain volume and metabolism in fetuses with congenital heart disease: Evaluation with quantitative magnetic resonance imaging and spectroscopy. *Circulation* **2010**, *121*, 26–33. [CrossRef]
36. Paladini, D.; Finarelli, A.; Donarini, G.; Parodi, S.; Lombardo, V.; Tuo, G.; Birnbaum, R. Frontal lobe growth is impaired in fetuses with congenital heart disease. *Ultrasound Obstet. Gynecol.* **2021**, *57*, 776–782. [CrossRef]
37. Masoller, N.; Sanz-Corté, S.M.; Crispi, F.; Gómez, O.; Bennasar, M.; Egaña-Ugrinovic, G.; Bargallo, N.; Martinez, J.M.; Gratacos, E. Mid-gestation brain Doppler and head biometry in fetuses with congenital heart disease predict abnormal brain development at birth. *Ultrasound Obstet. Gynecol.* **2016**, *47*, 65–73. [CrossRef]
38. Zeng, S.; Zhou, Q.C.; Zhou, J.W.; Li, M.; Long, C.; Peng, Q.H. Volume of intracranial structures on three-dimensional ultrasound in fetuses with congenital heart disease. *Ultrasound Obstet. Gynecol.* **2015**, *46*, 174–181. [CrossRef]
39. Peyvandi, S.; Kim, H.; Lau, J.; Barkovich, A.J.; Campbell, A.; Miller, S.; Xu, D.; McQuillen, P. The association between cardiac physiology, acquired brain injury, and postnatal brain growth in critical congenital heart disease. *J. Thorac. Cardiovasc. Surg.* **2018**, *155*, 291–300.e3. [CrossRef]
40. Marino, B.S.; Lipkin, P.H.; Newburger, J.W.; Peacock, G.; Gerdes, M.; Gaynor, J.W.; Mussatto, K.A.; Uzark, K.; Goldberg, C.S.; Johnson, W.H.; et al. American Heart Association Congenital Heart Defects Committee, Council on Cardiovascular Disease in the Young, Council on Cardiovascular Nursing, and Stroke Council. Neurodevelopmental outcomes in children with congenital heart disease: Evaluation and management: A scientific statement from the American Heart Association. *Circulation* **2012**, *126*, 1143–1172.
41. Seed, M. In utero brain development in fetuses with congenital heart disease: Another piece of the jigsaw provided by Blood Oxygen Level-Dependent Magnetic Resonance Imaging. *Circ Cardiovasc Imaging* **2017**, *10*, e007181. [CrossRef]
42. Khalil, A.; Bennet, S.; Thilaganathan, B.; Paladini, D.; Griffiths, P.; Carvalho, J.S. Prevalence of prenatal brain abnormalities in fetuses with congenital heart disease: A systematic review. *Ultrasound Obstet. Gynecol.* **2016**, *48*, 296–307. [CrossRef] [PubMed]
43. Ng, I.H.X.; Bonthrone, A.F.; Kelly, C.J.; Cordero-Grande, L.; Hughes, E.J.; Price, A.N.; Hutter, J.; Victor, S.; Schuh, A.; Rueckert, D.; et al. Investigating altered brain development in infants with congenital heart disease using tensor-based morphometry. *Sci. Rep.* **2020**, *10*, 14909. [CrossRef] [PubMed]
44. Paladini, D.; Alfirevic, Z.; Carvalho, J.S.; Khalil, A.; Malinger, G.; Martinez, J.M.; Rychik, J.; Ville, Y.; Gardiner, H.; ISUOG Clinical Standards Commite. ISUOG consensus statement on current understanding of the association of neurodevelopmental delay and congenital heart disease: Impact on prenatal counseling. *Ultrasound Obstet. Gynecol.* **2017**, *49*, 287–288. [CrossRef] [PubMed]
45. Vena, F.; Donarini, D.; Scala, C.; Tuo, G.; Paladini, D. Redundancy of foramen ovale flap may mimic fetal aortic coarctation. *Ultrasound Obstet. Gynecol.* **2020**, *56*, 857–863. [CrossRef]

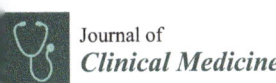

Article

Detection of Coronary Artery and Aortic Arch Anomalies in Patients with Tetralogy of Fallot Using CT Angiography

Zsófia Kakucs [1,*], Erhard Heidenhoffer [2,*] and Marian Pop [3,4]

1. Mures County Clinical Emergency Hospital, 540136 Targu Mures, Romania
2. Clinical County Hospital Mures, 540103 Targu Mures, Romania
3. ME1 Department, "George Emil Palade" University of Medicine, Pharmacy, Science and Technology of Targu Mures, 540142 Targu Mures, Romania
4. Emergency Institute for Cardiovascular Disease and Transplant of Targu Mures, 540136 Targu Mures, Romania
* Correspondence: kakucs_zsofia@yahoo.com (Z.K.); heiden.erhard@gmail.com (E.H.)

Abstract: Background: Tetralogy of Fallot (TOF) is the most common form of cyanotic congenital heart disease (CHD). Furthermore, the prevalence of anomalous origin of a coronary artery is higher in patients with TOF than in the general population (6% vs. ≤1%). Preoperative assessment of cardiovascular anatomy using computed tomography (CT) angiography enables the adaptation of the surgical approach to avoid potentially overlooked anomalies. Our purpose was to determine the prevalence of coronary artery and aortic arch anomalies in a cohort of TOF patients. **Methods:** In this retrospective analysis, data were collected from CT reports (2015–2021) of 105 TOF patients. All images were acquired using a 64-slice multi-detector CT (MDCT) scanner. **Results:** The median age of the patients was 38.7 months, with a male-to-female ratio of 1.39. The overall prevalence of coronary artery anomalies (CAAs) was 7.61% (8 of 105 cases). The anomalous origin and course of coronary arteries across the right ventricular outflow tract (RVOT; prepulmonic course) were defined in 5.71% of cases (six patients). In four of these, the left anterior descending artery (LAD) originated from the right coronary artery (RCA), while in two cases, the RCA arose from the LAD. In the remaining two patients, the coronary arteries followed an interarterial course. The most frequent anomalous aortic arch pattern in the overall TOF population was the right aortic arch (RAA) with mirror image branching, seen in 20% of patients (21 cases). The most frequent anomaly of the supra-aortic trunks was bovine configuration, found in 17.14% (18 cases). **Conclusions:** The prevalence of CAAs and aortic arch anomalies detected by CT angiography was in line with the data reported in anatomical specimens. Therefore, this technique represents a powerful tool for the evaluation of congenital cardiovascular anomalies.

Keywords: CT angiography; Fallot tetralogy; coronary arteries; aortic arch anomalies

1. Introduction

Tetralogy of Fallot (TOF) is the most common form of cyanotic congenital heart disease (CHD), consisting of a ventricular septal defect, stenosis, or atresia of the pulmonary outflow; biventricular origin of the aorta; and right ventricular hypertrophy as a secondary feature (Figure 1C,D). This combination of defects occurs in 421 cases per million live births, constituting around 7–10% of all congenital cardiac malformations [1,2]. Echocardiography is the initial modality of choice for making the diagnosis and follow-up. Useful secondary diagnostic tools are electrocardiogram (ECG) and chest radiography. Findings from these tests are often suggestive but not definitive for the diagnosis of TOF. Invasive angiography is sometimes needed to establish the diagnosis and to provide detailed anatomy and hemodynamic characterization. As a good alternative to invasive cardiac catheterization, multi-detector computed tomography (MDCT) with high spatial and temporal resolution plays an important role in the evaluation of complex anatomical findings [3].

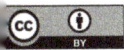

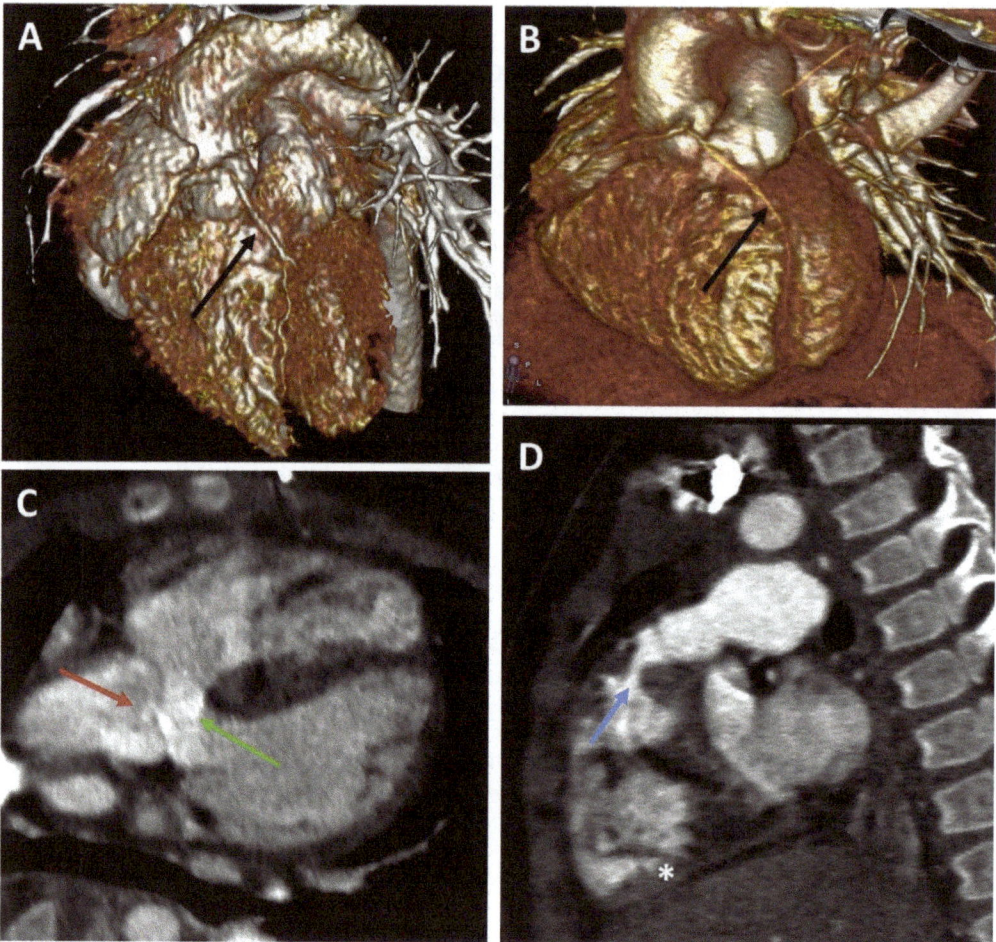

Figure 1. Representative CT angiography images. (**A,B**) Volume-rendering technique (VRT) reconstructions for CT images of 2 patients with Fallot tetralogy (ages: 7 and 14 months). Black arrow: anomalous course of the left anterior descending artery over the right ventricle outflow tract (RVOT). (**C,D**) Double oblique reconstruction of CT images in an infant with Fallot tetralogy. Red arrow: Mildly dilated aortic root overlapping the interventricular septum. Green arrow: Ventricular septal defect. Blue arrow: Narrowing of the right ventricular outflow tract (subpulmonary stenosis). The right ventricle (star) is mildly hypertrophied.

Coronary artery anomalies (CAAs) are a diverse group of congenital conditions with highly variable clinical presentation and pathophysiological mechanisms usually observed in the context of complex CHDs [4]. The prevalence of the anomalous origin of a coronary artery is higher in patients with TOF than in the general population (6% vs. ≤1%), as described by Koppel et al. [5].

Right aortic arch (RAA) anomalies are known to occur in association with cardiac outflow malformations, of which the most common type is TOF [6]. The prevalence of RAA varies between 13% and 34% in TOF patients, as opposed to 0.1% in the general population [7,8]. While the appearance of CAAs and RAA in TOF has been intensively analyzed, the number of studies describing the variety of branching patterns in patients with the left aortic arch (LAA) configuration is limited.

Preoperative identification of the coronary tree and aortic arch anatomy in patients with TOF is relevant to enable the adaptation of the surgical approach and avoid potentially overlooked anomalies. Some cases of CAAs crossing the right ventricular outflow tract (RVOT) are not detectable intraoperatively due to their intramyocardial course, overlying epicardial fat, or pericardial–epicardial adhesions from previous palliative surgery [9].

Consequently, preoperative computed tomography (CT) angiography may be essential in coronary assessment to minimize the risk of negative postoperative outcomes such as myocardial infarction and patient death. Furthermore, knowledge of aortic arch morphology is of crucial importance in deciding the appropriate access to palliative interventional procedures (e.g., constructing a systemic to pulmonary artery shunt), placement of monitoring lines, and cannulation for extracorporeal life support [7].

In the present study, our goal was to determine the prevalence of coronary artery and aortic arch anomalies in a cohort of TOF patients and to compare our results with findings from previous studies. The majority of studies were based on invasive coronary angiography (ICA) for assessing coronary anatomy; therefore, we also aimed to highlight the role of CT angiography in preoperative evaluation.

2. Materials and Methods

This retrospective analysis included 105 TOF patients who underwent CT angiography examinations between 2015 and 2021 for the evaluation of cardiovascular anatomy at a single tertiary care hospital. All examinations were performed using a 64-MDCT scanner (Definition AS, Siemens, Erlangen, Germany or Revolution HD, GE Healthcare, Milwaukee, WI, USA) using ECG gating and power injectors, with contrast volumes and flow rate according to local protocols.

The institutional reports database was queried to identify Fallot tetralogy patients who underwent CT examinations, and the reports were further analyzed. All reports were provided by a radiologist with 5+ years of experience in cardiovascular imaging (EACVI Level 3). The data were collected retrospectively from the CT report protocols, with variables being recorded in an MS Excel database (see Figures 1 and 2 for representative images). We included all patients with a diagnosis of TOF, including those with extreme variants (pulmonary atresia with major aortopulmonary collateral arteries (MAPCAs) or Fallot type double outlet right ventricle (DORV)). For patients with multiple examinations, the data were recorded only once. We recorded the following variables: gender, age, thoracic vessels anatomical course, and variants, as well as coronary arteries' course. CAAs and aortic arch anomalies were assessed in both unrepaired and repaired TOF patients. This is a small sample size and a single-center study; therefore, neonates, children, and adults were also included. Patients who underwent surgical repair in our center before 2015 were evaluated preoperatively through ICA as the golden standard. In this subgroup, CT angiography was executed as part of a preoperative screening protocol for later interventions if any acute cardiovascular event or late postoperative TOF complication arose. With the emergence of newer-generation CT-scanners and software, CT angiography was preferred to ICA due to its non-invasive approach, and, as such, it was the predominantly used evaluation method, preceding primary TOF repair after 2015, in our center.

From these data, the incidences of both surgically critical (prepulmonic course) and non-critical CAAs and aortic arch anomalies were calculated.

All statistics were performed using GraphPad InStat. Associations were tested using Chi-test with a significance level $p < 0.05$. The Emergency Institute for Cardiovascular Diseases and Heart Transplant ethics committee approved the tertiary analysis of data through address 8984/2020.

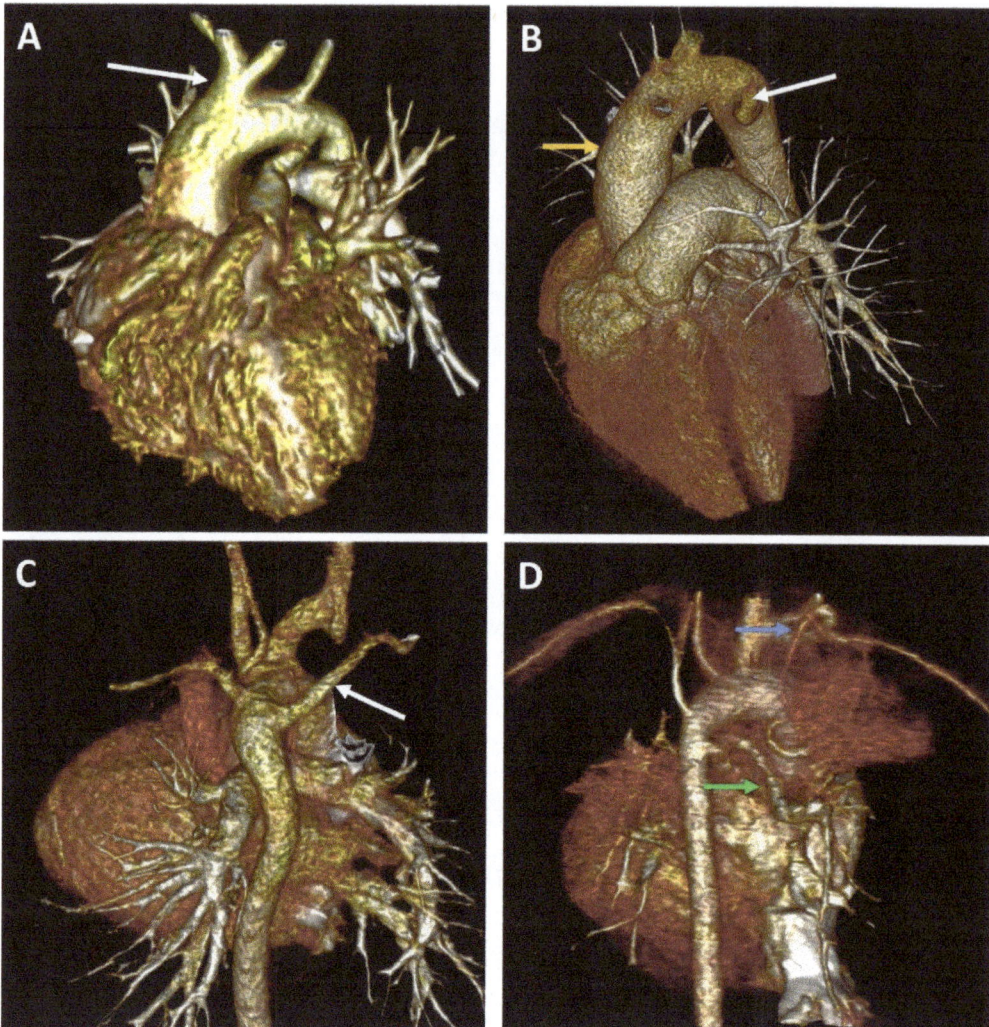

Figure 2. Representative image for aortic arc anomalies. (**A**) Left-sided aortic arch with left carotid artery (white arrow) from brachiocephalic trunk ("bovine arch"). (**B**) Right-sided aortic arch (yellow arrow) with anomalous left subclavian artery (white arrow). (**C**) Left-sided aortic arch with aberrant right subclavian artery (white arrow). (**D**) Major aortopulmonary collateral arteries (MAPCAs) feeding the left pulmonary artery (green arrow) and the apical portion of the left upper lobe (blue arrow).

3. Results

In this study, a comprehensive CT angiography evaluation was performed on 105 TOF patients, of whom 61 (58.1%) were male (male/female ratio of 1.39). The median age of this population was 38.7 months (interquartile range 6.9–179.4), with a broad age distribution ranging from 0 months to 47 years. The majority of participants were under 18 years of age, and more than one-third were neonates and infants (35.2%). Table 1 summarizes the demographic characteristics of these patients.

Table 1. Demographic characteristics.

Gender	Male	58.1% (61/105)
	Female	41.9% (44/105)
	M:F ratio	1.39
Age distribution	Range	0 month to 47 years
	Median	38.7 months (IQR 6.9–179.4)
	<1 year	35.2% (37/105)
	1–18 years	47.6% (50/105)
	≥18 years	17.1% (18/105)

IQR = interquartile range (IQR); M:F ratio = male to female ratio.

The overall prevalence of CAAs was 7.61% (8 of 105 cases). Anomalous origin and course of the coronary arteries across the RVOT (prepulmonic course) were defined in 5.71% of cases (six patients), representing 75% of CAAs. Within this group, the left anterior descending artery (LAD) emerging from the right coronary artery (RCA) was found in four patients (Figure 1A,B), while RCA originating from the LAD was seen in two cases. In the remaining two patients, the CAAs followed an interarterial course, with one case of LAD arising from the RCA and one case of RCA originating from the left main coronary artery (LM). Additional anatomical findings were noted, namely four other cases with a prominent conus artery similar in caliber to the RCA (Table 2).

Table 2. Coronary artery anomalies and prominent conus artery.

Course	Origin	Overall Prevalence
Prepulmonic	LAD from RCA	3.8% (4/105)
	RCA from LAD	1.9% (2/105)
Interarterial	LAD from RCA	0.95% (1/105)
	RCA from LM	0.95% (1/105)
Other coronary findings	Coronary pattern	Overall prevalence
	Prominent conus artery	3.8% (4/105)

LAD = left anterior descending artery; LM = left main coronary artery; RCA = right coronary artery.

Of 105 patients with TOF, CAAs following a prepulmonic course were found in five patients in addition to aortic arch anomalies. Of these, LAD emerging from the RCA and bovine arch was observed in three patients, while LAD originating from the RCA and RAA with mirror image branching was seen in one. Another patient had RCA arising from the LAD in addition to RAA with mirror-image supra-aortic trunks. No statistically significant association was found between the prevalence of CAAs and anomalous aortic arch patterns ($p > 0.9999$).

The variation in aortic arch position and branching pattern is summarized in Tables 3 and 4. In total, 76.2% of patients (80) had LAA, while RAA was seen in 23.8% of cases (25 patients). As determined using the classification of Popieluszko et al. [10]—see Table 3—the most common aortic arch pattern among these patients was type 1 (normal configuration), which occurred in 40.95% of all cases. The second most frequently observed configuration was RAA (23.8%), followed by the bovine arch variant (16.19%; Figure 2A). Equal proportions of aberrant branching of the left vertebral artery (LV) and right subclavian artery were observed (2.85%; Figure 2C). Only one patient had both a bovine arch and an aberrant LV branching pattern (0.95%).

Table 3. Different types of aortic arch variations.

	Prevalence in LAA	Overall Prevalence	Characteristics
Popieluszko classification			
Type 1—normal	53.75% (43/80)	40.95% (43/105)	-
Type 2—bovine arch	21.25% (17/80)	16.19% (17/105)	One patient had PDA
Type 3—LV from aortic arch	3.75% (3/80)	2.85% (3/105)	-
Type 4—bovine arch and LV	1.25% (1/80)	0.95% (1/105)	-
Type 5—common carotid trunk	-	-	-
Type 6—ARSA	3.75% (3/80)	2.85% (3/105)	-
Type 7—RAA	-	23.8% (25/105)	-
Unclassified branching pattern			
LCC from anterior aspect of aortic arch	1.25% (1/80)	0.95% (1/105)	-
LCC and LSA from anterior aspect of aortic arch	1.25% (1/80)	0.95% (1/105)	The patient had MAPCAs
RSA from aortic arch	1.25% (1/80)	0.95% (1/105)	-

ARSA = aberrant right subclavian artery; LAA = left aortic arch; LCC = left common carotid artery; LSA = left subclavian artery; LV = left vertebral artery; MAPCAs = major aortopulmonary collateral arteries; PDA = patent ductus arteriosus; RAA = right aortic arch; RSA = right subclavian artery.

Table 4. Types of RAA according to the Edwards classification.

	Prevalence in RAA	Overall Prevalence	Characteristics
Type I—RAA with mirror image	84% (21/25)	20% (21/105)	Two patients had PDA
Type II—RAA with ALSA	12% (3/25)	2.85% (3/105)	-
Type III—Isolated LSA	-	-	-
Unclassified RAA with bovine arch	4% (1/25)	0.95% (1/105)	-

ALSA = aberrant left subclavian artery; LSA = left subclavian artery; PDA = patient ductus arteriosus; RAA = right aortic arch.

During the evaluation of LAA patterns, we found three unclassified arch anatomy features. In one patient, both the left common carotid artery (LCC) and left subclavian artery (LSA) arose from the anterior aspect of the aortic arch, while in another patient, only the LCC had an anterior origin. A separate origin of each supra-aortic trunk was also noted in one case. None of the patients in this series had a type 5 (common carotid trunk) branching configuration.

In Table 4, we present the various forms of RAA. Within this group, 84% (21 of 25 patients) had RAA with mirror image branching of the main vessels, 12% (three patients) had RAA with an aberrant left subclavian artery (ALSA; Figure 2B), and 4% (one patient) had RAA with a bovine arch. Three types of RAA exist in the literature, as defined by the Edwards classification scheme [11,12]. However, none of the CT scans showed obliteration or isolation of the LSA with collateralization (type III).

The most frequent anomalous aortic arch pattern found in the overall TOF population was RAA with mirror image branching, identified in 20% of cases (21 patients). The most frequent anomaly of the supra-aortic trunks was bovine configuration, found in 17.14% of cases (eighteen patients, one of them in association with RAA), followed by an aberrant course of the subclavian artery in 5.71% of cases (six patients, equal numbers of left and right subclavians).

Other vascular anomalies were detected using CT angiography: patent ductus arteriosus (PDA; eight patients, 7.61% of all cases), major aortopulmonary collateral arteries (MAPCAs; four patients, 3.8%; Figure 2D), prominent sinoatrial nodal artery (one patient, 0.95%), and ductal diverticulum (one patient, 0.95%). PDA was associated with RAA in two cases, while the remaining six patients had a left-sided aortic arch (Table 5).

Table 5. Other vascular findings.

	Prevalence in LAA	Overall Prevalence	Characteristics
PDA	7.5% (6/80)	7.61% (8/105)	One patient had bovine arch
MAPCAs	5% (4/80)	3.8% (4/105)	One patient had LCC and LSA arising from the anterior aspect of the arch
Prominent sinoatrial nodal artery	1.25% (1/80)	0.95% (1/105)	-
Ductal diverticulum	1.25 (1/80)	0.95% (1/105)	-

LAA = left aortic arch; LCC = left common carotid artery; LSA = left subclavian artery; MAPCAs = major aortopulmonary collateral arteries; PDA = patent ductus arteriosus.

4. Discussion

The survival rate of neonates with TOF has increased over the years due to highly sophisticated imaging techniques and successful management of patients with CHDs. The treatment strategies currently used in TOF have improved, offering excellent long-term survival (30-year survival rate of 68.5% to 90.5%). However, reintervention procedures are still often required [13]. Diagnostic imaging findings provide key information about the anatomical relationships of cardiac and extracardiac structures and hemodynamic features prior to surgical repair. The goals of preoperative imaging in TOF are to establish the severity of the primary anatomical lesions and the degree of functional alterations, as well as identify associated anomalies (such as variants of aortic arch patterning, CAAs, PDA, and MAPCAs). Moreover, the assessment of the presence and extent of lesions is required to determine the optimal timing and approach of surgical interventions—either definitive early repair or a palliative interventional procedure followed by surgery at a later stage [14].

Inadvertent division of coronary vessels crossing the RVOT during right ventriculotomy or transannular repair can lead to serious complications. Thus, clear delineation of the origin and course of these arteries is vital for the selection of a suitable surgical approach. Alternative surgical techniques must be chosen individually for this subset of anomalies (e.g., transatrial-transpulmonary repair, RVOT stenting) [15,16]. Cases have been described where a CAA crossing the RVOT was not identified during the preoperative assessment and did not become clear during surgical repair, causing it to be damaged, followed by myocardial infarction [5].

Different methods of visualization of the coronary tree anatomy can be used during the surveillance of patients with TOF. ICA was considered the gold standard imaging modality to identify and classify CAAs. However, a potential complicating factor during ICA examination is the counterclockwise rotation of the aortic root, which causes overlapping of the right and left coronary arteries in anteroposterior projection [17]. The possible utility of ICA has been reappraised, and this technique is being progressively replaced by coronary computed tomography angiography (CCTA). As CCTA is non-invasive, it is more widely applicable for diagnosis [4].

Multi-detector CCTA offers a detailed characterization of cardiac structures and small vessels using static images as well as 3D reconstructions. Although no studies have compared coronary angiography and CT scanning directly, CCTA has been shown to be a promising substitute for ICA as a method of identifying aberrant coronary patterns [5]. The main limitations of CT angiography are the dose of ionizing radiation given to the patients and the potential induction of contrast-induced nephrotoxicity. However, the patient's radiation dose is higher during ICA when an appropriate pediatric protocol is used [18]. Moreover, invasive angiography also involves the administration of an intravascular contrast agent, leading to iatrogenic renal injury in susceptible individuals. It is important to note that the introduction of ECG gating and postprocessing techniques has resulted in significant improvements in image resolution, as well as reductions in acquisition time and radiation dose [4].

In adults, cardiac magnetic resonance (CMR) imaging has an established role in the diagnosis of CAAs. However, this method has had limited success in the evaluation of children as the smaller heart size and faster heart rate in pediatric patients lead to poor spatial and temporal resolution. Moreover, additional sedation may be needed for adequate image quality. In a recent study, CMR angiography did not perform well in patients younger than 4 months; diagnostic image quality was obtained in only 17% of cases, even though all examinations were performed under general anesthesia [19].

There is also increasing evidence for the successful identification of anatomical evidence by transthoracic echocardiography, which can be a suitable method of primary investigation in children that avoids radiation exposure. However, echocardiography is not routinely used for the visualization of coronary vessels in the adult population because of its lower spatial resolution and suboptimal acoustic windows [4].

Due to many possible anatomic variants, which are not considered anomalies, the term CAA, as a definition, has historically been restricted to those occurring in less than 1% of the general population [4]. The reported prevalence of CAAs in patients with TOF is between 2% and 23%. The overall prevalence of these congenital malformations was 6% in a meta-analysis including 28 studies, which was similar to our results (7.61%). In our TOF patients, the proportion of surgically significant anomalies with coronary arteries passing across the RVOT was 75% of all CAAs; again, this was similar to the percentage (72%) calculated in the previously mentioned large-scale meta-analysis [5]. Anomalous origin of the LAD from the RCA or the right sinus of Valsalva was the most common CAA in the majority of studies; this was also the vascular anomaly most frequently encountered in conjunction with prepulmonic course in TOF patients [5,14]. Our results correlated with these findings.

Solitary coronary arteries arising from one of the sinuses of Valsalva are also frequently reported CAAs in patients with TOF [9,17,20]. The prevalence varies between 0.0240% and 0.066% in the general population, whereas these anomalies are reported between 1.5% and 3.7% in TOF patients [21,22]. In the present study, a single coronary artery was found in three cases (2.85%), which is in line with the reported frequency in TOF patients. This type of CAA may cause myocardial ischemia by different mechanisms, even in the absence of atherosclerotic coronary lesions. The abnormal vessel angulations or courses may affect the distribution of blood flow, leading to serious complications. Coronary classification systems are useful tools for providing detailed information about these anomalies; however, neither of them can be applied in all TOF cases. The Leiden Convention coronary coding system has been shown to be a feasible method for the characterization of single coronary arteries in the setting of complex CHD; however, this classification is not routinely used in patients with TOF. In this classification system, the aortic sinuses are described as left- or right-facing or non-facing relative to the pulmonary valve sinuses; therefore, the applicability is limited in cases of pulmonary atresia. In such cases, a detailed description of the coronary anatomy, as well as associated characteristics, should be provided for treatment planning [23].

By the classic definition, five CAA course subtypes exist: prepulmonic, interarterial, subpulmonic (intraconal or intraseptal), retroaortic, and retrocardiac [24]. As in the general population, not all variations in CAAs are of equal clinical importance. Coronary arteries following an interarterial course (between the ascending aorta and the pulmonary trunk) with high-risk anatomic features (e.g., intramural tract, slit-like ostium) are considered malignant and require additional corrective surgery. In this study, the morphological aspects of these arteries were deemed benign.

It should also be noted that a single coronary artery with an interarterial course may increase the risk of major adverse cardiac events [4]. In the case of subpulmonic course, the coronary vessel exits the aorta below the pulmonic valve and traverses the RVOT, pulmonary infundibulum, and interventricular septum. The differential diagnosis between the intraseptal and the intramural interarterial course of a coronary artery is especially relevant and can be difficult; however, an intraseptal CAA has a more inferior position [25]. In this study, none of the CT scans showed CAAs with subpulmonic, retroaortic, or retrocardiac courses in patients with TOF. In our sample population, represented mainly by preoperative

TOF patients with a median age of 3 years, the clinical impact of the "malignant" variant remains to be investigated in follow-up examinations.

The conus artery is a small branch that usually originates from the proximal portion of the RCA. A large conus artery (as identified in four cases in this study) may supply a larger area of myocardium and therefore should undoubtedly be preserved during corrective surgery [26]. Variants larger than the RCA have been described, crossing over the outflow tract of the right ventricle and reaching the heart apex. These variants could be easily mistaken for an accessory LAD on ICA examination in the anteroposterior projection [27]. Hence, the true prevalence remains uncertain [5].

Congenital aortic arch malformations embody a large group of anomalies that result from the disordered embryogenesis of the pharyngeal arches, including abnormal or incomplete regression of one or more embryogenic vascular segments [28]. The recognition of these aberrations is of paramount importance in TOF patients to ensure accurate preoperative surgical decisions. In this study, the classic branching pattern of the aortic arch (left-sided aorta giving rise to the brachiocephalic trunk, LCC, and LSA) was found in 40.95% of patients, whereas the prevalence of this pattern is significantly higher in the general population (80.9%) [10]. This finding suggests that the occurrence of atypical aortic arch patterns is higher in TOF patients. According to the Popieluszko classification, the most frequently seen anomalous arch pattern in our patients was the RAA variant (23.8%). The incidence of RAA has been reported as around 25% in previous studies [7,18,29]. Apart from the normal branching pattern, the most common left-sided aortic arch pattern was the bovine arch, including the common origin of the innominate artery and the LCC, which were seen in 40.95% and 16.19% of patients, respectively. These findings are in accordance with those of Moustafa et al. (40.4% and 22.8%) [29] and Tawfik et al. (36% and 16%) [30].

The aberrant origin of one of the subclavian arteries occurs with a higher incidence in patients with TOF than in the general population, where it is less than 2% [31,32]. Aberrancy of the subclavian artery can influence monitoring line placement—if this anomaly is recognized preoperatively, the arterial line should be placed in the contralateral radial or the femoral artery [33,34]. Different palliative procedures are offered depending on clinical presentation, although the procedure most often carried out remains the modified Blalock–Taussig shunt, which involves inserting an interposed graft between the subclavian artery and the ipsilateral pulmonary artery [35]. Failure to identify an aberrant subclavian artery prior to surgery might lead to incorrect insertion of the shunt between the carotid artery and the pulmonary circulation [7].

Within the RAA branching configuration, a mirror image of supra-aortic trunks was observed in 84% of patients, whereas RAA with ALSA was found in 12% of cases. These findings are in accordance with the results of Prabhu et al., who identified RAA with mirror image branching in 86.6% of 688 patients and RAA with ALSA in 10.6% [7].

Fallot-type DORV (where DORV means abnormal ventriculoarterial connection with both great vessels arising, entirely or predominantly, from the right ventricle, and Fallot-type means that DORV mimics elements of TOF) is an uncommon complex congenital heart anomaly in which early complete repair should be considered to avoid ventricular volume overload and progression of tricuspid valve regurgitation. The complex anatomy of Fallot-type DORV can make surgical correction a challenge; therefore, comprehensive preoperative assessment and planning are needed [36].

Tetralogy of Fallot with pulmonary atresia (TOF-PA) is a severe variant of TOF, characterized by a lack of antegrade flow into the pulmonary arteries. To provide additional blood flow to the pulmonary circulation, PDA is usually seen in association with TOF-PA. Stenting of PDA has gained acceptance for palliation in TOF-PA, although the PDA is usually elongated and tortuous, making the implantation of a rigid, straight stent challenging. Hence, advanced imaging with MDCT angiography is necessary for case selection and preprocedural planning [37]. The common carotid and axillary artery approaches are the most feasible routes for stent implantation. However, ductal stenting is contraindicated in the case of the common carotid trunk, as damage to the vessels during direct surgical or percutaneous approach could lead to neurological deficits [7].

Finally, MAPCAs are persistent tortuous fetal arteries branching from the aorta or systemic arteries that form in an attempt to compensate for the underdeveloped pulmonary circulation via multifocal supply. TOF-PA with MAPCAs is a severe and rare type of congenital heart defect [38]. We found this malformation in just 5% of cases. Surgical management to restore normal pulmonary blood flow is challenging due to the heterogeneity of arborization in these patients [35]. Therefore, preoperative imaging is necessary to achieve a complete understanding of cardiovascular anatomy.

The systematic use of CT angiography for preoperative identification of CAAs and aortic arch patterns in TOF was scarcely reported. Therefore, one of the main objectives of our study was to highlight the role of CT angiography in the evaluation of complex anatomical findings, as a good alternative to invasive cardiac catheterization. Moreover, the number of studies describing the variety of aortic arch and branching patterns in TOF patients is limited, and most provide incomplete information regarding the entire spectrum of aortic anomalies. This led to our aspiration to encompass all classifiable and non-classifiable aortic malformations in this specific population.

5. Study Limitations

There are several limitations to the design of this study. First, this is a single-center, small-sample observational study based on retrospective data analysis. Therefore, no comparison of diagnostic accuracy was performed for CT angiography and ICA in TOF patients. As mentioned previously, no prospective studies comparing these diagnostic imaging methods have been found in the literature [5]. However, Gorenoi et al. declared that CCTA with at least 64 slices should be used to identify coronary alterations in order to avoid invasive investigation in patients with CHD [39].

Second, the concordance of coronary artery patterns between the preoperative CCTA and corrective surgical findings was not evaluated. However, Goo et al. demonstrated that dual-source CCTA with a high temporal resolution was useful for the assessment of coronary artery anatomy before corrective surgery in TOF, exhibiting not only a high concordance rate (95.0%) with surgical findings but also a high level of diagnostic accuracy (96.9%) [9].

Technical limitations were also present. Not only was it possible that different contrast agents might have impacted the quality of the CT examination [40], but the results of this study were obtained using a 64-slice last-generation CT scanner. In order to reduce the number of misinterpreted cases, higher temporal resolution CCTA is needed. The second-generation 128-slice dual-source CT is one of the most frequently used imaging modalities for evaluating TOF patients, enabling high temporal resolution and scanning speed, as well as a low radiation dose. Moreover, diagnostic accuracy is expected to be further improved with the recently introduced third-generation 192-slice dual-source CT system, which provides even better image quality at lower radiation doses [41].

6. Conclusions

The prevalence of CAAs and aortic arch anomalies detected by CT angiography in this study is in line with the data reported in anatomical specimens. Therefore, CT angiography represents a powerful tool for the evaluation of congenital cardiovascular anomalies.

Author Contributions: Conceptualization, Z.K. and M.P.; methodology, M.P.; software, Z.K..; validation, Z.K. and M.P.; formal analysis, Z.K.; investigation, Z.K. and E.H.; resources, M.P.; data curation, Z.K.; writing—original draft preparation, Z.K.; writing—review and editing, Z.K. and E.H.; visualization, Z.K.; supervision, M.P.; project administration, M.P.; funding acquisition, M.P. All authors have read and agreed to the published version of the manuscript.

Funding: This research received no external funding.

Institutional Review Board Statement: This study was conducted in accordance with the Declaration of Helsinki and approved by the Ethics Committee of Emergency Institute for Cardiovascular Diseases and Heart Transplant of Tirgu Mures (4920/2020).

Informed Consent Statement: This is a data analysis using secondary sources. Informed consent was obtained from all subjects/legal guardians prior to CT examinations.

Data Availability Statement: Data are available upon reasonable request.

Conflicts of Interest: The authors declare no conflict of interest.

References

1. Bailliard, F.; Anderson, R.H. Tetralogy of Fallot. *Orphanet J. Rare Dis.* **2009**, *4*, 2. [CrossRef] [PubMed]
2. Hoffman, J.I.; Kaplan, S. The incidence of congenital heart disease. *J. Am. Coll. Cardiol.* **2002**, *39*, 1890–1900. [CrossRef]
3. Shaaban, M.; Tantawy, S.; Elkafrawy, F.; Haroun, D.; Romeih, S.; Elmozy, W. Multi-detector computed tomography in the assessment of tetralogy of Fallot patients: Is it a must? *Egypt. Heart J.* **2020**, *72*, 1–13. [CrossRef] [PubMed]
4. Gentile, F.; Castiglione, V.; De Caterina, R. Coronary Artery Anomalies. *Circulation* **2021**, *144*, 983–996. [CrossRef] [PubMed]
5. Koppel, C.J.; Jongbloed, M.R.; Kiès, P.; Hazekamp, M.G.; Mertens, B.J.; Schalij, M.J.; Vliegen, H.W. Coronary anomalies in tetralogy of Fallot—A meta-analysis. *Int. J. Cardiol.* **2020**, *306*, 78–85. [CrossRef] [PubMed]
6. Knight, L.; Edwards, J.E. Right Aortic Arch. *Circulation* **1974**, *50*, 1047–1051. [CrossRef] [PubMed]
7. Prabhu, S.; Kasturi, S.; Mehra, S.; Tiwari, R.; Joshi, A.; John, C.; Karl, T.R. The aortic arch in tetralogy of Fallot: Types of branching and clinical implications. *Cardiol. Young* **2020**, *30*, 1144–1150. [CrossRef]
8. Kanne, J.P.; Godwin, J.D. Right aortic arch and its variants. *J. Cardiovasc. Comput. Tomogr.* **2010**, *4*, 293–300. [CrossRef]
9. Goo, H.W. Coronary artery anomalies on preoperative cardiac CT in children with tetralogy of Fallot or Fallot type of double outlet right ventricle: Comparison with surgical findings. *Int. J. Cardiovasc. Imaging* **2018**, *34*, 1997–2009. [CrossRef]
10. Popieluszko, P.; Henry, B.M.; Sanna, B.; Hsieh, W.C.; Saganiak, K.; Pękala, P.A.; Walocha, J.A.; Tomaszewski, K. A systematic review and meta-analysis of variations in branching patterns of the adult aortic arch. *J. Vasc. Surg.* **2017**, *68*, 298–306.e10. [CrossRef]
11. Mark, A.L.; Jay, M. *Right Aortic Arches*; StatPearls Publishing: Tampa, FL, USA, 2022. Available online: https://www.ncbi.nlm.nih.gov/books/NBK431104/ (accessed on 24 August 2022).
12. Cinà, C.; Althani, H.; Pasenau, J.; Abouzahr, L. Kommerell's diverticulum and right-sided aortic arch: A cohort study and review of the literature. *J. Vasc. Surg.* **2004**, *39*, 131–139. [CrossRef]
13. van der Ven, J.; Bosch, E.V.D.; Bogers, A.J.; Helbing, W.A. Current outcomes and treatment of tetralogy of Fallot. *F1000Research* **2019**, *8*, 1530. [CrossRef]
14. Banderker, E.; Pretorius, E.; De Decker, R. The role of cardiac CT angiography in the pre- and postoperative evaluation of tetralogy of Fallot. *S. Afr. J. Radiol.* **2015**, *19*, 9. [CrossRef]
15. Luijten, L.W.; Bosch, E.V.D.; Duppen, N.; Tanke, R.; Roos-Hesselink, J.; Nijveld, A.; van Dijk, A.; Bogers, A.J.; Van Domburg, R.; Helbing, W.A. Long-term outcomes of transatrial–transpulmonary repair of tetralogy of Fallot. *Eur. J. Cardio-Thoracic Surg.* **2014**, *47*, 527–534. [CrossRef]
16. Afifi, A.R.S.A.; Mehta, C.; Bhole, V.; Chaudhari, M.; Khan, N.E.; Jones, T.J.; Stumper, O. Anomalous coronary artery in Tetralogy of Fallot—Feasibility of right ventricular outflow tract stenting as initial palliation. *Catheter. Cardiovasc. Interv.* **2022**, *100*, 105–112. [CrossRef]
17. Hussain, I.; Patel, N.; Ghaffar, A.; Kundi, A. Coronary anomalies in Pakistani children with tetralogy of Fallot. *J. Coll. Physicians Surg. Pak.* **2010**, *20*, 3–5.
18. Lapierre, C.; Dubois, J.; Rypens, F.; Raboisson, M.-J.; Déry, J. Tetralogy of Fallot: Preoperative assessment with MR and CT imaging. *Diagn. Interv. Imaging* **2016**, *97*, 531–541. [CrossRef]
19. Tangcharoen, T.; Bell, A.; Hegde, S.; Hussain, T.; Beerbaum, P.; Schaeffter, T.; Razavi, R.; Botnar, R.M.; Greil, G.F. Detection of Coronary Artery Anomalies in Infants and Young Children with Congenital Heart Disease by Using MR Imaging. *Radiology* **2011**, *259*, 240–247. [CrossRef]
20. Hrusca, A.; Rachisan, A.; Gach, P.; Pico, H.; Sorensen, C.; Bonello, B.; Ovaert, C.; Petit, P.; Fouilloux, V.; Mace, L.; et al. Detection of pulmonary and coronary artery anomalies in tetralogy of Fallot using non-ECG-gated CT angiography. *Diagn. Interv. Imaging* **2016**, *97*, 543–548. [CrossRef]
21. Beig, J.R.; Ahmed, W.; Hafeez, I.; Gupta, A.; Tramboo, N.A.; Rather, H.A. Pentalogy of Fallot with a Single Coronary Artery: A Rare Case Report. *J. Tehran Heart Cent* **2014**, *9*, 132–134.
22. Michalowska, A.M.; Tyczynski, P.; Pregowski, J.; Skowronski, J.; Mintz, G.S.; Kepka, C.; Kruk, M.; Witkowski, A.; Michalowska, I. Prevalence and Anatomic Characteristics of Single Coronary Artery Diagnosed by Computed Tomography Angiography. *Am. J. Cardiol.* **2019**, *124*, 939–946. [CrossRef]
23. Katekaru-Tokeshi, D.; Jiménez-Santos, M.; Koppel, C.; Vliegen, H.; Díaz-Zamudio, M.; Castillo-Castellón, F.; Jongbloed, M.; Kimura-Hayama, E. Applicability of the Leiden Convention and the Lipton Classification in Patients with a Single Coronary Artery in the Setting of Congenital Heart Disease. *J. Cardiovasc. Dev. Dis.* **2021**, *8*, 93. [CrossRef]

24. Cheezum, M.K.; Liberthson, R.R.; Shah, N.R.; Villines, T.C.; O'Gara, P.T.; Landzberg, M.J.; Blankstein, R. Anomalous Aortic Origin of a Coronary Artery from the Inappropriate Sinus of Valsalva. *J. Am. Coll. Cardiol.* **2017**, *69*, 1592–1608. [CrossRef]
25. Unzué, L.; García, E.; López-Melgar, B.; Agudo-Quilez, P. Percutaneous treatment of an anomalous left main arising from the opposite sinus with subpulmonic course. *Cardiovasc. Revasc. Med.* **2018**, *19*, 632–637. [CrossRef]
26. Sasaki, S.; Mishima, A.; Asano, M.; Nomura, N. Surgical Repair of Tetralogy of Fallot with Large Conus Artery. *Pediatr. Cardiol.* **2003**, *24*, 601–603. [CrossRef]
27. Dabizzi, R.P.; Caprioli, G.; Aiazzi, L.; Castelli, C.; Baldrighi, G.; Parenzan, L. Distribution and anomalies of coronary arteries in tetralogy of fallot. *Circulation* **1980**, *61*, 95–102. [CrossRef]
28. Priya, S.; Thomas, R.; Nagpal, P.; Sharma, A.; Steigner, M. Congenital anomalies of the aortic arch. *Cardiovasc. Diagn. Ther.* **2018**, *8*, S26–S44. [CrossRef]
29. Moustafa, S.A.E.F.; Hussein, M.M.; Sultan, A.A.; Bilal, M.M.Z.; El Gamal, M.A.F.; Sobh, D.M. Three steps approach for preoperative evaluation of tetralogy of Fallot patients: Role of 128 MDCT. *Egypt. J. Radiol. Nucl. Med.* **2021**, *52*, 1–14. [CrossRef]
30. Tawfik, A.M.; Sobh, D.M.; Ashamallah, G.A.; Batouty, N.M. Prevalence and Types of Aortic Arch Variants and Anomalies in Congenital Heart Diseases. *Acad. Radiol.* **2018**, *26*, 930–936. [CrossRef] [PubMed]
31. Rao, B.S.; Anderson, R.C.; Edwards, J.E. Anatomic variations in the tetralogy of Fallot. *Am. Heart J.* **1971**, *81*, 361–371. [CrossRef] [PubMed]
32. Kuribayashi, T.; Roberts, W.C. Tetralogy of fallot, truncus arteriosus, abnormal myocardial architecture and anomalies of the aortic arch system induced by bis-diamine in rat fetuses. *J. Am. Coll. Cardiol.* **1993**, *21*, 768–776. [CrossRef]
33. Hastreiter, A.R.; D'Cruz, I.A.; Cantez, T.; Namin, E.P.; Licata, R. Right-sided aorta. I. Occurrence of right aortic arch in various types of congenital heart disease. II. Right aortic arch, right descending aorta, and associated anomalies. *Heart* **1966**, *28*, 722–739. [CrossRef]
34. Krishnan, K.S.; Theodore, S.; Sai Kiran, K.V.S.S.; Neelakandhan, K.S. Embryologic and surgical considerations in tetralogy of Fallot with right arch and aberrant left subclavian artery from the ascending aorta. *J. Thorac. Cardiovasc. Surg.* **2005**, *130*, 215–216. [CrossRef]
35. Wise-Faberowski, L.; Asija, R.; McElhinney, D.B. Tetralogy of Fallot: Everything you wanted to know but were afraid to ask. *Pediatr. Anesthesia* **2018**, *29*, 475–482. [CrossRef]
36. Raju, V.; Burkhart, H.M.; Hedberg, N.R.; Eidem, B.W.; Li, Z.; Connolly, H.; Schaff, H.V.; Dearani, J.A. Surgical Strategy for Atrioventricular Septal Defect and Tetralogy of Fallot or Double-Outlet Right Ventricle. *Ann. Thorac. Surg.* **2013**, *95*, 2079–2085. [CrossRef]
37. Rehman, R.; Marhisham, M.C.; Alwi, M. Stenting the complex patent ductus arteriosus in tetralogy of Fallot with pulmonary atresia: Challenges and outcomes. *Futur. Cardiol.* **2018**, *14*, 55–73. [CrossRef]
38. Bauser-Heaton, H.; Borquez, A.; Han, B.; Ladd, M.; Asija, R.; Downey, L.; Koth, A.; Algaze, C.A.; Wise-Faberowski, L.; Perry, S.B.; et al. Programmatic Approach to Management of Tetralogy of Fallot with Major Aortopulmonary Collateral Arteries. *Circ. Cardiovasc. Interv.* **2017**, *10*, e004952. [CrossRef]
39. Gorenoi, V.; Schönermark, M.P.; Hagen, A. CT coronary angiography vs. invasive coronary angiography in CHD. *GMS Heal. Technol Assess* **2012**, *8*, Doc02. [CrossRef]
40. Pop, M. Cardiothoracic CTA in Infants Referred for Aortic Arch Evaluation—Retrospective Comparison of Iomeprol 350, Ioversol 350, Iopromide 370 and Iodixanol 320. *Children* **2021**, *8*, 949. [CrossRef]
41. Linsen, P.V.M.; Coenen, A.; Lubbers, M.M.; Dijkshoorn, M.L.; Ouhlous, M.; Nieman, K. Computed Tomography Angiography with a 192-slice Dual-source Computed Tomography System: Improvements in Image Quality and Radiation Dose. *J. Clin. Imaging Sci.* **2016**, *6*, 44. [CrossRef]

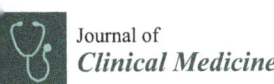

Journal of
Clinical Medicine

Article

Atrial Function Impairments after Pediatric Cardiac Surgery Evaluated by STE Analysis

Massimiliano Cantinotti [1], Pietro Marchese [1,2], Marco Scalese [3], Eliana Franchi [1], Nadia Assanta [1], Martin Koestenberger [4], Alessandra Pizzuto [1], Vitali Pak [1], Giuseppe Santoro [1], Vivek Jani [5], Shelby Kutty [5] and Raffaele Giordano [6,*]

1. Fondazione G. Monasterio CNR-Regione Toscana, 54100 Massa, Italy; cantinotti@ftgm.it (M.C.); pitrino91@gmail.com (P.M.); efranchi@ftgm.it (E.F.); assanta@ftgm.it (N.A.); apizzuto@ftgm.it (A.P.); pakv2001@yahoo.com (V.P.); giuseppe.santoro@ftgm.it (G.S.)
2. Institute of Life Sciences, Scuola Superiore Sant'Anna, 56127 Pisa, Italy
3. Institute of Clinical Physiology, 56124 Pisa, Italy; scalese@ifc.cnr.it
4. Division of Pediatric Cardiology, Department of Pediatrics, Medical University Graz, 8036 Graz, Austria; martin.koestenberger@medunigraz.at
5. Taussig Heart Center, Department of Pediatrics, Johns Hopkins Hospital, Baltimore, MD 21287, USA; vpjani@ucsd.edu (V.J.); shelby.kutty@gmail.com (S.K.)
6. Adult and Pediatric Cardiac Surgery, Department Advanced Biomedical Sciences, University of Naples "Federico II", 80131 Naples, Italy
* Correspondence: r.giordano81@libero.it; Tel./Fax: +39-0817464702

Abstract: Background: Applications of atrial speckle tracking echocardiography (STE) strain (ε) analysis in pediatric cardiac surgery have been limited. This study aims to evaluate the feasibility of atrial STE ε analysis and the progression of atrial ε values as a function of post-operative time in children after pediatric cardiac surgery. **Methods:** 131 children (mean 1.69 ± 2.98; range 0.01–15.16 years) undergoing cardiac surgery were prospectively enrolled. Echocardiographic examinations were performed pre-operatively and at 3 different post-operative intervals: Time 1 (24–36 h), Time 2 (3–5 days), Time 3 (>5 days, before discharging). The right and left atrium longitudinal systolic contractile (Ct), Conduit (Cd), and Reservoir (R) ε were evaluated with a novel atrial specific software with both P- and R-Gating methods. One hundred and thirty-one age-matched normal subjects (mean 1.7 ± 3.2 years) were included as controls. **Results:** In all, 309 examinations were performed over the post-operative times. For each post-operative interval, all STE atrial ε parameters assessed were significantly lower compared to controls (all $p < 0.0001$). The lowest atrial ε values were found at Time 1, with only partial recovery thereafter (p from 0.02 to 0.04). All atrial ε values at discharge were decreased compared to the controls (all $p < 0.0001$). Significant correlations of the atrial ε values with cardio-pulmonary-bypass time, left and right ventricular ε values ($p < 0.05$), and ejection fraction ($p < 0.05$) were demonstrated. **Conclusions:** Atrial ε is highly reduced after surgery with only partial post-operative recovery in the near term. Our study additionally demonstrates that post-surgical atrial and ventricular ε responses correlated with each other.

Keywords: congenital heart disease; STE echocardiography; atria; pediatric cardiac surgery

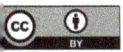

1. Introduction

Speckle tracking echocardiography (STE)-derived myocardial strain (ε) analysis has demonstrated a significant prognostic value in pediatric cardiology [1–4]. Preliminary studies have reported both the feasibility and post-operative trends of left [4,5] and right [6] ventricular ε in children with congenital heart disease (CHD) after cardiac surgery. Atrial function has been shown to be an important predictor of cardiovascular outcomes in the adult population [1,2]. Atrial ε indices enable a better understanding of the overall function of the atrium, and there is increasing evidence to support the additional role of atrial ε as a sensitive parameter of ventricular diastolic dysfunction [1,2]. Investigation of STE-derived atrial ε [1,2] to evaluate post-surgical outcomes in pediatric cardiology has been limited. While some studies [7,8] evaluated differences in the atrial ε response a few months after percutaneous versus surgical closure of atrial septal defects on small cohorts (10–30 subjects), no large-scale analysis has been performed in the pediatric population [7,8]

The recent availability of pediatric nomograms for atrial [9–11] ε values, including those obtained with dedicated atrial strain software [12], may allow for the comparison of post-operative atrial ε values with normal values, consequently enabling further understanding of the degree of alteration in atrial mechanics. The primary aims of this investigation were to (1) assess the feasibility of atrial STE ε analysis in a large cohort of children after biventricular cardiac surgery, (2) evaluate the progression of STE derived atrial ε as a function of post-operative time, and (3) to compare these findings to atrial ε values in normal age-matched controls.

2. Methods

From May 2018 to May 2019, children undergoing biventricular cardiac surgery for CHD were prospectively enrolled at a Single Institution (Fondazione CNR-Regione Toscana, G. Monasterio, Massa, Italy). Demographic data are reported in Table 1. Echocardiographic examinations were performed at three different post-operative times according to institutional protocols: Time 1 ($n = 131$) 24–36 h, Time 2 ($n = 108$) 3–5 days, Time 3 ($n = 70$) 6–9 days, and at the immediate pre-operative time ($n = 95$). In complicated patients, echocardiograms were repeated whenever required for clinical management, and no examinations other than those necessary for treatment were performed. Only subjects in which atrial strain analysis was deemed feasible for at least 80% of the parameters evaluated were included in this study. A group of 131 age-matched normal subjects (mean 1.7 ± 3.2 years old) were used as controls from a pool of 721 healthy children collected in a previous study [9]. Echocardiograms were performed on Philips iE33 systems (Philips Medical Systems, Bothell, WA, USA) using 8 Mhz and 5 Mhz transducers [9,13]. All studies were performed with simultaneous electrocardiographic monitoring. Images were obtained in the apical four-chamber (4Ch), three-chamber (3Ch), and two-chamber (2Ch) views for the evaluation of left ventricular strain, and in apical four-chamber (4Ch) for the evaluation of right and left atrium speckle tracking analysis. The following parameters were calculated off-line: LA and RA longitudinal reservoir ε (SR), conduit ε (SCd.), and contractile ε (SCt) [9,13–16]. A dedicated atrial ε package was used for analysis on a computer workstation (QLAB 10; Philips Medical Systems, Andover, MA, USA) according to recent guidelines [9–13]: interatrial septum was included, and the atrial appendages were excluded. Feasibility is meant as the capacity of the software to recognize and define all the atrial wall segments. Atrial ε analysis was validated when at least $\geq 80\%$ of the atrial segments were recognized correctly.

After semi-automatic placement of basic markers (lateral and septal mitral/tricuspid annulus and septal roof) in end-diastole, the software automatically generated atrial contours and performed STE analysis in seven segments through the cardiac cycle [9]. Minimal manual adjustment of tracking was performed when required. For each parameter, the mean value of three consecutive measurements was obtained. The P waves (P-P gating) were used as the initiation of the ε calculation (Figure 1). The analysis was then repeated by using QRS complex (R-R gating) for the initiation of the ε calculation (Figure 2). End-diastole and onset of atrial contraction were checked and manually corrected according to mitral inflow profile. Two experienced pediatric cardiologists (M.C., E.F.) acquired the images and performed the measurements. Rates of intra-observer and inter-observer variability were calculated from 20 subjects, randomly selected.

Table 1. Patients demographics.

	Older (nr 64)	Infant (nr 37)	Neonates (nr 30)	Total (nr 131)	
	Mean	Mean	Mean	Mean	p
Age (years)	3.23 ± 3.64	0.28 ± 0.13	0.03 ± 0.03	1.69 ± 2.98	<0.0001 *
BSA (m^2)	0.57 ± 0.31	0.28 ± 0.06	0.21 ± 0.02	0.41 ± 0.28	<0.0001 *
CPB (min)	1.52 ± 0.75	1.6 ± 0.85	2.24 ± 1.16	1.69 ± 0.91	<0.0001 *
STAT-score	95.82 ± 46.38	93.97 ± 59.22	134.11 ± 99.79	103.96 ± 66.8	0.043 *
Extubation Time (days)	1.09 ± 1.22	2.74 ± 2.46	5.16 ± 5.77	2.48 ± 6.54	0.0389 *
ICU LOS (days)	10.19 ± 48.14	7.24 ± 7.15	10.67 ± 8.05	9.5 ± 34.75	0.023 *
Major complications	1 §	2 °	3 *	6	
CHD Numerosity					
LVVO (nr)	18	17	2	37	
RVPO (nr)	20	9	1	30	
TGA (nr)	0	3	18	21	
LVPO (nr)	8	2	9	19	
RVVO (nr)	12	3	0	15	
AVSD (nr)	6	2	0	7	
Others (nr)	0	1	0	1	
Total	64	37	30	131	

AVSD = Atrioventricular Septal Defect; BSA = body surface area; CHD = congenital heart disease; CPB = cardio-pulmonary bypass; ICU = intensive care unit; LUS = lung ultrasound; LOS = length of stay; min = minutes; LVPO = Left Ventricle Pressure Overload; LVVO = Left Ventricle Volume Overload; RVPO = Right Ventricle Pressure Overload; RVVO = Right Ventricle Volume Overload; TGA = transposition of the great arteries; STAT-score = Society of Thoracic Surgeons/European Association of Cardio-Thoracic Surgery-STS/EACTS. § 1 tamponed, ° 1 tamponed, 1 Av block, * 1 AV block, 2 diaphragmatic paralyses.

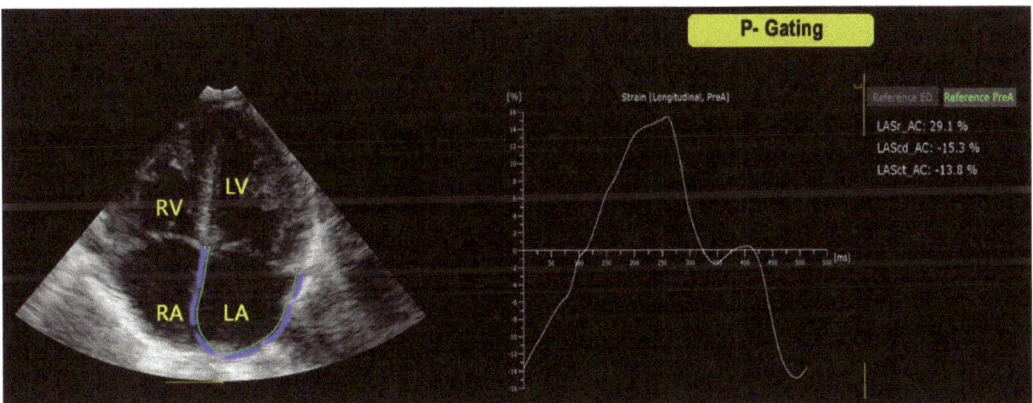

Figure 1. Left atrial ε analysis in the four-chamber view by using the atrial specific software for strain STE analysis with P-gating method. LA = Left atrium, LV = Left Ventricle, RA = Right Atrium, RV = Right Ventricle, Sr = strain reservoir, Sct = strain contractile, Scd = strain conduit.

The ejection fraction was calculated by the biplane Simpson method. Approval for this study was obtained from the Local Ethics Committee (Comitato Etico Meyer no. 62/2016). Parents or legal guardians of all the children were informed and provided written consent for participation in this study.

Images were acquired only in cooperative babies or in those who were sedated for clinical reason. No sedations just for image acquisition were performed. Only patients in sinus rhythm during the echocardiography were included in the present study.

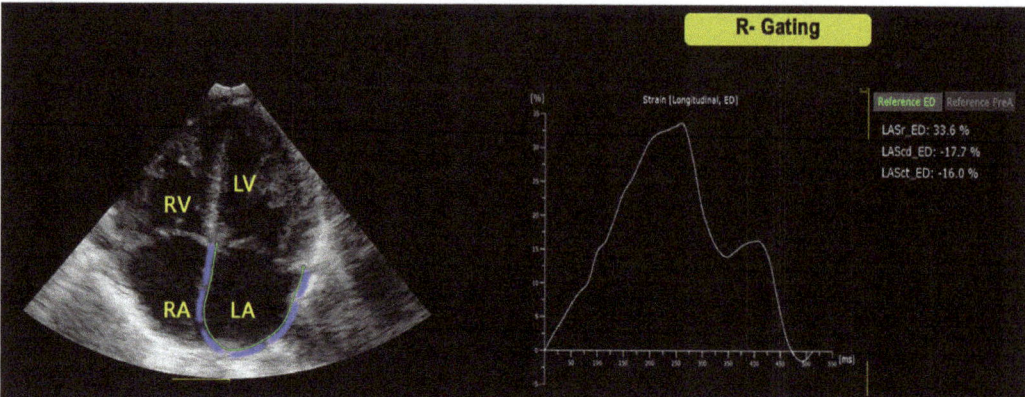

Figure 2. Left atrial ε analysis in the four-chamber view by using the atrial specific software for strain STE analysis with R-gating method. LA = Left atrium, LV = Left Ventricle, RA = Right Atrium, RV = Right Ventricle, Sr = strain reservoir, Sct = strain contractile, Scd = strain conduit.

All images and measurements were acquired by two independent and experienced pediatric cardiologists (M.C., E.F.). The low rate of intra- and inter-observer variability in atrial [9] ε measurements has been described in the previous reports [9].

Statistical Analysis

All continuous variables and categorical variables were expressed as mean standard deviation (SD) and a number of cases and percentage, respectively. Comparison of continuous variables at different time points was performed using Wilcoxon test and nonparametric test for trends, as appropriate. Comparison of categorical variables at different time points was performed using a chi-square (Cochran–Armitage) test for trends in proportions. Comparison of age class was performed using a Mann–Whitney U test and a chi-square test as appropriate. Additionally, Pearson correlation coefficients (r) between strain values, operative data, and outcome parameters were determined. The control group of normal subjects was selected by 1:1 propensity score matching. Propensity score matching was calculated for each group with bivariate logistic regression analysis by age. All calculations were done by using SPSS v23 (SPSS Inc, Chicago, IL, USA) and STATA v13 software. A $p < 0.05$ was considered significant.

3. Results

3.1. Population

In all, 621 examinations were performed from May 2018 to May 2019 in 210 children (mean 2.25 ± 3.62 years; range 0.01–17.68 years). Seventy-nine patients were excluded for incomplete examinations (of these, 52 were not cooperative children and 27 had a poor acoustic window due to wounds and medications), leaving 309 examinations in 131 children (mean 1.69 ± 2.98 years; range 0.01–15.16 years) for final analysis. Among these children, 30 were neonates (0–31 days), 37 were infants (1–6 months), and 64 were >6 months. All demographic data are summarized in Table 1.

One hundred and thirty-one age-matched normal subjects (mean age 1.71 ± 2.94 years; range 0.03–14.12 years; mean BSA 0.43 ± 0.25) were included as controls. No differences in both age and BSA among healthy and CHD children were found ($p = 0.94$ and $p = 0.657$, respectively).

3.2. Feasibility

Feasibility, as assessed by the total number of studies from which relevant atrial ε parameters were acquired, ranged from 62 to 85% for all parameters. Feasibility was similar between all age groups, although at Time 1 and Time 2, it was marginally higher in neonates (≥80%) ($p = 0.15$ and $p = 0.7$). These results are summarized in Table 2.

Table 2. Feasibility at different post-operative times and in different age groups.

%		Time 1			Time 2			Time 3	
	Neonates	Infant	Older	Neonates	Infant	Older	Neonates	Infant	Older
LARε	80.0%	85.2%	72.1%	84.8%	80.0%	76.0%	70.4%	82.1%	61.9%
LACTε	80.0%	82.0%	72.1%	84.8%	80.0%	74.7%	70.4%	75.0%	61.9%
RARε	80.0%	78.7%	70.6%	75.8%	80.0%	77.3%	63.0%	75.0%	64.3%
RACTε	80.0%	75.4%	70.6%	75.8%	76.7%	74.7%	63.0%	67.9%	61.9%
Feasibility	80.0%	80.3%	71.3%	80.3%	79.2%	75.7%	66.7%	75.0%	62.5%

ε = strain, LAR = left atrial reservoir, LACT = left atrial contractile, RAR = right atrium reservoir, RACT = right atrium contractile.

3.3. Comparison vs. Normal Subjects

Pre-operative atrial ε values, obtained with either P-P or R-R gating methods, were significantly lower (p all < 0.0001), compared with normal subjects, with the only exception being the RA and LA contractile functions which were comparable with normal subjects.

3.4. The Post-Operative Trend for Atrial STE ε

Post-operatively, all atrial ε values decreased with the lower values observed at Time 1 with a progressive recovery thereafter (p ranging from <0.0001 to 0.027). At discharge, however, all atrial ε parameters remained significantly lower compared to the control group (p ranging <0.0001 to 0.004), with the only exception being the LA Ct ε function, which was similar to healthy subjects' values, as reported in Table 3. From Time 1 to Time 2, only the reservoir function, for both LA and RA, reported a significant increase (p from 0.007 to 0.022). From Time 2 to Time 3, the reservoir ε function, for the LA and RA, and the LA Cd ε function, reported a significant increase (p from 0.010 to 0.022). The remaining atrial functions showed a slower, however, significant, upward trend from Time 1 to Time 3 (p from 0.0009 to 0.002, p 0.0066 and 0.027, respectively). All these results are summarized in Table 3 and Supplementary Table S1, and Figures 3 and 4.

Table 3. Mean and standard deviations of examinations at different pre-/post-operative times and in control group.

	Normal Subjects	Pre	Time 1	Time 2	Time 3
	Mean	Mean	Mean	Mean	Mean
(R-Gating) LA ε R	52.07 ± 15.87	35.21 ± 11.63	25.44 ± 12.17	29.94 ± 11.24	35.29 ± 13.57
(R-Gating) LA ε Cd	37.82 ± 13.8	20.85 ± 10.17	15.94 ± 8.48	18.21 ± 7.85	21.58 ± 9.23
(R-Gating) LA ε Ct	14.74 ± 7.27	13.95 ± 6.28	10.65 ± 7.46	12.31 ± 7.65	13.85 ± 8.79
(P-Gating) LA ε R	45.19 ± 13.03	30.72 ± 9.34	22.69 ± 9.62	26.46 ± 8.58	30.58 ± 10.21
(P-Gating) LA ε Cd	33.25 ± 12.57	18.37 ± 8.87	14.7 ± 7.92	16.41 ± 7.3	19.05 ± 7.82
(P-Gating) LA ε Ct	12.6 ± 5.41	12.36 ± 4.89	9.36 ± 5.89	10.61 ± 5.65	11.68 ± 6.45
(R-Gating) RA ε R	47.84 ± 16.6	38.49 ± 12.77	18.96 ± 9.49	22.4 ± 8.38	28.2 ± 14.71
(R-Gating) RA ε Cd	31.14 ± 13.66	22.72 ± 9.06	11.37 ± 6.72	13.49 ± 7.92	16.59 ± 10.27
(R-Gating) RA ε Ct	17.25 ± 9.09	15.84 ± 7.82	8.81 ± 6.64	10.19 ± 6.83	12.51 ± 7.86
(P-Gating) RA ε R	40.7 ± 13.15	33.22 ± 9.48	17,23 ± 7.92	20.26 ± 6.93	24.56 ± 11.13
(P-Gating) RA ε Cd	27.04 ± 12.4	19.9 ± 7.98	10.35 ± 6.55	12.64 ± 8.2	14.86 ± 9.22
(P-Gating) RA ε Ct	14.31 ± 6.52	13.38 ± 5.8	8.15 ± 5.72	8.98 ± 5.41	10.59 ± 5.8

ε = strain, R = reservoir, Ct = contractile, Cd = conduit.

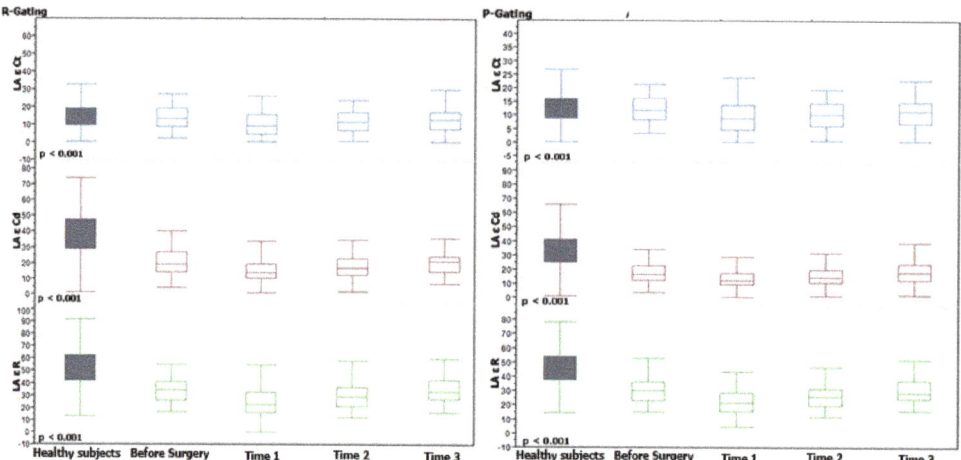

Figure 3. Left Atrial Strain trends at different pre-/post-operative times and in comparison to the control group. Median and interquartile range of ε values over time are shown. *p* values in the patient group were determined relative to strain from Time 1 to Time 3. Horizontal line = median; Box = interquartile range.

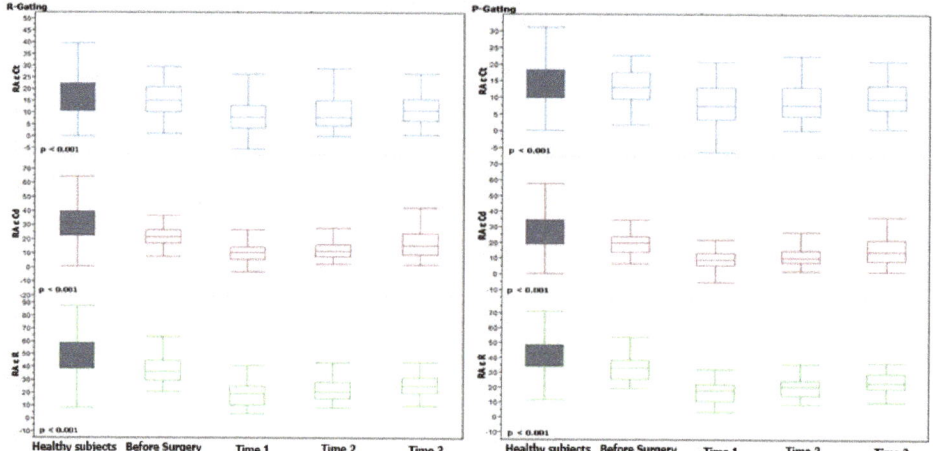

Figure 4. Right Atrial Strain trends at different pre-/post-operative times and in comparison to the control group. Median and interquartile range of ε values over time are shown. *p* values in the patient group were determined relative to strain from Time 1 to Time 3. Horizontal line = median; Box = interquartile range.

3.5. Comparison of Post-Operative Trend for Atrial STE ε with Pre-Operative Values

Time 1 reported lower values in all LA and RA functions than the pre-operative data. Concerning Time 3, all LA ε values were totally recovered with values comparable with the pre-operative data ($p > 0.05$ each one), but, contrariwise, all RA ε values were still lower than the pre-operative data.

All these results are summarized in Table 3 and Supplementary Table S1.

3.6. Differences among P- and R-Gating Post-Operative ε Values

No significant differences in the post-operative time for the atrial ε trends were observed among values calculated with the P- and R-gating methods. Surgery atrial strain values calculated with P-gating, however, were constantly lower than those obtained with R-gating ($p < 0.001$).

3.7. Differences among Age Groups

Children younger than 6 months reported no significant differences from Time 1 to Time 2 in atrial STE ε with both gating methods. Children older than 6 months reported a significant increase from Time 1 to Time 2 only for the LA ε R function, through P-Gating (p 0.04), and for RA ε Cd through the two Gating methods, R and P (p 0.015 and p 0.017).

3.8. Correlation of Atrial Strain with Operative Data and Outcome Parameters

Strain parameters correlated with a CPB and cross-clamp time. At Time 1 (12–36 h post-surgery), CC inversely correlated with the RA conduit function in both the P- and R-gating methods (beta -0.04 p 0.009 and beta -0.004 p 0.045, respectively). Furthermore, a CPB is inversely related with the conduit function of both LA and RA (p all < 0.05), while it is inversely related with the reservoir function only for RA. Moreover, the LA reservoir function demonstrated an inverse correlation with the STAT-score (beta -3.78 p 0.008 for P-gating and beta -2.98 p 0.008 for R-gating).

No significant correlations were observed between the atrial STE ε values and the additional outcome parameters. Furthermore, no significant correlation was observed between the atrial STE values, body surface area (BSA), and age. These results are summarized in Supplementary Tables S2 and S3.

3.9. Correlation of Atrial Strain with Left and Right Ventricular STE

The atrial ε values correlated with the right/left ventricular ε and left ventricle ejection fraction (LVEF).

At Time 1 (12–36 h post-surgery), univariate regression analysis demonstrated that LV Longitudinal 4c, 2c, 3c, and global longitudinal (GL) ε values all positively correlated with all the LA longitudinal systolic ε with the R-gating method only (Supplementary Table S4). Right Ventricular ε, instead, did not correlate with LA and RA longitudinal systolic ε with both gating methods. Additionally, EF positively correlated only with LA ε R in both the R- and P-gating method ($\beta = 0.28$, $p = 0.03$ and $\beta = 0.22$, $p = 0.03$, respectively).

At Time 2, approximatively all atrial longitudinal systolic ε parameters positively related with all LV ε in the univariate regression analysis. Right Ventricular ε, instead, positively correlated only with RA ε R in both the R- and P-gating method ($\beta = 0.44$, $p = 0.044$ and $\beta = 0.41$, $p = 0.023$, respectively). Lastly, EF remained positively related with almost all atrial longitudinal systolic ε parameters. These results are summarized in Supplementary Table S4.

4. Discussion

In this study, we prospectively investigated atrial ε using STE and examined trends in atrial ε as a function of time after pediatric cardiac surgery. Defects assessed in this study included atrial septal defects, ventricular septal defects, atrioventricular septal defects, tetralogy of Fallot, transposition of the great arteries (TGA), and aortic stenosis. Our data demonstrate that STE-derived atrial ε analysis is feasible for various surgical indications of CHD across different ages.

By using a novel software specifically designed for atrial STE analysis [12], we report the feasibility of 62–85%, which is slightly lower than that presented in similar studies assessing ventricular ε analysis in a similar population (87–93% feasibility) [4,5]. Feasibility in this study was also lower than that observed for atrial ε analysis in a normal cohort (feasibility from 96.8% to 98.9%) [12].

Our study has demonstrated that all atrial ε parameters evaluated were significantly reduced compared to atrial ε in normal subjects [9]. As expected, the lowest atrial ε values were recorded at the first post-operative sample time (e.g., 12–36 h), with progressive recovery thereafter. However, at discharge, STE atrial ε values remained depressed compared to that observed in normal subjects ($p < 0.0001$). To our knowledge, this is the first study to assess the STE atrial ε response after pediatric cardiac surgery. Few studies have assessed atrial ε response in the medium-term for children undergoing percutaneous versus surgical closure of atrial septal defects [7,8]. Di Salvo and colleagues [7] evaluated color doppler LA and RA atrial ε in 15 subjects (mean age: 9 ± 3 years) 6 months after surgical ASD closure and compared these data with 15 age-matched patients who underwent percutaneous closure, along with 15 age-matched controls. In this particular study, patients who had undergone surgical AS closure had significantly lower LA and RA atrial ε compared to the percutaneous group and to normal subjects [7]. In another study, adults [8] (30 subjects; age 34.4 ± 8.3 years) > 1 year from surgical closure (range 1–5 years) were more likely to have an impaired RA strain and LA conduit strain compared to age-matched controls.

The trend of atrial ε response, we found, is similar to what has been described in the limited studies available for STE ventricular ε response after pediatric cardiac surgery [5,6,17]. In a study of over 117 children (mean age: 2.4 ± 3.9; range: 0–16 years), evaluated at different times pre-operatively and post-surgery, STE ε analysis revealed a significant LV systolic impairment after surgery with amelioration thereafter, but incomplete normalization at discharge [12]. In one retrospective study, De Boer et. al [17] showed in children ($n = 204$; median age: 3.7 ± 5.1 years) undergoing cardiac surgery for different CHD variants that LV and RV global longitudinal strain at the discharge echocardiography (median 7, range 6–14 days post-op) were significantly lower compared to age-matched controls ($n = 78$). Another study in 37 children (median age 19 months, interquartile range 5–63 months) demonstrated that RV peak systolic strain significantly decreased compared to the baseline (−10.5 ± 2.9% vs. −19.5 ± 4.8%; $p < 0.0001$). In this same study, RV peak systolic strain remained depressed compared with pre-operative values (−13.5 ± 4.0% vs. −9.5 ± 4.8%; $p < 0.0001$) [6]. The results from our study support these observations.

The degree of impairment in ε correlated with the duration of the cardio-pulmonary bypass and cross-clamp time. Our results support what has been published on ventricular ε response after pediatric cardiac surgery. In a study with over 33 children (4.2 ± 2.5 years) undergoing bypass cardiac surgery [5], LV longitudinal strain (ε) values were correlated to the aortic cross-clamp duration on post-operative day 0 ($r = 0.47$, $p = 0.016$) and post-operative day 1 ($r = 0.53$, $p = 0.010$) [5].

Of note, atrial ε values correlated with RV and LV ε, and LVEF. While similar correlations between atrial ε and LV strain [18,19] have been demonstrated in adult populations, data on children are lacking. In general, impaired atrial ε is more reflective of diastolic dysfunction [20,21]. The impaired atrial function observed in the present study may be indicative of abnormal ventricular diastolic properties. This is clinically relevant because traditional echocardiographic parameters for ventricular diastolic function assessment are poorly validated in children. Indeed, our data suggest that both the systolic and diastolic function are impaired after pediatric cardiac surgery, and that the dysfunction in the systole is correlated with dysfunction in the diastole.

We present data with a novel atrial specific software, calculated with both the P- and R-gating method. Although the R-wave method of gating is the one currently recommended, the P-gating method may be more appropriate for assessing the atrial function. Significant differences among the two methods have been demonstrated in healthy children where all atrial ε values were lower with P- than R-gating ($p < 0.001$) [9]. Similar differences were noted even in children with CHD after surgery, where atrial strain values calculated with P-gating were constantly lower than those obtained with R-gating. Feasibility and time trends of atrial strain values, however, did not change among the P- and R-gating methods. Thus, under a clinical point of view, both methods may be used; however, measurements obtained with the two different methods cannot be used interchangeably and, during the follow-up, values should be compared with those obtained with the same gating method (and with the same vendor) [13]. Atrial strain analysis with the novel semi-automatic software is very easy and fast, requiring just a few seconds for processing and automated reporting. Thus, considering data acquisition and data analysis, atrial strain analysis may be routinely introduced in the follow-up of children with CHD undergoing cardiac surgery, without big efforts or a loss of time.

Limitations

We used STE software developed for the left atrium's deformation only, which has been used for measuring right atrial ε. The use of vendor-specific software represents another limitation. Atrial ε was measured only in the four-chamber view, and not in the two- and three-chamber views [5,6]. Our study assessed longitudinal ε, including components of atrial contraction, reservoir, and conduit function, but did not include indices of atrial electromechanical coupling [1]. Examination times were slightly variable between patients depending on the institutional protocols for single CHD and the clinical indications. However, all 12–36 h examinations corresponded with the time of the first post-operative echocardiographic examination. Around half of the patients, including most older children assessed in our study, were extubated at the time of the examination, while most neonates and infants were intubated.

In addition, patients included in this investigation were heterogeneous and included a wide range of ages and cardiac defects. The relatively limited number of subjects enrolled did not allow for a sufficiently powerful sub-group analysis of patients (e.g., age, corrected vs. palliated, CHD groups), which may have constituted some bias in the final analysis. Nonetheless, despite the heterogeneity of the patient population assessed, significant trends in the ε response after cardiac surgery were observed, across different ages and different CHD variants. Age-related differences for LA and RA strain values were too limited and heterogenous to draw definitive conclusions. Parameter acquisition was incomplete at different sample times, reflecting an additional limitation. A comparison with pre-operative STE data is lacking; however, in uncorrected CHD, when significant shunts are present, the value of the ε data may be limited.

5. Conclusions

We report the progression of STE-derived atrial ε values after pediatric cardiac surgery as a function of the post-operative time. Our study observed that after pediatric cardiac surgery, all atrial ε parameters were significantly reduced compared to normal subjects. Atrial ε progressively recovered during the post-operative time; however, despite this improvement, atrial values remained significantly depressed compared with normal subjects upon discharge. The degree of atrial ε reduction seems to reflect the duration of the cardio-pulmonary bypass. Furthermore, the atrial and ventricular ε response appears to be correlated with each other. Additionally, the atrial ε response significantly correlated also with the left ventricular ejection fraction. Further studies in a larger cohort are required to validate and reinforce these observations.

Supplementary Materials: The following supporting information can be downloaded at: https://www.mdpi.com/article/10.3390/jcm11092497/s1, Table S1. Mean differences of examinations at different pre-/post-operative times and in control group. Table S2. Atrial STE ε mean values at different post-operative times for the entire cohort and in different age groups. Table S3. Correlations of Atrial STE ε with outcome predictors at Time 1. Table S4. Correlation between Atrial and ventricular STE ε at Time 1 and Time 2.

Author Contributions: All authors contributed to the study conception and design. Material preparation, data collection and analysis were performed by R.G., P.M., M.S., E.F. and N.A. The first draft of the manuscript was written by M.C. and all authors commented on previous versions of the manuscript. All authors have read and agreed to the published version of the manuscript.

Funding: The authors declare that no funds, grants, or other support were received during the preparation of this manuscript.

Institutional Review Board Statement: This study was performed in line with the principles of the Declaration of Helsinki. Approval was granted by the Ethics Committee of the Meyer Hospital CE62/2016.

Informed Consent Statement: Informed consent was obtained from all individual participants/parents included in the study.

Data Availability Statement: The data presented in this study are available on request from the corresponding author.

Conflicts of Interest: The authors have no relevant financial or non-financial interest to disclose There is no potential conflict of interest, real or perceived, by the author.

References

1. Avesani, M.; Borrelli, N.; Krupickova, S.; Sabatino, J.; Donne, G.D.; Ibrahim, A.; Piccinelli, E.; Josen, M.; Michielon, G.; Fraisse, A.; et al. Echocardiography and cardiac magnetic resonance in children with repaired tetralogy of Fallot: New insights in cardiac mechanics and exercise capacity. *Int. J. Cardiol.* **2020**, *321*, 144–149. [CrossRef] [PubMed]
2. Cheung, Y.-F.; Yu, C.K.; So, E.K.; Li, V.W.; Wong, W.H. Atrial Strain Imaging after Repair of Tetralogy of Fallot: A Systematic Review. *Ultrasound Med. Biol.* **2019**, *45*, 1896–1908. [CrossRef] [PubMed]
3. Bárczi, A.; Lakatos, B.K.; Szilágyi, M.; Kis, É.; Cseprekál, O.; Fábián, A.; Kovács, A.; Szabó, A.J.; Merkely, B.; Salvi, P.; et al. Subclinical cardiac dysfunction in pediatric kidney transplant recipients identified by speckle-tracking echocardiography. *Pediatr. Nephrol.* **2022**, 1–13. [CrossRef] [PubMed]
4. Pletzer, S.A.; Atz, A.M.; Chowdhury, S.M. The Relationship between Pre-operative Left Ventricular Longitudinal Strain and Post-operative Length of Stay in Patients Undergoing Arterial Switch Operation Is Age Dependent. *Pediatr. Cardiol.* **2018**, *40*, 366–373. [CrossRef]
5. Perdreau, E.; Séguéla, P.-E.; Jalal, Z.; Perdreau, A.; Mouton, J.-B.; Nelson-Veniard, M.; Guillet, E.; Iriart, X.; Ouattara, A.; Roubertie, F.; et al. Postoperative assessment of left ventricular function by two-dimensional strain (speckle tracking) after paediatric cardiac surgery. *Arch. Cardiovasc. Dis.* **2016**, *109*, 599–606. [CrossRef]
6. Karsenty, C.; Hadeed, K.; Dulac, Y.; Semet, F.; Alacoque, X.; Breinig, S.; Leobon, B.; Acar, P.; Hascoet, S. Two-dimensional right ventricular strain by speckle tracking for assessment of longitudinal right ventricular function after paediatric congenital heart disease surgery. *Arch. Cardiovasc. Dis.* **2017**, *110*, 157–166. [CrossRef]
7. Di Salvo, G.; Drago, M.; Pacileo, G.; Rea, A.; Carrozza, M.; Santoro, G.; Bigazzi, M.C.; Caso, P.; Russo, M.G.; Carminati, M.; et al. Atrial function after surgical and percutaneous closure of atrial septal defect: A strain rate imaging study. *J. Am. Soc. Echocardiogr.* **2005**, *18*, 930–933. [CrossRef]
8. Hajizeinali, A.; Iri, M.; Hosseinsabet, A. Assessment of the Right and Left Atrial Functions at Midterm after Surgical and Device Atrial Septal Defect Closure: A 2-Dimensional Speckle-Tracking Echocardiographic Study. *J. Ultrasound Med.* **2019**, *38*, 1979–1993. [CrossRef]
9. Cantinotti, M.; Scalese, M.; Giordano, R.; Franchi, E.; Assanta, N.; Molinaro, S.; Iervasi, G.; Santoro, G.; Koestenberger, M.; Kutty, S. Left and Right Atrial Strain in Healthy Caucasian Children by Two-Dimensional Speckle-Tracking Echocardiography. *J. Am. Soc. Echocardiogr.* **2019**, *32*, 165–168.e3. [CrossRef]
10. Kutty, S.; Padiyath, A.; Li, L.; Peng, Q.; Rangamani, S.; Schuster, A.; Danford, D.A. Functional Maturation of Left and Right Atrial Systolic and Diastolic Performance in Infants, Children, and Adolescents. *J. Am. Soc. Echocardiogr.* **2013**, *26*, 398–409.e2. [CrossRef]
11. Ghelani, S.J.; Brown, D.W.; Kuebler, J.D.; Perrin, D.; Shakti, D.; Williams, D.N.; Marx, G.R.; Colan, S.D.; Geva, T.; Harrild, D.M. Left Atrial Volumes and Strain in Healthy Children Measured by Three-Dimensional Echocardiography: Normal Values and Maturational Changes. *J. Am. Soc. Echocardiogr.* **2018**, *31*, 187–193.e1. [CrossRef] [PubMed]
12. Marchese, P.; Scalese, M.; Giordano, R.; Assanta, N.; Franchi, E.; Koestenberger, M.; Ravaglioli, A.; Kutty, S.; Cantinotti, M. Pediatric ranges of normality for 2D speckle-tracking echocardiography atrial strain: Differences between p- and r-gating and among new (Atrial Designed) and conventional (Ventricular Specific) software's. *Echocardiography* **2021**, *38*, 2025–2031. [CrossRef] [PubMed]
13. Badano, L.P.; Kolias, T.J.; Muraru, D.; Abraham, T.P.; Aurigemma, G.; Edvardsen, T.; D'Hooge, J.; Donal, E.; Fraser, A.G.; Marwick, T.; et al. Standardization of left atrial, right ventricular, and right atrial deformation imaging using two-dimensional speckle tracking echocardiography: A consensus document of the EACVI/ASE/Industry Task Force to standardize deformation imaging. *Eur. Heart J. Cardiovasc. Imaging* **2018**, *19*, 591–600. [CrossRef] [PubMed]
14. Cantinotti, M.; Scalese, M.; Giordano, R.; Franchi, E.; Assanta, N.; Marotta, M.; Viacava, C.; Molinaro, S.; Iervasi, G.; Santoro, G.; et al. Normative Data for Left and Right Ventricular Systolic Strain in Healthy Caucasian Italian Children by Two-Dimensional Speckle-Tracking Echocardiography. *J. Am. Soc. Echocardiogr.* **2018**, *31*, 712–720.e6. [CrossRef] [PubMed]
15. Moustafa, S.; Zuhairy, H.; Youssef, M.A.; Alvarez, N.; Connelly, M.S.; Prieur, T.; Mookadam, F. Right and Left Atrial Dissimilarities in Normal Subjects Explored by Speckle Tracking Echocardiography. *Echocardiography* **2015**, *32*, 1392–1399. [CrossRef]
16. Atas, H.; Kepez, A.; Tigen, K.; Samadov, F.; Ozen, G.; Cincin, A.; Sunbul, M.; Bozbay, M.; Direskeneli, H.; Basaran, Y. Evaluation of left atrial volume and function in systemic sclerosis patients using speckle tracking and real-time three-dimensional echocardiography. *Anatol. J. Cardiol.* **2016**, *16*, 316–322. [CrossRef]
17. De Boer, J.M.; Kuipers, I.M.; Klitsie, L.M.; Blom, N.A.; Ten Harkel, A.D. Decreased biventricular longitudinal strain shortly after congenital heart defect surgery. *Echocardiography* **2017**, *34*, 446–452. [CrossRef]

18. Fung, M.J.; Thomas, L.; Leung, D.Y. Left atrial function: Correlation with left ventricular function and contractile reserve in patients with hypertension. *Echocardiography* **2018**, *35*, 1596–1605. [CrossRef]
19. Ramkumar, S.; Yang, H.; Wang, Y.; Nolan, M.; Negishi, T.; Negishi, K.; Marwick, T.H. Association of the Active and Passive Components of Left Atrial Deformation with Left Ventricular Function. *J. Am. Soc. Echocardiogr.* **2017**, *30*, 659–666. [CrossRef]
20. Loar, R.W.; Pignatelli, R.H.; Morris, S.A.; Colquitt, J.L.; Feagin, D.K.; Denfield, S.W.; Tunuguntla, H.P. Left Atrial Strain Correlates with Elevated Filling Pressures in Pediatric Heart Transplantation Recipients. *J. Am. Soc. Echocardiogr.* **2020**, *33*, 504–511.e1. [CrossRef]
21. Sabatino, J.; Di Salvo, G.; Prota, C.; Bucciarelli, V.; Josen, M.; Paredes, J.; Borrelli, N.; Sirico, D.; Prasad, S.; Indolfi, C.; et al. Left Atrial Strain to Identify Diastolic Dysfunction in Children with Cardiomyopathies. *J. Clin. Med.* **2019**, *8*, 1243. [CrossRef] [PubMed]

MDPI
St. Alban-Anlage 66
4052 Basel
Switzerland
www.mdpi.com

Journal of Clinical Medicine Editorial Office
E-mail: jcm@mdpi.com
www.mdpi.com/journal/jcm

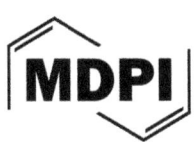

Disclaimer/Publisher's Note: The statements, opinions and data contained in all publications are solely those of the individual author(s) and contributor(s) and not of MDPI and/or the editor(s). MDPI and/or the editor(s) disclaim responsibility for any injury to people or property resulting from any ideas, methods, instructions or products referred to in the content.

www.ingramcontent.com/pod-product-compliance
Lightning Source LLC
LaVergne TN
LVHW070631100526
838202LV00012B/778